TEXTBOOK OF ORTHOPAEDICS AND FRACTURES

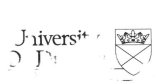

TEXTBOOK OF ORTHOPAEDICS AND FRACTURES

S P F Hughes

MS FRCS Ed Orth FRCS FRCS I

*Professor of Orthopaedic Surgery, Royal Postgraduate Medical School
and Chief of Orthopaedic Service, Hammersmith Hospitals NHS Trust, London, UK*

R W Porter

MD FRCS Ed FRCS

*Director of Education and Training, Royal College of Surgeons of Edinburgh,
and formerly Professor of Orthopaedic Surgery, University of Aberdeen, Scotland*

616.7
HUG

A member of the Hodder Headline Group
LONDON • SYDNEY • AUCKLAND
Co-published in the USA by Oxford University Press, Inc., New York

First published in Great Britain in 1997 by Arnold,
a member of the Hodder Headline Group,
338 Euston Road, London NW1 3BH

Co-published in the United States of America by
Oxford University Press, Inc.,
198 Madison Avenue, New York, NY10016
Oxford is a registered trademark of Oxford University Press

Whilst the advice and information in this book is believed to be true and
accurate at the date of going to press, neither the authors nor the publisher
can accept any legal responsibility or liability for any errors or omissions
that may be made. In particular (but without limiting the generality of the
preceding disclaimer) every effort has been made to check drug dosages;
however it is still possible that errors have been missed. Furthermore,
dosage schedules are constantly being revised and new side-effects
recognized. For these reasons the reader is strongly urged to consult the
drug companies' printed instructions before administering any of the drugs
recommended in this book.

British Library Cataloguing in Publication Data
A catalogue record for this book is available from the British Library

Library of Congress Cataloging-in-Publication Data
A catalog record for this book is available from the Library of Congress

ISBN 0 340 61381 5

Typeset in 9/11pt Palatino by Scribe Design, Gillingham, Kent, UK
Printed and bound in Great Britain by Alden Press

CONTENTS

PREFACE

This is a new edition of an established undergraduate book on orthopaedics and fractures

As well as rewriting the text and providing new illustration I have combined authorship with Professor Richard Porter who has had extensive experience in undergraduate teaching.

The book has been enhanced with trauma and knee sections by Mr Robin Strachan, who has brought up-to-date information to this area. The section on physiotherapy has been rewritten by Miss Sue Griffith.

The late Professor Douglas Miller's chapter on head injuries has been included because of its clear approach to the management of these conditions.

The whole emphasis of this book has been to provide information on the rapidly changing face of orthopaedics.

There are increased chapters on examination and basic sciences and an overall revision of the layout of the original Ashton chapters.

It is hoped that by this fresh approach, this book will remain a useful aid to undergraduates in medicine who require a clear account of the orthopaedic conditions that affect the musculo-skeletal system.

INTRODUCTION

The branch of medicine referred to as 'orthopaedics' is primarily concerned with the locomotor system of the body. This consists of the bones, joints, muscles and the peripheral nervous system as they affect the limbs and spine.

In considering orthopaedics, it is important for the student to appreciate that, first, while a localized lesion is the presenting feature it usually affects the mechanics of the body as a whole and this must constantly be borne in mind. Second, if any operation is contemplated, this is merely the first incident (albeit a major one) in a course of treatment.

The success of any surgical measure is intimately bound up with the aftercare, and this in turn is greatly dependent upon the patient themselves.

DESCRIPTIVE TERMS

Various specialist words are employed in orthopaedics, and it may be helpful if they are mentioned at the outset.

OPERATIONS

In operations upon joints, *arthrodesis* means that the joint is fused. This in practice implies that an artificial fracture has been made, and it must there-fore be supported, either internally or externally, until it has united and the two bones concerned have become one. When a diseased joint fuses spontaneously, this is *ankylosis*, which can be either bony – a natural arthrodesis – or fibrous, if a jog of movement still remains.

Arthroplasty means that the joint has been remade, often by the employment of an implant (prosthesis) to replace one or more of the joint components.

Arthrotomy implies that the joint has been opened and, probably, explored.

In operations upon bones, *osteotomy* is division of a bone. This is usually employed either to correct a deformity or, in the lower limb, to alter the line of weight-bearing.

Tenotomy is used to describe simple operative division of a tendon. *Tenodesis* is an operation to anchor a tendon at a new site. Tendons may also be *transferred* or *transplanted*. This is employed when one group of muscles cannot function, either because they are paralysed or as a result of previous injury. *Tenolysis* means freeing a tendon from adhesions, usually caused by earlier trauma or infection.

MOVEMENTS AND DEFORMITIES

Flexion implies bending a joint; in the case of the shoulder this is used to describe elevation of the arm in the forward plane. *Extension* describes straightening the joint and in hyperextension means that the joint is extended beyond the straight line. *Abduction* is the movement away from the midline – of the body in the case of the hip and shoulder, and of the individual limb in the case of fingers or toes. *Adduction* is the opposite, meaning movement towards the midline of the body or the limb, depending upon the joint concerned. *Circumduction* is a combination of flexion, abduction, adduction and extension, permitting the limb to be moved in a circular direction. Rotation, which may be internal or external, also takes place in many joints.

In addition, if there is limitation of movement in a joint, so that it cannot reach the neutral position, an adduction, abduction, flexion or rotational deformity is said to be present. If there is an angular deformity, so that the distal component points towards the midline of the body, this is described as *varus*, whereas if it is directed away from the midline, this is described as *valgus*.

Individual parts

These are often given their latin names – thus *cubitus* is used to describe the elbow, *coxa* the hip, *genu* the knee and *pes* the foot.

In the case of the spine, *kyphosis* is used to describe a flexion deformity at one level. *Lordosis* means the spine is extended. A lateral curve is described as *scoliosis*.

In the foot, an *equinus* – 'horse-like' – deformity is said to be present when the heel cannot be brought down to the ground easily.

EXAMINATION OF THE JOINTS

Examination of the locomotor system is often only part of the overall assessment of the patient, which should include a general history as well as relevant past history and systemic enquiry.

The physical examination of the locomotor system can be conducted under three headings: posture; gait; and movement of the limbs and spine.

POSTURE

For an adequate assessment of posture the patient should be able to stand and walk. When this is not possible, posture can be assessed by examining the patient in the supine and prone positions.

Posture varies with age. In the neonate there is a generalized convexity of the spine or kyphosis. As the child loses its primitive reflexes and is able to sit and pivot, the cervical spine develops a lordosis. When the child starts to walk lordosis develops in the lumbar spine and is often exaggerated, with the result that the hips and knees are flexed and abducted. In the child and adolescent the typical erect posture is reached. It is interesting that as we proceed through age we reverse this posture, so that by old age the infant's flexed posture is returned to.

GAIT

Normal gait is a complex phenomenon and is on the whole a smooth process dependent on movements occurring between the spine and pelvis, at the hip, knee and ankle.

Interference with proper action of any of these movements will alter the gait cycle and may result in a limp.

There is a great variation in normal gait and in the degree of abnormality, which can be considered under the headings painful gait and painless gait.

Stance phase

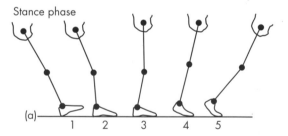

Swing phase

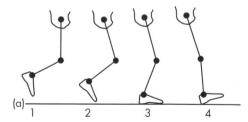

FIG. 1.1 The gait cycle: (a) Stance phase 60% – 1, heel strike; 2, foot flat; 3, midstance; 4, heel off; 5, toe off. (b) Swing phase 40% – 1, acceleration; 2, midswing; 3, deceleration; 4, heelstrike

Painful gait

In this type, the gait rhythm is disturbed and the patient takes weight off the painful limb as quickly as possible.

Painless gait

These may be due to

■ bony causes
■ joint deformities
■ muscle weakness
■ neurological disease.

MOVEMENT OF THE LIMBS AND SPINE

Examination of the limbs and spine includes an assessment of posture and gait and is by inspection, palpation and movement of the joints.

Inspection

This entails looking for deformity, the presence of scars, sinuses or swellings, changes in the skin structure and the presence of muscle wasting.

Palpation

Palpation includes feeling for swellings, be they bony or soft tissue, such as synovium, and also detecting the vascular status of the limb.

Movement

This entails moving the joint through the normal range. Excess movement can occur in children and is associated with hypermobility, possibly due to muscle disorder.

The upper limb

The principles of clinical examination include:

■ posture – paying particular attention to deformity and wasting
■ movement – the whole upper limb may be involved in a postural abnormality.

SHOULDER JOINT

The shoulder joint is a ball and socket joint involving the head of the humerus and the glenoid fossa of the scapula. It is important to consider that shoulder movement incorporates sternoclavicular rotation and scapulothoracic movement.

The most useful functional movements of the shoulder joint are internal rotation and flexion –

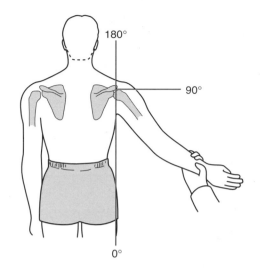

FIG. 1.2   Abduction of the shoulder, showing glenohumeral involvement

feeding – and external rotation and adduction – toilet.

The described movements are

■ abduction   0–90° glenohumeral
                90–150° scapulothoracic
■ flexion   0–120°
■ extension   0–30°
■ rotation   45° internal
                45° external.

ELBOW JOINT

The elbow joint is complex and consists of the articular portion of the humerus with the head of the radius and the coranoid fossa of the ulna.

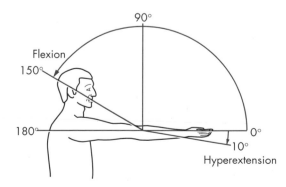

FIG. 1.3   Flexion and extension movements of the elbow joint

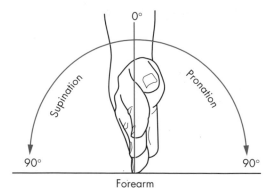

FIG. 1.4   Movements of the forearm

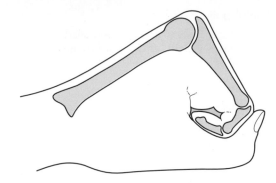

FIG. 1.6   Flexion of the metacarpal and phalangeal joints

Movement of the elbow joint includes

- flexion/extension   10–150°
- supination and pronation 90°: achieved with the elbow flexed and held to the patient's side, so as not to incorporate shoulder movement.

WRIST AND HAND

The wrist and hand are important structures that are essential for normal activity. The hand produces grasp, pinch and sensation.

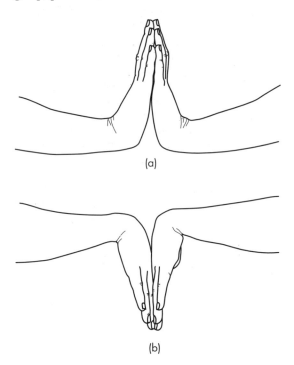

(a)

(b)

FIG. 1.5   (a) Dorsiflexion of the wrist; (b) palmarflexion of the wrist

If any part of the upper limb is affected, hand function is impaired.

Movement of the wrist includes

- dorsiflexion
- palmarflexion.

In the hand, in order to achieve full grasp the long flexors and the intrinsics need to function.

Movement occurs at the metacarpal phalangeal joints of flexion/extension with a range of 0–90°. The same is applicable to the interphalangeal joints.

For pinch grip the limb must be stable and it is against the thumb that all activity occurs.

The hand more than any other part of the locomotor system depends on full movement of the proximal joints, and also its own joints. Hand stiffness is a major disability. The sensation is also a vital part of hand function and nerve damage leads to severe disability.

The lower limb

HIP JOINT

The hip joint, made up of the femoral head and the acetabulum, is a ball and socket joint. The femoral neck is angled on the shaft at 130° and anteverted from 70° in the infant reaching 30° in adult life. It lies in the acetabulum, which faces outwards, downwards and forwards in the infant, changing to the adult shape of downwards, outwards and backwards. In the infant therefore, the hip joint is stable in flexion and abduction and can be at risk of dislocation in extension and adduction.

The movements occurring at the hip joint are flexion, extension, abduction, adduction and rotation.

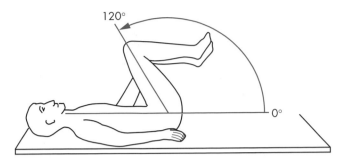

FIG. 1.7   Flexion of the hip

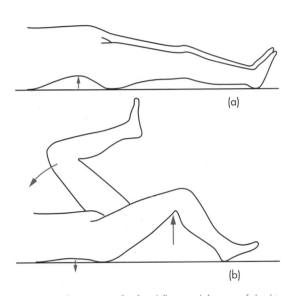

FIG. 1.8   Thomas' test for fixed flexion deformity of the hip

Examination

■ Gait – to note whether there is a limp;
■ posture – this can be assessed standing. If there is femoral neck anteversion, there will be a significant degree of deformity.

Shortening of the limb can be due to a deformity in the bone or contracture of the joint.

If there is true shortening caused by bone loss, it is measured from the anterior superior iliac spine to the medial malleolus.

Apparent shortening is measured from a fixed point, that is the xiphisternum, to the medial malleolus, and reflects joint contractures.

Movement

The movements of the hip joint are performed with the patient lying flat.

Flexion is from 0 to 120°.

Thomas' test is performed to see whether any fixed flexion is present. This is done by flexing the normal hip until the lumbar lordosis has been flattened. The degree of flexion of the abnormal hip is then assessed and this gives the fixed flexion.

Extension is from 0 to 30°.

Abduction: with the pelvis fixed, the leg is abducted 30° from the midline.

Adduction is to the midline, 30°.

Rotation is performed with the patient lying flat and their feet held in the examiner's hands.

Internal rotation and external rotation are about 45°. If the hip is sharply internally rotated and the opposite external obliques contract this is highly suggestive of hip disease and is known as Gervain's sign.

In children it is particularly useful to lie the child flat on the couch with the knees over the end of the bed in order to assess the degree of internal rotation.

FIG. 1.9   Extension of the hip

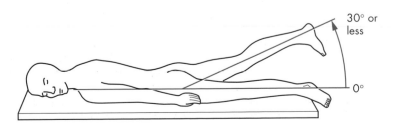

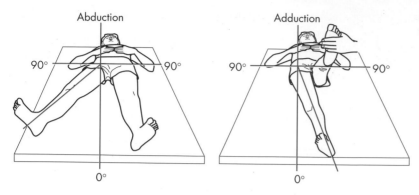

FIG. 1.10   Abduction and adduction of the hip

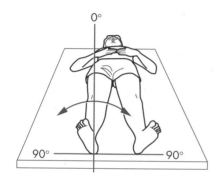

FIG. 1.11   Rotation of the hip

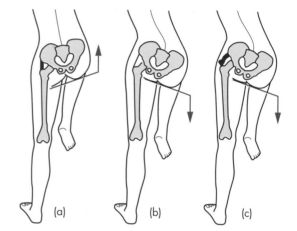

FIG. 1.12   Trendelenburg's sign: (a) negative in a normal hip; (b) positive because of abductor muscle weakness; (c) positive because of joint instability

Trendelenburg's sign is a test that assesses the function of the abductors of the hip, the gluteii. It is useful in disorders of the hip, in which instability, muscle weakness, joint destruction or bone loss occur.

The test is performed by asking the patient to stand, put weight on their normal hip and flex the knee of the affected side while keeping the affected hip extended. The gluteii of the normal hip contract causing the pelvis on the opposite side to be raised.

The test is then applied to the abnormal hip in which there is gluteal weakness and loss of stability to that hip. When weight is taken on this hip joint the opposite side of the pelvis is not elevated and indeed tilts down. This is accentuated when the patient walks causing a dip or lurching effect on the abnormal hip.

KNEE JOINT

The knee is a complex joint, formed by the femoral condyles and the tibial plateau, on which are the meniscii.

The whole joint, which is capable of rotatory movement as well as flexion and extension, is linked by strong medial and lateral ligaments and by the anterior and posterior cruciate ligaments.

The muscles around the knee include the powerful quadriceps muscle, inserted into the tibial tubercle by means of the patellar ligament.

Examination

- Gait: particular attention should be paid to gait (as for the hip), as to whether there is evidence of a painful limp caused by disorder of the knee joint.
- Posture is examined with the patient standing and lying flat. *Genu valgum*, *varum* and *tibial torsion* are clearly demonstrable with the patient standing.

When the joint is inspected deformity, particularly flexion deformity, should be noted.

Swelling of the knee joint can be due to an effusion or synovial thickening. An effusion elicited by pushing the fluid from the suprapatella pouch and demonstrating a patella tap is always symptomatic of some disorder, be it infection, inflammation, trauma, degenerative conditions, or rarely in response to a tumour.

Synovial thickening may be found in rheumatoid arthritis or chronic infections such as tuberculosis or brucellosis.

Movement

The ranges of knee movement are 0–150° flexion, although in a few, hyperextension is possible.

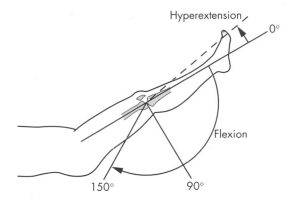

FIG. 1.13   Movements of the knee joint

Stability is assessed through the collateral ligaments; for these to be tested the knee needs to be fully extended. This tests the ligaments along with the capsule and the cruciates. Flexing the knee 10° allows for true medial and lateral ligament assessment.

Cruciate stability is assessed with the knee flexed to 90° and the hamstrings relaxed. Anterior and posterior glide can be achieved.

McMurray's test is a method for assessing the presence of a torn or displaced meniscus. The principle of the test is that the torn portion of the meniscus is caught between the tibia and femur reproducing pain and eliciting a 'clunk' noise. Holding the foot of the flexed knee, the joint is fully flexed as far as possible and then extended while the tibia is rotated internally and externally.

Stability of the patella is assessed by side to side movement with the knee fully extended and the patella compressed against the femoral condyles to reproduce retropatellar pain.

FOOT AND ANKLE

The foot is an important structure that articulates with the tibia at the ankle joint. The ankle joint movements of dorsiflexion and extension occur with a degree of rotation based upon the shape of the talus.

In the foot, inversion and eversion occur at the talonavicular, calcaneocuboid and subtalar joints.

In the forefoot, dorsiflexion and plantar flexion of the metatarsophalangeal joints are dependent on the long flexors and extensors in combination with the intrinsic muscles.

Examination

- Gait: the foot and ankle are integral parts of the gait cycle and any disorder of these structures will affect gait. For example, neurological deformity will affect the gait pattern.
- Posture: the position the foot is held in is of vital importance in examining the foot.

The complex talipes equinovarus deformity demonstrates total joint involvement.

In flat feet the full medial arch demonstrates the deformity. In this the heel of the foot is in valgus, in distinction to the varus deformity seen in pes cavus, the latter being invariably due to a neuromuscular condition commonly associated with calf muscle wasting. Indeed, the shape of the foot may be significantly altered.

Movement

The ankle joint moves through 20° dorsiflexion and 20° plantar flexion.

The subtalar joint is examined by holding the heel at right angles to the leg and examining for adduction and abduction.

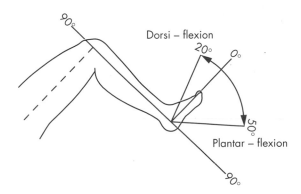

FIG. 1.14   Movements of the ankle joint

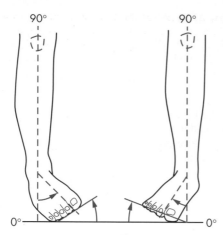

FIG. 1.15   Movements of the midtarsal and subtalar joints

Inversion and eversion occur at the midtarsal joints and these movements are elicited while stabilizing the hindfoot. Active inversion and eversion are usefully performed to demonstrate whether there is a painful flat foot.

Dick's test in infants is a useful means of reproducing the medial arch of the foot and correcting the mobile painless flat foot. In this test, the big toe is dorsiflexed and this will cause the plantar arch to appear.

The spine

LUMBAR SPINE

The lumbar spine consists of five vertebrae articulating with the sacrum below and the thoracic spine above. In between each vertebral body is the intervertebral disc contained within the annulus fibrosus. Articulation between vertebrae occurs between the facet joints, supported on the pedicles. Interspinous and supraspinous ligaments contribute to stability. Lying within the spinal canal of the lumbar vertebrae is the spinal cord up to the level of second lumbar vertebrae with the cauda equina below.

The lamina of the vertebral arch are separated from each other by a strong elastic tissue, the ligamentum flavum.

Examination

■ Gait: examination of the patient walking gives some indication of the balance of the pelvis and the presence or absence of a scoliosis.

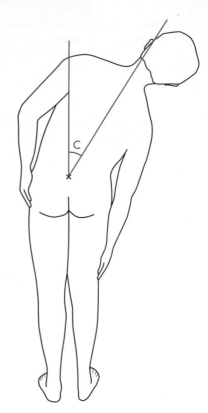

FIG. 1.16   Lateral bending of the thoracic spine

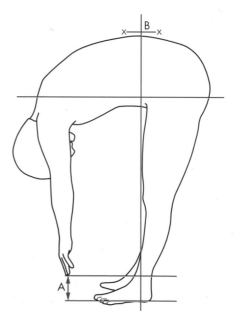

FIG. 1.17   Flexion of the lumbar spine: (a) fingertip to the floor; (b) movement of the lumbar spine

■ Posture: the lumbar spine should be examined with the patient standing, and particular attention paid to the presence of a postural scoliosis or a defect from spondylolisthesis.

Movement

The lumbar spine is examined standing, for flexion and extension. Movement is detected by marking the spinous processes of two vertebrae and measuring the movement that occurs in flexion and extension. Hamstring tightness associated with a spondylolisthesis restricts movement.

Patients with local causes for low back pain (excluding such general causes as infection, tumours and inflammatory disorder) can present with low back pain on its own, or low back pain with nerve root signs. In the latter evidence needs to be sought for nerve root compression, such as in a disc prolapse; L4–5 posterolateral disc prolapse produces L5 nerve root signs, and L5–S1 produces S1 nerve root signs.

Examination

Back

Firm pressure over the affected structure will elicit pain – 'doorbell' sign.

Nerve root signs in the leg

Sciatic nerve root Involvement of the sciatic nerve is tested by straight-leg raising. Normally 90° of straight-leg raising can be achieved with the knee straight. When the nerve roots are stretched over a prolapsed disc there is a reduction in straight-leg

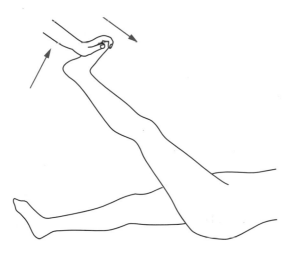

FIG. 1.18 'Straight-leg raising' test for sciatica (Lasègue's test)

raising. When the limit of straight-leg raising is reached the foot is then dorsiflexed aggravating the pain and eliciting a positive sciatic stretch test.

Lasègue's sign is performed for the same condition. In this test straight-leg raising is performed to its limit, the knee is then flexed and the hip flexed further. The knee joint is then extended again producing pain if the test is positive.

Femoral nerve Disc prolapses higher up in the lumbar spine, that is L3–4 or higher, will alter the anterior nerve roots of L2, L3 and L4. If the patient is placed prone and the knee of the affected leg flexed, pain may be elicited and will be accentuated, if the response is positive, when the hip is also extended.

Motor power and sensory involvement need to be carefully examined in patients with nerve root involvement.

Motor power
The following is a general guide:

■ S1 – weakness – Flexor hallucis longus (FHL) Flexor digitorum longus (FDL)
■ L5 – weakness – Extensor hallucis longus (EHL) Extensor digitorum longus (EDL)
■ L4 – weakness tibialis anterior; quadriceps
■ L3 – weakness quadriceps
■ L2 – weakness hip flexors; psoas.

Sensation
The following indicates rough distribution:

■ S1 – back of the calf and lateral side of the foot;
■ L5 – outside of the calf and in first web space;
■ L4 – inside of the calf;
■ L3 – inside of the thigh;
■ L2 – groin and upper area of the thigh.

Reflexes
■ knee jerk – L4
■ ankle jerk – S1.

THORACIC SPINE

This segment of the spine is the least mobile, because of the rib cage, and consists of twelve thoracic vertebrae.

■ Gait: patients' walking should be assessed, including the degree of spinal movement.
■ Posture: scoliosis is visible on direct inspection or on forward flexion, which produces a rib hump. The patient should also be examined from the side to detect a kyphosis.

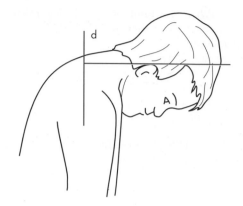

FIG. 1.19   Flexion of the cervical spine

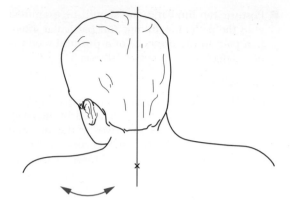

FIG. 1.20   Rotation of the cervical spine

Movement

Flexion and extension of the spine occurs, as does rotation. Lateral bending is also possible.

CERVICAL SPINE

The cervical spine is the most mobile part of the spine and consists of seven vertebrae, which articulate with the occiput and the atlas and the thoracic spine at C7.

The action of nodding occurs at the atlantoaxial joint and the most mobile segment is C5–6.

Examination

- Posture: the position of the head needs to be noted.

Movement

- Flexion (Fig. 1.19)
- extension
- lateral bending
- rotation (Fig. 1.20).

Motor power should also be assessed in the upper limbs.

Power
- Shoulder abduction – C3/4
- elbow flexion – C5–6
- wrist and hand stability – C6/7
- abduction/adduction of fingers – T1.

Sensation
- C6 – outer arm
- C6 – outer forearm
- C7 – hand

- C8 – inner forearm
- T1 – inner arm.

Reflexes
- Biceps – C5/6
- triceps – C6/7
- supination – C7/8.

TISSUES IN THE MUSCULOSKELETAL SYSTEM

Bone

Bone is a highly specialized connective tissue that consists of organic and inorganic constituents. The organic component consists of collagen, mucopolysaccharides, water and bone cells. The inorganic component is made up of hydroxyapatite and contains the solutes carbon, citrate, magnesium, fluorine, sodium, potassium, strontium and lead. Each bone is ensheathed by a relatively tough membrane, the periosteum. This consists of mainly white fibrous tissue with a small amount of elastic tissue, and there is a highly vascular layer containing active osteoblasts.

BONE CELLS

Osteoblasts

Osteoblasts (specialized fibroblasts) synthesize collagen, which makes up the matrix, and concentrate

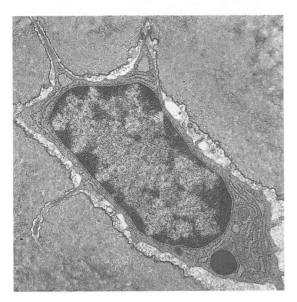

FIG. 1.21 Electron micrograph of an osteocyte within the bone matrix, showing the cytoplasmic processes (prepared by Mr. S. Robertson, Princess Margaret Rose Orthopaedic Hospital, Edinburgh)

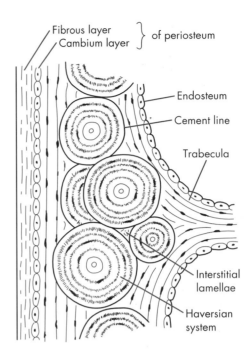

FIG. 1.22 Diagram of the arrangement of mature cortical bone

the ions to produce the amorphous calcium precipitate, the precursor of hydroxyapatite. Osteoblasts convert to osteocytes.

Osteocytes

Osteocytes are the single most numerous type of bone cell. Osteocytes are derived from osteoblasts and do not form collagen. They undergo progressive structural and functional change with age. The osteocytes are involved in the control of mineralization and are the target cells for the action of Parathyroid Hormone (PTH) and calcitonin.

Osteoclasts

Osteoclasts are of haemopoietic origin, contain high concentrations of acid phosphatase and can undergo change into other cell types, transforming even into osteoblasts. They are intimately related to the mineralized bone surface and they are complex cells.

COLLAGEN

Collagen accounts for about 90 per cent of the dry weight of the organic matrix. It provides the strength of the bone in tension and provides resistance to bending. In mature bone the collagen fibres are arranged in regular layers, the lamellae. Woven

bone, in contrast, has an irregular pattern of collagen distribution. Woven bone is found in both the fracture callus and also in Paget's disease of bone.

TYPES OF BONE

Cortical bone

Cortical bone contains primary osteons, which are sheets of lamellar bone wrapped around a central osteon, and are found in newly formed bone. Cortical bone undergoes continuous resorption and renewal; this leads to the primary osteons being replaced by secondary osteons; this is the haversian system.

Each Haversian system consists of a capillary surrounded by osteocytes or osteoblasts that separate it from the hydroxyapatite and collagen.

Trabecular bone

Trabecular bone is found in the medullary cavities of short bones and the metaphyses of long bones. It is arranged in a three-dimensional lattice-work of plates and columns to provide maximum strength and minimum weight.

Periosteum

Periosteum is a membrane that covers cortical bone except on the articular surface or where

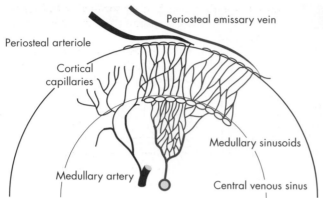

FIG. 1.23   The blood supply of bone (adapted from Murray Brookes)

tendons are inserted. It blends with joint capsules, ligaments and tendons at their attachment to bone and is firmly attached to the periphery of growth plates when they are extra-articular.

In childhood the periosteum is thick and vascular, but in adults it is less vascular, and is thin and adherent. It is attached to bone by Sharpey's fibres, fibrous tissue passing from periosteum to bone.

The periosteum has two layers: an outer fibrous layer and an inner osteogenic cambrium layer.

THE BLOOD SUPPLY OF BONE

The blood supply of bone is of major importance for bone growth, development and formation. Long bones receive their afferent blood supply from nutrient, metaphyseal, epiphyseal and periosteal arteries. Efferent veins drain the bone. The movement of solutes from the capillaries to the bone is a passive event and the flow is centrifugal in direction. Control of bone flow is by neurohumoral and local mechanisms, including such factors as calcitonin gene related peptide (CGRP) and nitric oxide.

Cartilage

Hyaline cartilage contains type II collagen and ground substances – proteoglycans. Fibrocartilage contains more fibres relative to the ground substance and elastic cartilage contains elastic and collagen fibrils.

Articular cartilage covers the bones in synovial joints and is mainly hyaline cartilage. The thickness of articular cartilage varies from over 3 mm in large joints to less than 0.05 mm in the joints of the middle

ear. The thickness does not normally diminish with age. There are four zones of articular cartilage:

- Zone I: nearest to the joint cavity. It contains an abundance of collagen.
- Zone II: intermediate zone. It contains thicker fibrils and single cells are apparent.
- Zone III: deep zone. It contains a fibrous mesh in which the fibrils run radial to the surface. In this layer there are more cells, which appear in groups.
- Zone IV: calcified zone. Here few chondrocytes are found; hydroxyapatite is present, which bonds the cartilage to the subchondral zone.

Cartilage is devoid of blood vessels and neural tissue. The chondrocytes are derived from undifferentiated mesenchyme and the metabolic activity of mature cartilage is low. The nutrition of cartilage is primarily by means of passive diffusion.

Articular cartilage is actively involved in joint lubrication; fluid is expressed through pores in the articular cartilage surface. Hyaluronic acid present in the synovial fluid affects the viscosity of the fluid in the joint. Injury to cartilage produces a variable result, depending partly on the thickness of the defect and also the cause, for example infection in the joint.

A full thickness injury exposing the bone results in the release of inflammatory products. These deeper injuries can initially heal with hyaline cartilage, but frequently transform to fibrocartilage, which disintegrates with load. Superficial injuries to cartilage do not heal completely, but do not appear to proceed to excessive joint destruction.

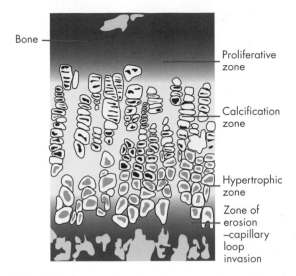

Bone

Proliferative zone

Calcification zone

Hypertrophic zone

Zone of erosion –capillary loop invasion

FIG. 1.24   The growth plate of a mammalian metatarsal bone showing the four layers that give rise to longitudinal growth of the developing bone

GROWTH

Growth occurs at the epiphysis during development. In the epiphysis, the cartilage cells arrange themselves in a radical fashion, so that growth results in a spherical form. The epiphysis has zones of hypertrophy, degeneration, calcification and ossification.

The whole is the growth plate, which closes on maturity (Fig. 1.24).

Muscle

Skeletal muscle is a highly differentiated structure that contracts with great rapidity and easily becomes fatigued. It is under the control of the central nervous system and, as well as its main function in providing active movement, it also produces heat.

Skeletal muscle is composed of individual cylindrical fibres bound together by a matrix of connective tissue. The surface of each muscle fibre is covered by a sarcolemma, which forms a resistant sheath enclosing the tendons. Each fibre is in turn multinucleated. The function of muscle in providing contraction is performed by the interaction of actin on myosin, which gives rise to the cross-striated patterns characteristic of striated muscle. Within the connective tissue of muscle are the

muscle spindles, which are associated with coordination of muscle activity and the maintenance of muscle tone.

On reaching the appropriate muscle fibre the nerve fibres lose their myelin and become continuous with the sarcolemma sheath. The axons of the nerve pierce the sheath and break up into terminal ramifications forming the motor end plate.

The range of movement through which a muscle can go is proportional to the length of the muscle fibres. Tendons allow the line of a muscle to be changed, by passing over a bony prominence or being held in a fibrous retinaculum.

Muscle action depends upon the contraction of individual fibres. As the force of the contraction of the whole muscle increases, more and more individual fibres come into action.

Muscles act as synergists or antagonists as well as producing prime movement. Hence, when a muscle contracts to produce a movement in one direction, synergists act to prevent movement that is antagonistic. Antagonists oppose the prime mover and thus allow a controlled smooth action – as the prime mover contracts the antagonist relaxes actively.

There are two main types of muscle fibres. Type I, which produce a slow contractile response, and type II, which produce a faster contraction. There are further subdivisions of type II into A and B. Muscle injury frequently occurs, especially following sports and after surgery. Myofibrils have the ability to regenerate, although frequently scar tissue forms in place of muscle. At its extreme, this can be seen in Volkmann's ischaemic contracture of muscle, when after a vascular injury to muscle extensive scar tissue will appear.

Nerves

The conducting elements of peripheral nerves are the axons, which are cytoplasmic extensors of the cell bodies in the dorsal root ganglia and the central horn of the spinal cord. These axons can be small (less than 2 µm in diameter), transmitting touch, pain and temperature, or large, surrounded by columns of Schwann cells to form the myelin sheath and ranging from 2 to 20 µm, transmitting impulses to skeletal muscle and specialized receptors in skin, muscle and joints.

The myelin sheath is segmented, narrowing at the nodes of Ranvier, where adjacent Schwann cells meet. A basement membrane is found outside the Schwann cytoplasm, which forms the boundary

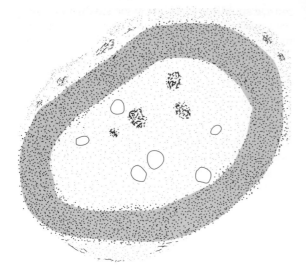

FIG. 1.25   A single myelinated axon. Rat sciatic nerve

BIOMECHANICS

Biomechanics is an expanding discipline that is closely allied to orthopaedics. Certain terms are in frequent use and are examined below.

Terms used

FORCE

Force is a vector and has magnitude, direction and a point of application. There are different types of force.

- Tension, in which molecules are pulled away from each other.
- Compression, in which molecules are pushed together in the direction of the force.
- Shear, in which one layer of molecules tries to slide sideways across the layer below them.

DYNAMICS

The velocity of an object is the distance it moves in a given direction in a given time.

KINETICS

Kinetics is the study of the forces, without considering the movement producing it; kinematics is the study of movement without considering the forces producing it. Both these concepts are used in gait analysis.

STATICS

Stress analysis

Stress is the internal response to an externally applied load and is measured in Newtons per square metre (N/m^2) or Pascals (Pa).

$$Stress = \frac{Force}{Unit\ area}$$

between the Schwann cell membrane and the endoneurium. Bundles of axons together are ensheathed by the perineurium. A nerve trunk is composed of numbers of such bundles, which form the epineurium.

Axons do not pass down nerve trunks in a direct line, as a telephone cable, but in a wavy pattern, in order to protect nerve fibres against the effect of traction. The numbers of nerve fibres vary in their course down a limb. For example, the median nerve has 12 bundles in the arm and 25–40 in the wrist, increasing further in the fingers.

After a complete injury to the nerve, the distal part typically undergoes Wallerian degeneration, as does the proximal stump to some degree. However, if the axons are preserved, as in a compression injury, recovery is probable. The muscle fibres are dependent on the nerve input, so that disruption of the nerve will be associated with muscle atrophy.

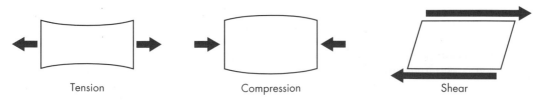

Tension   Compression   Shear

FIG. 1.26   The three types of force: tension, compression and shear

Strain

This is a measure of deformation of a solid body when in a state of stress:

$$\text{Strain} = \frac{\text{Change in length}}{\text{Original length}}$$

measured in microstrain units.

Bending

Most surgical implants are subject to bending stresses and fail when they are unable to withstand repeated bending.

All three types of stress are involved – tensile, compression and shear stress.

STRENGTH OF MATERIALS

Elasticity

Normally Hooke's law is obeyed and there is a linear relationship between stress and strain for the material, after which the elastic limit is reached, producing a large increase in strain for a little increase in stress (Fig. 1.27). Biological materials are not uniform and do not demonstrate non-linear elasticity.

Plastic behaviour

When a material is stressed beyond the elastic limit it becomes permanently deformed and will not return to its starting dimensions. This is plastic behaviour. It is seen in heavy patients who repeatedly stress the femoral component of a hip prosthesis, causing the material to fail and fracture.

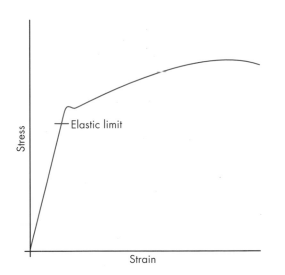

FIG. 1.27 The relationship between tensile stress and strain in steel. Beyond the elastic limit the material stretches, producing a large increase in strain for a little change in stress

Materials used

POLYMERS

Ultra-high molecular weight polyethylene, which is used for the acetabular component in total hip replacement or the tibial plateau of the knee joint, is biologically inert and articulates with smooth metal surfaces at low frictional resistance. The plastic is affected by constant wear, and can lead to long-term loosening of the components. Silicone rubbers are also used and are resilient materials, although they too tend to degrade *in situ*. Silicone rubber is used in metacarpal/phalangeal replacements in the hand and also in the foot.

METAL IMPLANTS

Metal implants, which are used for internal fixation of fractures or joint replacements, are made of substances such as stainless steel, cobalt chromium alloys or titanium and its alloys. These are inert and highly resistant to fatigue and corrosion. Corrosion of the metal can occur either from stress after a passage of time or when an electric circuit is set up from the metal, which will gradually corrode it and is a cause for screw head failure years after insertion. High quality manufacturing has reduced the problem of corrosion and fatigue to a degree.

CEMENT

Bone cement is a self-curing poly methylmethacrylate and matches the shape of the bone into which it is inserted. It is a brittle material that can penetrate the trabecular structure of cancellous bone and provide a degree of adhesion. This process strengthens the bonding of the prosthesis to the bone, reducing tension and stress.

REHABILITATION

TERMS

Rehabilitation is concerned with the physical, social and organizational aspects of the aftercare of patients. This may involve definitive treatment to regain locomotor function, retraining for a new job or modification of existing work, adaptation to the home environment in order to cope with progressive disability and the coordination of all the various departments that can help a disabled person.

Rehabilitation for the patient who may be expected to become independent can be considered as planned withdrawal of support. However, for the patient in whom there is likely to be severe restriction of activity it requires the deployment of a variety of skills and expertise to ensure that he or she lives as purposeful a life as is possible.

It is the responsibility of every doctor to make sure that his patient is fully rehabilitated, but there are now so many aspects of rehabilitation that there is often a specialist in each major hospital who coordinates the various rehabilitation services. In practice, rehabilitation can be considered under the headings:

- preoperative;
- postoperative;
- restoration of the patient to their social surroundings.

PREOPERATIVE

In orthopaedics in particular, definitive surgery is elective and there is time before surgery to assess in detail exactly what is required to improve the patient's function so that the appropriate operative procedure may be performed. This is particularly true in patients with rheumatoid arthritis, suffering from multiple joint involvement. Careful functional assessment by the physiotherapist and occupational therapist will help to elucidate the problems and suggest the most suitable order of surgery.

POSTOPERATIVE

Once activity is permitted, the aim is to restore the range of joint movement and to develop muscle power and coordination. The surgeon relies on the expertise of the physiotherapist together with the help of the occupational therapist to develop the programme.

REHABILITATION

The restoration of the patient to his or her own environment requires the skills of the physiotherapist, the occupational therapist, the rehabilitation specialist and the medical social worker. Occasionally a patient needs to be treated in a special rehabilitation centre.

Physiotherapy

The physiotherapist has available a variety of treatment modalities for rehabilitating the patient. These are described below.

SPINAL AND PERIPHERAL JOINT MOBILIZATIONS

Such mobilizations are used to restore specific joint motion or to relieve pain.

EXERCISE

Individual exercise programmes, or group sessions, can be used to mobilize or strengthen muscles in acute and chronic conditions.

NEURAL MOBILIZATIONS

These are used to mobilize nervous tissue when adverse neural tension is a component of the problem.

TRACTION

Traction is used in conjunction with other techniques in the treatment programme. It is most effective in the treatment of lumbar and cervical disorders, applied by manual technique or a mechanical unit, in either a sustained or intermittent mode.

ELECTROTHERAPY

- Ultrasound: therapeutic frequencies used in the treatment of soft tissue injuries to promote healing and relieve pain;
- interferential: used to relieve pain, decrease swelling and stimulate muscle contractions;
- pulsed shortwave: useful for reabsorption of effusion, healing tissue with minimal heating effect;
- transcutaneous nerve stimulator (TNS): based on the pain/gate theory. It is useful as a non-invasive pain relieving treatment;
- laser: useful for acute wound healing and pain relief.

SOFT-TISSUE MASSAGE

A traditional physiotherapy technique still used in the treatment of haematomas or for injuries to ligaments, tendons and other tissue.

HYDROTHERAPY

Exercises in a heated pool, utilizing the properties of water to assist and resist movement.

HOT OR COLD THERAPY

Ice packs and hot packs are useful for reducing swelling and promoting healing by removal of tissue irritants.

SPLINTING AND STRAPPING

Serial splints can be used to reduce deformity and may be made out of plaster of Paris or a thermoplastic material. Collars or corsets may also be used in the acute stages of cervical or lumbar disorders.

Strapping tape can be used as a temporary support, usually when the patient is strengthening the muscles and requires support.

ADVICE

Advice, relating to posture, neck and back care; ergonomics; and exercise is an important factor in preventing recurrence of the condition.

Occupational therapy

The occupational therapist's role is to maintain and maximize a patient's functional performance in the activities of daily living and hence improve their overall quality of life. The occupational therapist works together with the patient, their family and the community services in order to achieve this.

The occupational therapist's role in orthopaedics involves assessment of:

- the patient's functional ability, in terms of daily living, such as personal hygiene·and domestic tasks;
- the patient's psychosocial function;
- the patient's physical ability, such as joint movement, muscle power and activity tolerance.

Treatment includes:

- restoration and maintenance of muscle power, coordination and joint motion;
- energy conservation and improving activity;
- education and provision of appropriate equipment in order to enhance the surgical treatment, for example providing a raised toilet seat and perching stool after hip joint replacement;
- optimizing functional performance and independence by the provision of appropriate equipment and adaptations of the home, for example bath rails;
- facilitating the patient's return to work.

Medical social worker

The medical social worker is an important member of the rehabilitation team. His or her role is to explore all the social and economic problems that affect the patient and their family. In order to do this the medical social worker has access to a wide range of statutory and voluntary bodies who help the disabled.

The local social services department provides aids and appliances, home helps, meals on wheels, day and residential care, and also provides advice on local clubs. The local housing department and health authority assist the medical social worker in organizing rehousing.

Rehabilitation centres

Rehabilitation is usually performed in the general hospital, with one consultant designated to lead the rehabilitation team. However, there are certain complex disabilities that are best treated in special rehabilitation centres. These may be specific disabilities such as those that follow multiple injuries, spinal injuries or cerebrovascular accidents. In these centres intensive forms of rehabilitation can be conducted on a personal basis.

The introduction of a team spirit with an overall atmosphere of enthusiasm and obvious progress of the patients make ideal conditions for motivation and more rapid recovery.

2 TRAUMA

INTRODUCTION

Various types and amounts of energy can damage tissue to differing degrees. However, even low velocity trauma, for example resulting from a simple fall, can cause severe consequences, such as a hip fracture, in an elderly osteoporotic patient. Complications from the resulting surgery can be just as life threatening as the high velocity injury to a younger patient. However, the majority of trauma cases are not life-threatening and do not require intensive resuscitation.

All trauma should be treated with respect and careful assessment of the whole patient, rather than just the obviously injured parts, and there must be a well rehearsed routine by trained staff in a dedicated trauma assessment area. It has been well demonstrated that identification of patients at high risk can dramatically reduce mortality and morbidity.

After severe trauma the first peak of death occurs within minutes of injury. Causes of death include aortic rupture, brain injury and massive rapid blood loss. Very few of these patients survive to reach hospital. The second death peak is known as the 'Golden Hour' when skilled treatment can save lives from injuries such as skull haematomas, pneumothorax, ruptured spleen, and severe blood loss from, for example, multiple fractures and soft tissue damage. The third death peak occurs from complications many days after the injury from such events as infection and organ failure, for example respiratory distress syndrome. Effective initial resuscitation, however, has been shown to influence the incidence of even these late complications significantly.

The size of the problem

With the increase in road traffic accidents, trauma is approaching near epidemic proportions. At the same time, as a result of improved social and medical care, more people are reaching old age. In the elderly, in whom there is osteoporosis and loss of function, falls become more frequent and the resulting effects of these falls are more serious.

PRINCIPLES OF FIRST AID

The main purpose of first aid is to save the person's life and to prevent further immediate damage. On arriving at the scene of a road traffic accident the priorities are:

- to enlist help and, if need be, call for an ambulance;
- to ensure that traffic is controlled to prevent a further accident;
- to maintain the airway (A = airway);
- maintain breathing (B = breathing);
- to control obvious haemorrhage (C = circulation);
- to splint the neck, back or a fractured limb.

Initial assessment

Assessment and management priorities are part of the formal structured teaching included in the 'Advanced Trauma Life Support' (ATLS) courses that are readily available today.

The 'primary survey' consists of:

- A airway maintenance with cervical spine control;
- B breathing and ventilation is maintained by use of inspection and airways;
- C circulation and haemorrhage control;
- D disability assessment by neurological examination;
- E exposure must be complete by removal of clothing.

The airway is maintained by opening the mouth, removing anything that is blocking the free flow of air and, if possible turning the patient on their side to prevent the tongue occluding the trachea. If necessary, mouth-to-mouth resuscitation can be initiated, in combination with external cardiac massage, in order to maintain oxygenation of vital organs. Oropharyngeal airways can be useful.

If practical, obvious haemorrhage should be controlled, by the application of firm pressure. Unless haemorrhage is life threatening, tourniquets should not be used because extensive tissue necrosis may occur.

Splintage of the neck and careful handling of suspected spinal injuries are essential. Splintage of a limb, although ideal, may not be possible, but should be practised if feasible in order to prevent any further painful movement.

At this stage it is invaluable to obtain a story of the accident from other witnesses, to note the pulse, the pattern of respiration, level of consciousness and state of the pupils. Medical and paramedical staff are now frequently in attendance to initiate resuscitation, safe handling and splintage. The patient is then transferred to an accident centre at a hospital as soon as possible and treatment is continued.

MANAGEMENT OF THE PATIENT IN HOSPITAL

On arrival in the accident and emergency department the immediate priorities for the multiply injured patient include assessment and resuscitation. Once again, before any detailed examination of the patient is commenced, a clear airway must be established and the control of blood loss must be attempted. ATLS principles are once again applied in terms of a further 'Primary Survey'.

Shock management should be started immediately, including intravenous access, oxygenation and haemorrhage control. Only once these life-threatening problems have been adequately attended to, can the so-called 'Secondary Survey' begin.

During the Secondary Survey monitoring of the vital life-signs must continue. Teamwork and good leadership is essential. This phase of examination should therefore include a region by region search, palpation and auscultation. Head, chest, abdomen and the limbs must be carefully inspected, including assessment of the local circulation and neurological status. Finally an assessment of the Glasgow Coma Scale (GCS) is carried out. Chest, pelvis and cervical radiographs are performed during this early phase because of the serious nature of any potential injuries.

Any life-threatening problems identified during the surveys must of course be addressed immediately. Techniques such as cricothyroidotomy, chest drain insertion and improved immobilization of the spine must therefore be carried out quickly but safely.

'Special Procedures' can now be performed during the next phase of assessment, which can include peritoneal lavage, further radiographs and catheterization. X-ray examination should include chest, spine, skull, pelvis, abdomen and appropriate limb views. Improved venous and arterial access, further immobilization and splintage can then take place. Once the patient is fully stabilized then other investigations such as computed tomography (CT) scanning can be carried out.

The so-called 'Definitive Care Phase' can then begin in which individual specialties of medicine and surgery can be consulted to agree upon a plan of action. Often this will involve several teams such as 'general', 'neuro', 'cardiac', 'oral' and orthopaedic surgeons working simultaneously.

Treatment of shock

If there is or there has been significant haemorrhage, it will be necessary to restore the circulating blood volume. The peripheral tissues need adequate perfusion by well oxygenated blood, and after a fracture blood is lost from the bone and from the damaged tissues. The amount of blood loss can be estimated as follows:

- the type of fracture:
  (a) displaced fracture = 1 litre;
  (b) comminuted fracture of the pelvis = 2 litres;
  (c) open fracture of the lower limb = 1 litre;
- examining the patient and taking recordings.

Table 2.1 gives approximate values for clinical readings and overall fluid requirements (reproduced with kind permission from the ATLS® manual).

The recommendations in the table for the actual amounts of different fluids used in the resuscitation are based on the premise that most patients in shock will require more electrolyte solution than the actual volume of blood lost. If the patient is shocked, they are pale, restless and sweating profusely. Central venous pressure (CVP) is a good monitor of the circulation. The normal CVP is 4–8 cmH$_2$O, and sudden changes in the pressure are significant. In well equipped accident departments and intensive care units, low blood pressure can also be measured by an intra-arterial catheter.

This allows continuous readings of the systolic and diastolic pulse pressures. The catheter can be inserted via the radial artery. Pulmonary capillary wedge pressure can also be used as a more accurate guide to fluid deficit. A Swan–Ganz flotation balloon is inserted into the pulmonary artery via the subclavian or internal jugular vein. The tip of the catheter wedges in a terminal branch of the pulmonary artery and records pressure, giving a good index of the heart function.

Urine output should also be monitored and the urea and electrolytes estimated. Serial arterial blood gases are also vital for monitoring shock.

Fluid loss can be replaced by:

- physiological (0.9%) saline or Ringer's lactate;
- colloids such as dextran 70;
- plasma protein (human albumin) 5%;
- whole blood, which should be as fresh as possible; for every 2 litres, give 10 ml of calcium gluconate.

If multiple transfusions are required, fresh-frozen plasma and platelets may be needed as well.

Immediate treatment of fractures and dislocations

The definitive classification and treatment of individual fractures will be discussed in more

	Mild	Moderate	Severe	Pre-morbid
Blood loss (ml)	<750	750–1500	1500–2000	>2000
% Blood volume	<15%	15–30%	30–40%	>40%
Pulse rate (per min)	<100	>100	>120	>140
Blood pressure	Normal	Normal	Decreased	Decreased
Respiratory rate (per min)	14–20	20–30	30–40	>35
Urine output (ml/h)	>30	20–30	5–20	<5
CNS mental state	Calm	Slight anxiety	Anxious and confused	Lethargic
Fluid replacement	Crystalloid	Crystalloid	Crystalloid and blood	Crystalloid and blood

TABLE 2.1 Estimated fluid and blood losses based on patient's initial presentation. Source: *Advanced Trauma Life Support® Student Manual*, ACS Committee on Trauma (1993)

detail elsewhere. However, a major fracture is usually obvious. There is pain, swelling, deformity and loss of function. It is important to note whether the skin overlying the fracture is broken. If it is, the fracture is 'open' and hence liable to infection. It is sensible at this stage to take a photograph and cover the wound with antiseptic soaked dressings. The state of the muscle damage, particularly in open fractures, should be noted. It is essential to check the arterial blood supply beyond the site of the injury because if this is impaired it must be restored as soon as possible to prevent permanent damage to the limb from ischaemia. The peripheral nerves should be examined as the baseline for future recovery.

Splintage has been carried out since ancient times in order to reduce pain and improve long-term recovery. However, since the First World War it has been known that splintage of, for example, a fractured femur in a 'Thomas splint' will improve mortality by reducing shock. This principle is particularly true in the fractured pelvis in which huge amounts of blood can be lost.

Pain

Injuries are painful. Regional nerve blocks will provide considerable relief from pain and Entonox® (50% N_2O/50% O_2) may be used without interfering with the assessment of head or intra-abdominal injuries. However, if an adequate diagnosis has been made and the peripheral circulation is not collapsed, pain can be relieved by morphine or pethidine.

Antibiotics and infection

In open fractures in which the tissues and bone are contaminated with potentially infected material the administration of intravenous antibiotics to treat infection is essential. The antibiotics of choice are benzylpenicillin combined with a cephalosporin such as cefuroxime.

Antitetanus

Measures to treat tetanus must be taken in all patients brought to hospital with open wounds. In superficial wounds contaminated with soil, tetanus toxoid 0.5 ml is given. It produces an active immunity. In clean but larger, deeper wounds without a great quantity of devitalized tissue and in which early surgical toilet is practised, both tetanus toxoid and an antibiotic may be effective.

However, in large, heavily contaminated wounds with a great deal of devitalized tissue it is best to give human antitetanus serum, antibiotics and tetanus toxoid. Whenever antitetanus serum is given, a preliminary test dose should be injected subcutaneously to see whether a reaction occurs. If active immunity is required, booster doses will be needed to be given at 6 weeks and at 6 months.

Polytrauma and triage

The term 'triage' dates from the times of the Napoleonic Wars when casualties were divided into three groups based upon their likelihood of survival. Such triage is essential, particularly during mass casualty situations. However, any multiply injured patient can now be assessed by means of the 'CRAMS' scale, which makes it possible to decide whether the patient should be transferred to a special trauma centre. A score of 6 or less is said to warrant such transfer.

TABLE 2.2 CRAMS scale

System	Clinical finding	Points
Circulation	normal capillary filling; systolic BP >100 mmHg	2
	delayed filling; systolic BP <100 mmHg	1
	no capillary filling; systolic BP <85 mmHg	0
Respiration	normal	2
	shallow/laboured	1
	respiratory rate >35/min	0
Abdomen and thorax	non-tender	2
	rigid abdomen or flail chest	1
	penetrating injury	0
Motor function	normal	2
	responds to pain	1
	posturing or no response	0
Speech	normal	2
	confused	1
	nil or unintelligible	0

For retrospective analysis the Abbreviated Injury Scale (AIS) introduced by the Committee on Injury Scaling of the American Association for Automotive Medicine in 1976 is more widely used.

This is based upon a scoring system for injuries in different regions of the body with the Injury Severity Score (ISS) being obtained from the sum of the squares of the three most severely injured areas. A non-linear, quadratic type of relationship between the score and mortality is found.

0 – no injury
1 – minor injury
2 – moderate injury
3 – severe injury (not life-threatening)
4 – severe injury (life-threatening)
5 – critical injury (survival uncertain)
6 – fatal/maximum injury (currently untreatable)

However, the whole point of identifying 'at risk' patients is to alert clinicians immediately to the need for expert care, including urgent operations, cardiorespiratory support, advanced investigations and well planned courses of 'delayed' surgery. Such so-called 'delayed' surgery has to be carried out within 24–48 hours of admission. In the case of long-bone fracture fixation in particular, such early intervention has been shown to reduce post-traumatic complications such as 'respiratory distress syndrome' and infection significantly.

COMPLICATIONS

Fat embolus

This condition is associated with multiple fractures. About 24 hours after injury the patient suddenly becomes breathless, develops multiple skin haemorrhages and there is an obvious fall in the PO_2. Treatment consists of giving oxygen by means of positive end-expiratory ventilation in the intensive care unit. Antibiotic cover and physiotherapy are essential. All fractures should be stabilized as soon thereafter as possible.

Shock lung

This condition can be related to fracture-related 'fat embolus', and is also known as respiratory distress syndrome or wet lung, and is associated with shock related to fluid overload or excess blood transfusion and septicaemia. The patient develops respiratory distress and there is a significant hypoxaemia. Essentially treatment is by giving oxygen and positive end-expiratory pressure (PEEP) ventilation support.

Disseminated intravascular coagulation

This probably occurs to some degree in all severely shocked patients and is diagnosed by a decrease in levels of fibrinogen, factor VIII and platelets. There is also evidence of enhanced fibrinolytic activity with high concentrations of the fibrin degradation products. Treatment aims to correct the underlying disorder, and to reduce bleeding by giving fresh-frozen plasma and platelet concentrates if necessary.

Summary
From much clinical evidence four principles emerge:

■ Medical and nursing personnel should all be ATLS® or equivalent trained.
■ There should be an effective triage system such as CRAMS to identify the patient at risk to be transferred to the appropriate hospital.
■ Specialist Trauma Centres are required.
■ Early internal fixation of fractures saves lives and if used in combination with adequate vascular volume control and PEEP, the majority of trauma deaths can be prevented.

3 HEAD INJURIES*

In the UK, 300 patients per 100 000 of the population are admitted to hospital each year because of head injury; 85 per cent of these are minor injuries, 10 per cent moderate and 5 per cent severe (in coma). In at least half of the severe cases there are one or more other major injuries, and in 40 per cent an intracranial haematoma, the major cause of brain compression, is present. More than 70 per cent of patients admitted to hospital with multiple injuries have some degree of head injury.

PATHOLOGY AND CLINICAL FINDINGS

Injuries to the head may be open (compound or penetrating) or closed (blunt or acceleration/deceleration). The skull may or may not be fractured, and the injury to the brain may in either circumstance be mild or severe according to the forces applied to the head. Brain injury may be classified as follows.

Concussion

Concussion is a transient paralysis of brain function, occurring at the moment of injury. The patient is therefore immediately unconscious, but recovers spontaneously within a short time. There is always a period of amnesia, and the duration of the post-traumatic amnesia is a useful guide to the severity of the concussion. Less than 1 hour signifies a minor concussional injury, 1–24 hours moderate concussion and more than 24 hours a severe concussional injury, with a prolonged time off work and likely occurrence of post-traumatic neuropsychological symptoms.

Diffuse white matter injury

When the head is subjected to a considerable force, as in a car crash, swirling movements of the brain occur within the skull, which result in shearing of nerve fibres diffusely in the subcortical white matter. This is microscopic damage, invisible to the naked eye, but it abruptly reduces the connections between the cortex and the reticular formation of the brainstem causing prolonged unconsciousness. There is also abnormal motor activity with abnormal flexor (decorticate) or extensor (decerebrate) responses.

Cerebral contusion and laceration

Contusion (bruising) and/or laceration of the brain may be localized under a depressed skull fracture, or may be more widespread, at the frontal and temporal poles consequent on the movement of the brain within the skull. The clinical correlates depend upon the area of the brain that has been injured – behavioural disturbance and anosmia when the frontal lobes are damaged, dysphasia

*Written by the late Professor Douglas Miller.

with damage to the dominant temporal lobe, motor or sensory deficit when those cortical areas are involved, and defects in the contralateral visual field when the occipital lobe is damaged.

Brain compression

This occurs nearly always as a result of haemorrhage into the middle or anterior fossa of the skull. Bleeding into the posterior fossa is less common, as is direct damage to the hindbrain. Rarely, brain compression is caused by abscesses, aeroceles or encysted collections of cerebrospinal fluid (hygromas) in the subdural or subarachnoid spaces.

Acute extradural haemorrhage occurs from meningeal arteries torn by an overlying fracture or severe bending of the infant skull. Subdural haematomas may form acutely from rupture of a single vein at the brain surface, or from cortical veins and arteries torn in a cerebral laceration. Chronic subdural haematomas are most common in the older age groups and in the very young, often after a trivial injury, and particularly when there is some cerebral atrophy. The source of bleeding is usually a cortical vein close to the superior sagittal sinus, and a slowly expanding fluid blood cyst forms over one or both cerebral hemispheres, quite different from the acute haematomas, which consist of clotted blood.

As any haematoma increases in size the underlying brain becomes progressively compressed and shifted in position. Displacement of the medial part of the temporal lobe into the tentorial hiatus distorts and damages the midbrain, resulting in deterioration of consciousness and often an oculomotor nerve palsy on the side of the lesion with a contralateral hemiparesis. If compression is not reversed the lower brainstem becomes ischaemic, resulting in the well known combination of a rising arterial pressure and bradycardia followed by respiratory arrest. At the same time, there is a rise in intracranial pressure from the normal upper limit of 10 mmHg to 60 mmHg or more. Other causes of brain compression are oedema or congestive swelling of the damaged brain itself.

MANAGEMENT

General principles

It is important to make an accurate neurological assessment as soon as life-threatening emergen-

cies, such as airway obstruction or severe haemorrhage, have been dealt with and a stable respiratory and circulatory status have been assured. The assessment must include the state of consciousness, pupillary size and reactions to light, eye movements and a comparison of the power of limb movements in response to command or to painful stimuli. When possible, a history of the patient's level of consciousness before admission to hospital should be obtained to determine whether the patient is improving, deteriorating or stable. The level of consciousness should be measured using the Glasgow Coma Scale (Table 3.1). In the acute phase these observations, together with measurements of heart rate, blood pressure, body temperature and respiration, should be repeated every 15 or 30 minutes and recorded on a head injury observation chart.

TABLE 3.1 Glasgow Coma Scale

Eye opening	Motor response	Verbal response
4 Spontaneous	6 Obeys commands	5 Orientated
3 To command	5 Localizes pain	4 Disorientated
2 To pain	4 Normal flexion	3 Words only
1 Nil	3 Abnormal flexion	2 Sounds only
	2 Extension	1 Nil
	1 Nil	

Most patients with concussion, contusion or laceration should improve steadily after admission. In contrast, in cerebral compression, after a variable period, deterioration in consciousness occurs, sometimes with dramatic rapidity, with or without localizing signs of neurological dysfunction such as unequal pupils or hemiparesis. In the intervening period, usually of not more than a few hours, the patient may have regained consciousness after the initial concussion – 'the lucid interval'.

In patients with summated coma scores of 9 or more, serial observation of the conscious level is a safe way to detect the deterioration that may herald intracranial haemorrhage requiring surgical decompression as a matter of urgency. In the patient who is in coma, defined on the coma scale as a state in which there is no eye opening, even to pain, no obedience to commands and no recognizable words uttered (a summated score of 8 or less), there is a 40 per cent probability that an

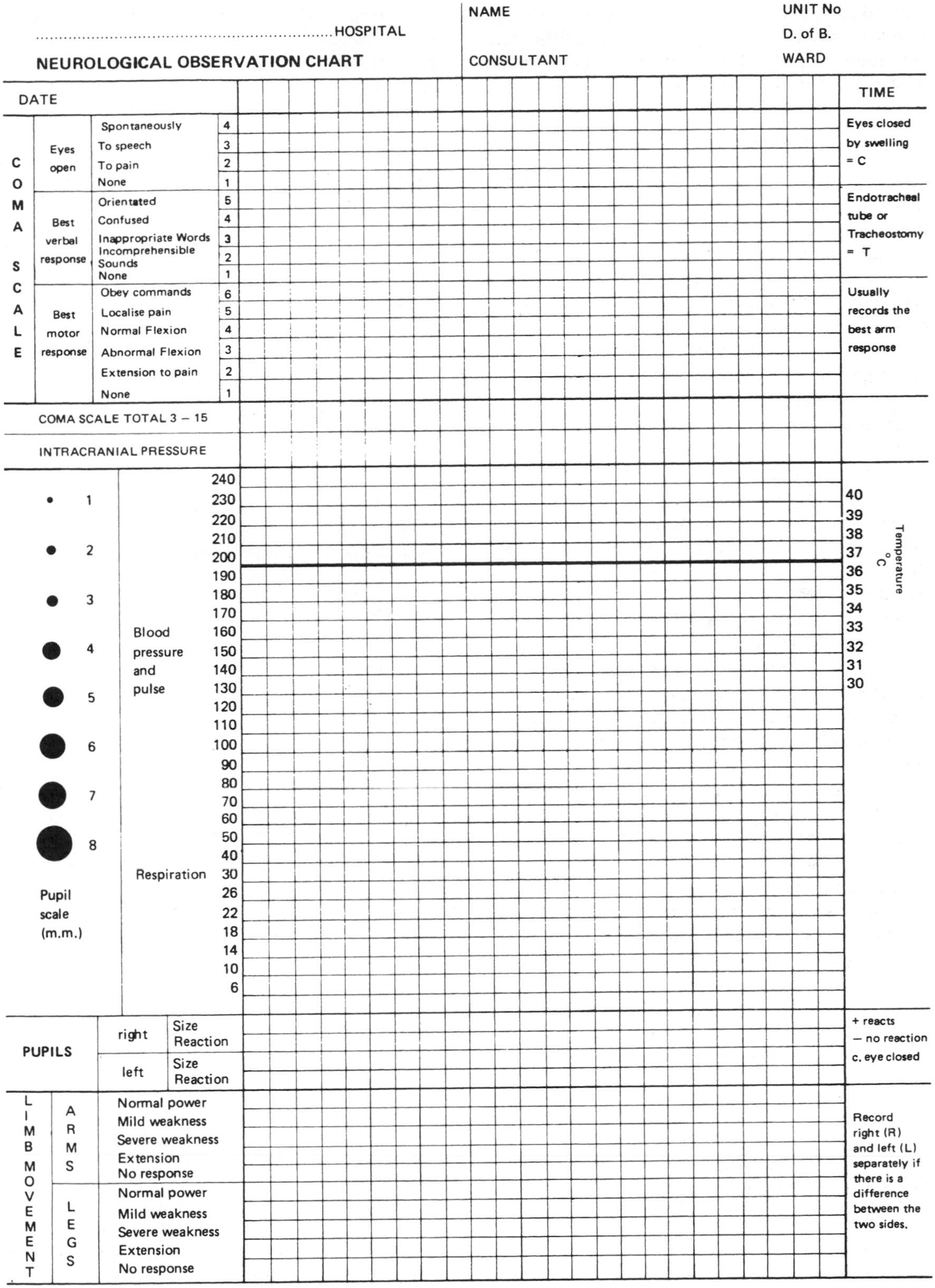

NAME

UNIT No

D. of B.

NEUROLOGICAL OBSERVATION CHART

CONSULTANT

WARD

DATE						TIME

COMA SCALE

	Eyes open	Spontaneously	4	Eyes closed by swelling = C
		To speech	3	
		To pain	2	
		None	1	
	Best verbal response	Orientated	5	Endotracheal tube or Tracheostomy = T
		Confused	4	
		Inappropriate Words	3	
		Incomprehensible Sounds	2	
		None	1	
	Best motor response	Obey commands	6	Usually records the best arm response
		Localise pain	5	
		Normal Flexion	4	
		Abnormal Flexion	3	
		Extension to pain	2	
		None	1	

COMA SCALE TOTAL 3 – 15

INTRACRANIAL PRESSURE

Pupil scale (m.m.)

- 1
- 2
- 3
- 4
- 5
- 6
- 7
- 8

Blood pressure and pulse

240 230 220 210 200 190 180 170 160 150 140 130 120 110 100 90 80 70 60 50 40

Respiration 30 26 22 18 14 10 6

Temperature °C: 40 39 38 37 36 35 34 33 32 31 30

PUPILS	right	Size		+ reacts
		Reaction		− no reaction
	left	Size		c. eye closed
		Reaction		

LIMB MOVEMENT	ARMS	Normal power		Record right (R) and left (L) separately if there is a difference between the two sides.
		Mild weakness		
		Severe weakness		
		Extension		
		No response		
	LEGS	Normal power		
		Mild weakness		
		Severe weakness		
		Extension		
		No response		

FIG. 3.1   Neuro-observation chart for use with head-injured patients

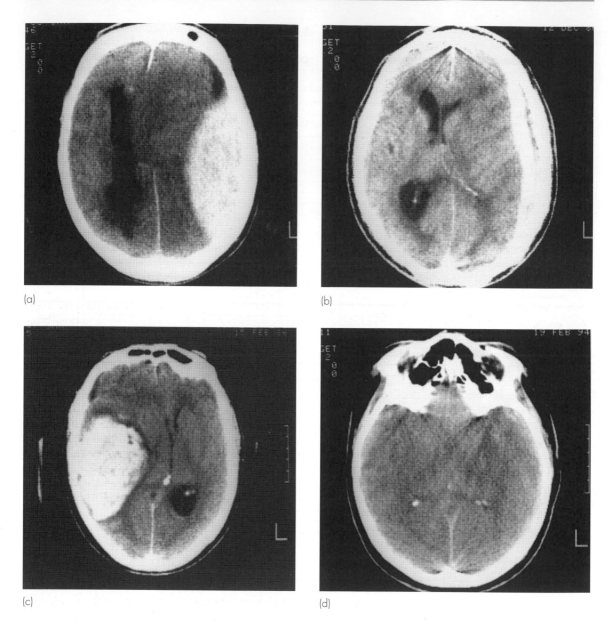

(a)

(b)

(c)

(d)

FIG. 3.2   CT images of common problems associated with head injury (a) top left, large left-sided extradural haematoma with shift and dilatation of opposite lateral ventricle indicating high intracranial pressure; (b) top right, extensive left-sided acute subdural haematoma with midline shift, compression of the ipsilateral ventricle and dilatation of the contralateral ventricle; (c) bottom left, large right-sided intracerebral haematoma with shift of the calcified pineal gland; (d) bottom right, post-traumatic swelling with loss of the image of any of the cerebrospinal fluid spaces

intracranial haematoma is present. It is inappropriate to await further neurological deterioration before taking measures to detect and localize the haematoma.

The most efficient means of diagnosing and localizing intracranial haemorrhage is computed tomography (CT). Because of the 40 per cent chance of finding an intracranial haematoma in a comatose patient, all such patients should be referred for immediate CT without awaiting further neurological deterioration. The presence of a skull fracture greatly increases the chance of a haematoma (extradural or subdural) being found. It is now recommended that in patients in whom skull fracture is accompanied by any impairment of consciousness (a score of 14 or less on the Glasgow Coma Scale), by focal neurological dysfunction (aphasia or hemiplegia, for instance) or by a seizure, CT should also be obtained without delay.

When CT is not available a plain skull X-ray may show on the anteroposterior view displacement of a calcified pineal gland away from the midline. More than 5 mm of shift strongly suggests a haematoma. As soon as an intracranial haematoma has been diagnosed, the patient should receive intravenous mannitol to reduce intracranial pressure and surgical decompression should be carried out without delay. If the exact location of the haematoma is not known, it is useful to remember that an extradural haematoma nearly always lies under the skull fracture, and an acute subdural haematoma nearly always lies over the anterior temporal lobe, often on the side opposite the fracture. Thus in the former case a burr-hole should be made close to the fracture line as identified on X-ray, and in the latter a burr-hole should be made just anterior to the top of the ear. Any delay in initiating surgical decompression in this way greatly increases morbidity and mortality. If there has been rapid neurological deterioration the operation may need to be started by the surgeon at hand, rather than transferring the patient to the neurosurgical unit.

Other causes of neurological deterioration that do not require surgery to the head, include respiratory embarrassment, epilepsy, meningitis, fat embolism, hyperthermia and hyponatraemia causing brain swelling and raised intracranial pressure. Hypoxaemia is sometimes signalled by increased agitation and confusion; under these circumstances there is a grave danger that sedative drugs may be given. These depress respiration further and death can ensue. If an epileptic fit has not been observed its occurrence can be suspected by the suddenness of the fall in conscious level and bilateral dilatation of the pupils, followed by spontaneous improvement. In the head-injured patient, the onset of meningitis may be insidious and require lumbar puncture for its diagnosis. Too often the diagnosis is made only at autopsy.

Care of the unconscious patient

In addition to the regular observations noted above, an unconscious patient requires special care of respiration, body temperature, fluid and electrolyte balance and nourishment.

A clear airway is absolutely essential. In many cases this can be achieved by positioning, sucking away excessive bronchial secretions and regular physiotherapy. If there is any doubt at all about the adequacy of respiration, an endotracheal tube should be inserted and the patient ventilated artificially. In prolonged coma, when artificial ventilation is required for days, the intracranial pressure becomes elevated at some point in the majority of patients. Continuous monitoring of the arterial and intracranial pressures is therefore required, with the facilities of a neuro-intensive care unit. The difference between arterial and intracranial pressure is a measure of the cerebral perfusion pressure. In head-injured adult patients, the perfusion pressure should be held at or above 70 mmHg.

Body temperature should not be allowed to rise above normal because this makes the injured brain swell. Removal of bed clothes, fanning and tepid sponging are the usual measures, sometimes aided by the use of aspirin suppositories.

An accurate measure of fluid output is essential; therefore the bladder must be catheterized and a nasogastric tube inserted. Intravenous fluids are given at first to take account of both observed and insensible fluid losses. Dehydration, with potential arterial hypotension, and overhydration, with hyponatraemia are both to be avoided. After the return of bowel sounds, fluids and nourishment are best provided via the nasogastric tube.

Cerebrospinal fluid fistulae: otorrhoea and rhinorrhoea

When a fracture of the base of the skull is combined with tearing of the dura mater, CSF may leak from the ear or from the nose via the paranasal air sinuses. In most patients this ceases spontaneously within a few days, but while it lasts and for 1 week afterwards there is a risk of meningitis. The role of prophylactic antibiotics is controversial, but if meningitis does occur, it must be treated vigorously with the appropriate antibiotics. Aeroceles sometimes complicate basal skull fracture and can be detected by a lateral skull X-ray in the brow-up position. If CSF rhinorrhoea persists for more than 1 week or if there is a large aerocele, fascial repair of the dural defect in the floor of the anterior cranial fossa should be considered by a neurosurgeon.

Depressed skull fracture

These fractures are usually open, the dura mater is torn in 50 per cent of patients and the damage to the brain is usually localized to the vicinity of the fracture. Consciousness is often preserved or lost only briefly, and so there is a real danger that the seriousness of the injury, which is often contaminated by indriven hair, is underestimated. Surgical treatment consists of careful debridement and cleaning of the wound, elevation of the indriven bone fragments, removal of hair, haematoma and necrotic brain, repair of the dura and replacement of the larger bone pieces followed by meticulous scalp closure.

Closed depressed fractures of the skull do not call for urgent treatment unless there is evidence of brain compression. The main indication for elevation of a closed fracture is cosmetic. This is in contrast to open fractures for which the indication for surgical treatment is the prevention of infection, and surgical treatment is needed within 6 hours of injury.

Outcome and sequelae of head injury

The mortality of head injury is closely related to the degree of depression of consciousness as observed after the patient reaches hospital. In comatose patients who score between 3 and 8 on the Glasgow Coma Scale, mortality is 40 per cent; in moderate injuries scoring 9–12, mortality is 4 per cent, whereas in minor cases scoring 13–15 on the scale it is only 0.4 per cent. Mortality is higher in older patients, in those with intracranial haematomas, in patients who are hypoxic and in those who have signs of brainstem damage (bilateral fixed pupils). Arterial hypotension is seldom, if ever, caused by brain injury but, because multiple injury is common in severely head-injured patients, it is seen on admission in one-sixth of cases. However, it occurs frequently thereafter, often in relation to administration of sedative or hypnotic drugs used to control raised intracranial pressure, and is a more likely complication in multiple-injury patients in whom volume replacement has been less than optimal. It is a most serious insult to the injured brain which greatly increases both mortality and morbidity. Raised intracranial pressure is also common and of equally adverse significance. Approximately one-half of the patients who die from their head injury do so because intracranial pressure rises to the level of the arterial pressure, cerebral perfusion ceases and brain death ensues.

In those who survive head injury, there may be late sequelae in the form of difficulty with memory and concentration, headaches and dizziness, and loss of social and sexual drive, leading to a change in personality all too evident to the family of the patient.

There is a risk of post-traumatic epilepsy in certain patients who have sustained a head injury. Factors that increase the risk of epilepsy include intracranial haemorrhage, infection, penetrating (missile) wounds of the brain and depressed skull fracture when associated with tearing of the dura mater. Most fits begin within 12 months of injury, but onset can be delayed for years. There is no convincing evidence that prophylactic anticonvulsant therapy prevents head-injured patients from developing post-traumatic seizures. In the UK, most neurosurgeons will await the occurrence of two post-traumatic seizures before commencing anticonvulsant therapy. Phenytoin is the most widely used drug; when used it should be given for 2 years and blood levels checked at regular intervals. If no fits have occurred, it can then be withdrawn gradually; if seizures have occurred, anticonvulsant therapy must be continued.

4 GENERAL PRINCIPLES OF BONE AND JOINT INJURIES

FRACTURES

When normal living bone is subjected to sufficient violence to cause it to break, considerable damage inevitably occurs to the soft tissue structures that surround it. The periosteum is stripped from the bone, and torn through on the side opposite to that to which the injuring force was applied. Blood vessels contained in the bone and periosteum are ruptured, and a haematoma forms round the fracture site. Blood also escapes through the rent in the periosteum into the surrounding muscles, and is associated with a variable degree of swelling. If the skin is broken, the fracture is open; if the skin is intact, the fracture is closed.

Skin

In any open fracture the skin, by definition, is damaged. In severe injuries the amount of skin loss may be extensive; as a result the wound does not heal, the bone does not unite and stiffness of the joints may occur.

Skin necrosis also occurs from pressure by a displaced bone fragment or an ill-fitting plaster. Blisters commonly occur at the fracture site and there is bruising and swelling. Usually this is of little importance, except as an indication of the extent of the damage to the deep tissues. Infection, however, may occur, and if the full thickness of the skin breaks down, deep tissue infection ensues. Then there is a grave risk to the integrity of the limb and even a risk to the life of the patient.

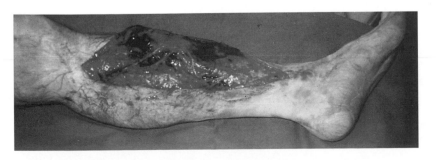

FIG. 4.1   Open fracture of left tibia

Gustillo and Anderson have introduced a practical classification of open fractures:

■ Grade I: when less than 1 cm skin is destroyed;
■ Grade II: more than 1 cm skin is involved;
■ Grade III: there is extensive damage to soft tissues, including muscle, skin and neurovascular structures.

Hence grade III open fractures are frequently associated with not only extensive skin damage but also other soft issue destruction and comminution to the bone. Grade III fractures carry by far the worst prognosis, and this group has been further divided into IIIa and IIIb depending upon whether the main vessel to part has been damaged, for example a grade IIIb fracture of the tibia involves division of the popliteal artery.

PRINCIPLES OF WOUND TREATMENT

Incisional wounds (uncomplicated by a fracture)

Unless there has been a delay of over 8 hours from the time of injury, incisional wounds may be treated by primary suture. The wound is cleaned and obviously devitalized tissue is excised, from both the skin edges and the deep layers, and haemostasis is secured, after which the wound is carefully closed.

Open fractures

In the presence of a fracture it is essential not to close the wound. As soon as the patient with an open fracture arrives in hospital, after thorough assessment and antibiotic therapy, they are taken to the operating theatre and a thorough wound toilet is performed in which all dead tissue, particularly dead muscle and foreign material, is removed. Copious irrigation with between 4 and 5 litres of saline is performed, and the wound may then be packed with moist antiseptic swabs or filled with antibiotic-containing bone cement beads. After this, the skin may be covered with a plastic dressing.

Meticulous inspection of the wound is carried out after 48 hours, in order to remove all remaining dead tissue and allow healthy granulation tissue to develop. If practical, a delayed primary suture may be performed. More often, though, skin grafting is necessary to cover the defect.

Crushing injuries

A minor crushing injury such as may follow a direct blow produces bruising, resulting in local swelling and a blue discoloration of the skin. A collection of blood in the tissues is known as a haematoma. Occasionally, suction drainage of the haematoma may be required.

When an injury is due to a more severe crushing force, extensive damage may be done to the underlying tissues. Such a crushing injury of the lower limb or forearm may or may not be associated with the development of the *compartment syndrome*. This condition, which is found in the forearm or in the calf, is the result of bleeding into tight fascial compartments. Fluid accumulates, cannot disperse and results in a rise in venous pressure. The capillaries in turn become more leaky, with the effect that the osmotic pressure falls. The overall result is that more fluid leaves the vascular system and enters the muscle compartments. Tissue death then follows, resulting in ischaemic contractures, gangrene and, if associated with superimposed clostridial infection, an overwhelming septicaemia and possible death.

The diagnosis *must* be made if the patient:

■ complains of persistent *pain* after a fracture has been reduced;
■ complains of *paraesthesia*; this occurs because the vascular supply to the nerves is reduced;
■ demonstrates signs of *loss in capillary filling*.

Assistance in making the diagnosis can be gained with catheters inserted into the calf or forearm muscles in those patients prone to develop this complication. Careful monitoring is then performed to detect sudden changes in pressure or if the pressure is high to begin with.

The treatment of compartment syndrome is urgent. As a first step the plaster is split down to and including the underlying wool bandage. If relief is not immediate, the patient is taken to the operating theatre for fasciotomy.

Skin grafts

There are two basic methods of replacing skin loss: free grafts or flap grafts. With free grafts, the skin is taken directly from the donor site and applied to the recipient area, with or without a vascular anastomosis. If a flap is employed, the skin for grafting remains attached to the area from which it has been raised by its base, thereby retaining its blood supply, the recipient site is detached from the donor area only when new vessels have grown into the flap.

Free grafts

These may be either split skin or full thickness skin.

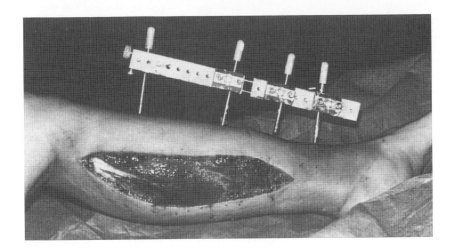

FIG. 4.2 Fasciotomy of the calf

Split skin grafts In split skin grafts, strips of partial thickness skin, consisting of epidermis and part of the dermal layer, but nowhere extending down to the subcutaneous fatty tissue, are cut using a special flat knife. These are then applied directly to the recipient area, which has been cleaned and 'rawed up' in preparation. The grafts are held in place by firm even pressure so that blood cannot collect beneath and raise them from the recipient site. Because part of the dermis remains, full regeneration of skin follows in the donor area.

Split skin provides a very satisfactory immediate treatment for areas of skin loss, but as sometimes there is no subcutaneous fat, the grafted part is adherent to deeper structures, and liable to injury, so it has no place as a permanent measure in the management of skin loss in areas subject to pressure. As it is cosmetically ugly, it also has no place in the definitive treatment of facial injuries. It has, however, a very useful function in the replacement of skin in donor areas from which flaps have been taken to provide full thickness skin elsewhere.

Full thickness (Wolfe) grafts Full thickness grafts are those in which the whole thickness of dermis down to the subcutaneous fat is included, thereby providing a slightly firmer cover. Their main use, therefore, is in replacing small areas of skin loss in the hand and face.

Flap grafts

Skin flaps may be used to provide full thickness skin cover to denuded areas in three ways. First, if the area to be covered is not very large, use may be made of the natural elasticity in the skin by turning one side of the raw area into a flap, and swinging it across to meet the opposite edge (rotation flap).

Second, in the extremities, a flap may be raised at one site and the affected limb brought to it. Thus,

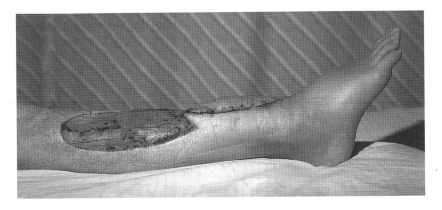

FIG. 4.3 Myocutaneous graft, left tibia

in the case of a hand, a flap may be raised from the abdominal wall, and sutured to the denuded area by approximating the limb to it. In the leg, a denuded area in one foot may be covered by raising a flap from the opposite calf (cross-leg flap).

Third, a flap may be raised from the chest or abdominal wall, remaining attached at either end, the two edges of the central portion being sutured together to form a tube. This can later be detached at one end and swung across to reach the recipient area, where it can be opened out once more (tubed pedicle graft). This method is of particular value in replacement of skin on the legs or arms. Occasionally the tube is moved by stages from the abdomen to the forearm, and then from the forearm to the face.

Vascularized grafts

These full thickness grafts, perhaps with muscle attached, are raised in their blood supply and transferred to the recipient site. It may be possible to swing this graft locally, as occurs in a combined skin and gastrocnemius graft to cover a defect in the tibia. In this case the blood vessels are dissected but do not require reanastomosis. On the other hand, a combined skin and latissimus dorsi flap transferred to the lower limb requires vascular reanastomosis, using an operating microscope.

Muscle and tendon

In most major fractures some damage occurs to the muscles and tendons in close proximity. The haemorrhage resolves and fibrous tissue forms, so the initial damage accounts for some of the stiffness that follows the removal of traction or of the plaster after the fracture has united. Occasionally in fractures of the shafts of major long bones, a length of muscle may become trapped between the bone ends, preventing anatomical reduction.

MYOSITIS OSSIFICANS

Myositis ossificans is ossification within muscle. It is liable to occur as a complication of a severe bony injury in the region of the larger joints and is fairly common around the elbow. The basic treatment for this condition is rest although radiotherapy and excision can be practised.

Nerves

Major nerves may be injured by the broken bone ends, particularly at sites where nerves are closely related to bone, for example the radial nerve where it lies in the spiral groove of the humerus. Many nerve lesions result from a sudden stretching of the nerve at the moment of injury. In these cases there is no permanent damage to the neurons and a full and rapid recovery usually follows: this is a *neurapraxia*.

In more severe injuries the axons and the myelin sheaths are damaged, leaving only the nerve sheath. The nerve has the ability to regenerate because the endoneural tubes can guide the outgoing streams of axoplasm. These are the usual nerve injuries associated with fractures and are known as *axon otmesis*.

If the nerve is completely severed or irreparably damaged by traction or ischaemia, it is known as a *neurotmesis*. In this case repair of the divided nerve is necessary.

Blood vessels

Major arteries are particularly liable to injury in the region of the elbow and knee joint, because at these levels the arteries bifurcate and are anchored by muscle attachments. The vessels may be completely divided, contused or compressed by swelling, within a tight compartment, such as the calf (see *Compartment syndrome* above). It may be difficult to diagnose acute traumatic ischaemia when a patient is in a state of shock; however, it should become apparent once the peripheral circulation has been restored. Ischaemic necrosis of muscle fibres occurs after traumatic ischaemia because the tissues are dependent on a good oxygen supply. The muscle fibres die and are replaced by fibrous tissue which in turn contracts. In the forearm, established muscle necrosis produces the typical clinical picture known as Volkmann's ischaemic contracture. Frequently, the nerves are involved as well and the result is a combined neurovascular injury. Patients with Volkmann's contracture present with an inability to extend the fingers with the wrist dorsiflexed. In the calf, the result of muscle necrosis is clawing of the toes and pes cavus. When occlusion of a vessel occurs, it is a matter of great urgency to restore the normal circulation as soon as possible. About 6 hours is the maximum time after which ischaemic muscle and nerve will recover.

All constricting bandages and dressings should be removed as soon as the diagnosis is considered. The patient is taken to theatre and decompression performed. The skin is divided, then the deep fascia, down to the vessel, which may be very thin as a result of constriction. The wound is left open and delayed primary skin graft performed after about 4 days. If the main artery has been divided, the fracture must first be stabilized, the ends of the vessel exposed, and a direct anastomosis or vein grafting undertaken; a fasciectomy is also essential. Once ischaemic changes have occurred in the muscle, meticulous dissection of all the destroyed muscle releases the contracture somewhat and reconstruction of the limb can then be undertaken, combined with tendon transfer to improve function.

BONE FRACTURES

Fractures result from direct or indirect violence. Those due to direct violence occur when the injury force is applied directly to the bone at the site of the fracture, either from a severe blow or from a crushing force. Open fractures therefore more often follow direct violence and may be either comminuted or transverse; fractures due to indirect violence usually follow rotational injuries and may be oblique or spiral.

Appreciating the shape of the fracture and the direction of the rotational force will help in the reduction of the fracture, which is achieved by applying the forces in the opposite direction.

Types of fractures

CLOSED

A closed fracture is one in which there is no communication between the fractured bone and the skin, so the bone is not exposed to contamination and infection. Skin damage may be present, but it does not actually link with the fracture site.

OPEN

An open fracture is one in which there is direct communication between the fracture and skin surface. It is therefore potentially infected. This type of fracture is graded from I to III, depending on the extent of skin damage (see above).

GREENSTICK

A greenstick fracture is an incomplete fracture occurring when a long bone is broken on the

(a)   (b)   (c)

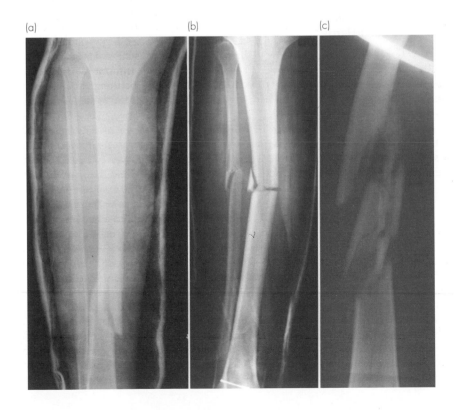

FIG. 4.4 Three types of fracture: (a) oblique; (b) transverse; (c) comminuted and segmental

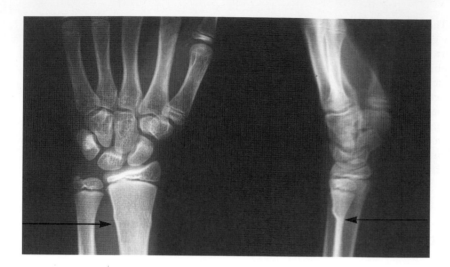

FIG. 4.5 A greenstick fracture of the radius

convex side, but buckled on the concave. A greenstick fracture occurs in the bones of growing children, where there is some springiness present.

EPIPHYSEAL INJURIES

Epiphyseal injuries occur in the growing child, in whom the epiphyseal plate is particularly vulnerable, that is at the zone of cartilage cell transformation (see Chapter 1, Fig. 1.21). Salter and Harris classified these injuries into five types:

I   a shear injury of the growth plate;
II   a shear injury of the growth plate with a fracture of the metaphysis;
III a fracture of the epiphysis at right angles to the articular surface;
IV   a single fracture plane running through the epiphyseal growth plate and the metaphysis;
V   a crushing injury to the growth plate.

In types IV and V the epiphyseal growth plate is damaged and premature growth plate fusion can occur, leading to subsequent deformity of the joint.

STRESS FRACTURE

A stress fracture may occur and is similar to fatigue fractures in metal caused by repeated strains in the same direction. It occurs in bones subject to abnormal stress, such as in the shaft of the second metatarsal, when it is called a march fracture.

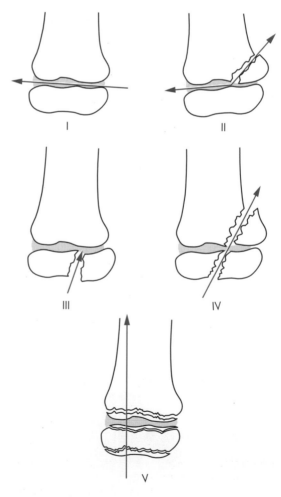

FIG. 4.6   Salter–Harris epiphyseal fractures

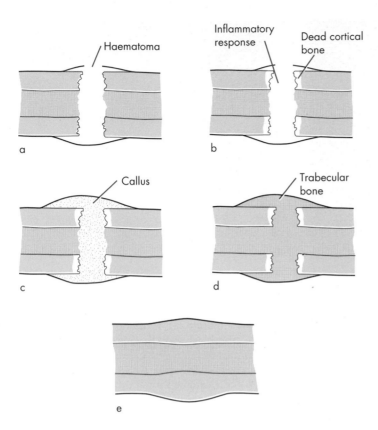

FIG. 4.7 The phases of healing in a fracture of the shaft of a long bone: (a) immediately after the fracture; (b) inflammatory phase; (c) formation of callus; (d) union with trabecular bone; (e) remodelling

PATHOLOGICAL FRACTURE

Pathological fractures occur through abnormal bone. They may be:

- congenital (e.g. osteogenesis imperfecta, fibrous dysplasia)
- inflammatory (e.g. osteomyelitis)
- neoplastic:
    benign (e.g. enchondroma)
    malignant:
        primary (e.g. osteosarcoma, myeloma)
        secondary (e.g. lung, breast, thyroid, kidney, prostate)
- metabolic (e.g. osteomalacia, osteoporosis, Paget's disease, hypercalcaemia)

Fracture healing

After a fracture there are three overlapping phases of healing: the inflammatory phase, the reparative phase: a) soft callus, b) hard callus and the remodelling phase.

INFLAMMATORY PHASE

The inflammatory phase occurs immediately after the fracture and is characterized by bleeding from the bone ends and the surrounding soft tissue, resulting in the formation of a haematoma. This is followed by a typical acute inflammatory reaction with vasodilatation and the arrival of polymorphonucleocytes and macrophages at the fracture site, and is thought to be influenced by nitric oxide. The fractured bone ends are sealed by blood clot, and bone and marrow death occurs. The degree of bone necrosis is dependent on the displacement and comminution of the fracture and may vary with the blood supply to the bone. Apart from osteocyte death in the bone, there is necrosis in the periosteum and marrow.

REPARATIVE PHASE

The reparative phase is the second stage of healing and is characterized by the formation of callus. External callus is derived from the periosteum and

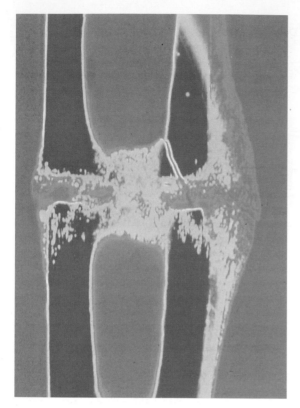

FIG. 4.8   Callus formation in fracture healing

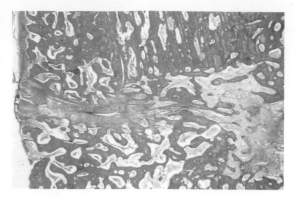

FIG. 4.9   Fracture healing, showing fracture gap (H+E staining)

develops to form a bridge between the fractured bones (Fig. 4.8). Internal callus also occurs and is derived from the endosteal cells. This soft callus, found in the reparative stage, is initially fibrous tissue.

The amount and composition of repair depends upon:

- whether it involves a metaphysis or a diaphysis;
- whether the fracture is stable or unstable;
- the extent of the soft-tissue disruption.

Bone healing is dependent on the development of specialized vascular and cellular tissue which goes on to form bone. The multipotential fibroblast that transforms into the osteoprogenitor cell may come from endothelial cells by the process of osteoinduction. During the early phase of fracture healing there is a marked increase in vascularity and this is associated with angiogenesis.

There are a variety of osteo-inductive factors, including cytokines, that are thought to be involved in the fracture healing process and act early and late through the phases of soft and hard callus.

- Platelet-derived growth factor (PDGF): derived from platelets; attracts inflammatory cells and stimulates bone cell formation.
- Basic fibroblast growth factor (BFGF): derived from intracellular and extracellular fibroblasts; promotes neovascularization and stimulates bone and cartilage formation with angiogenesis.
- Transforming growth factor β (TGFβ): derived from mesenchymal cells and osteoblasts; is thought to be the prime cytokine involved in regulating cartilage and bone' formation in fracture callus. There are several isoforms.
- Insulin-like growth factor (IGF): derived from bone cells and chondrocytes: stimulates bone cell proliferation and cartilage matrix production.
- Bone morphogenic protein (BMP): part of the TGF family, there have been 9 different types identified; BMP, originally isolated by Marshall Urist in California, is probably involved in all stages of bone formation.

Hard callus then forms as the cartilaginous soft callus is converted into woven bone. This occurs as endochondral bone formation or membranous ossification.

Endochondral ossification occurs in areas of cartilage formation and is the external callus. It is a relatively avascular structure and ossification occurs by the process of invasion from the surrounding tissues.

Membranous ossification is ossification from the mesenchymal cells in the periosteum and medulla.

Both these sources of repair are important to the fracture healing process and are influenced by many factors, including the cytokines already listed.

Local factors that influence the repair of a fracture include:

- velocity of the trauma
- interposition of soft tissue
- impaired blood supply
- types of bone: cancellous or cortical
- degree of bone loss
- adequacy of immobilization
- infection
- pathological conditions.

REMODELLING PHASE

Remodelling of the trabecular bone follows the formation of callus and restores the bone to its normal architecture. This is the longest stage of fracture repair. However, it must be clearly stated that these stages are not really distinct events but may overlap and all may occur at any time during the fracture healing process.

Clinical features of a fracture

The presence of a fracture should be suspected if after an injury the patient complains of pain in the region of a bone. Examination may reveal tenderness and swelling with deformity of the limb. Crepitus between the broken ends of the bone is pathognomonic of a fracture, though obviously this should not be invoked deliberately.

Clinically, union of the fracture can be tested by feeling the fracture and stressing the fracture site. There will be no discomfort once union has occurred, and the bone then feels rigid.

Radiologically, a fracture can be said to have united when the bone trabeculation can be seen crossing the fracture site. In addition, the shadow of a well defined fusiform callus beneath the periosteum can usually be seen.

The treatment of fractures

Basically, from the treatment point of view, fractures fall into three groups. First, those for which treatment is directed primarily towards dealing with the soft tissue lesions, the bony injury being largely ignored. Examples are the flat bones, such as the scapula or ilium, and avulsion or fractures of bony outgrowths, such as the transverse processes of vertebrae. In these fractures, treatment consists of managing the soft tissue problem, including extensive blood loss in the case of pelvic fractures. Second, fractures involving long bones, in which the main problems are non-union, delayed union and malunion. Third, fractures involving joints, in which the main problems are loss of joint surface integrity and the late onset of osteoarthritis.

The treatment of a fracture can be divided into three phases: reduction – to restore normal bony alignment; immobilization – to maintain the reduced position until union has occurred; and rehabilitation – to restore normal function to the injured part or, failing this, to assist the patient to cope with any residual disability.

REDUCTION

Reduction aims at restoring bone length and alignment to overcome both angular and rotatory deformities, and is achieved by closed manipulation or open operation.

Closed reduction consists first of traction to disengage the bony fragments or to overcome their overlap, followed by the manoeuvre required to restore normal alignment. The latter consists of manipulating the limb in the reverse direction to that which caused the fracture. Most injuries of the major long bones result from falls or other forms of indirect violence, with some rotation, and this must be taken into account at the time of reduction.

Open reduction is indicated if manipulative reduction fails, as when there is some soft tissue interposition between the bone ends, or if in the overall interests of the patient it is desirable to avoid external splintage of the part. Therefore, open reduction is always combined with some form of external or internal fixation. Examples of the latter method are applied in patients with multiple injuries, in whom internal fixation of one or more fractures will simplify the overall management, or when early mobilization of the part is desirable, as in elderly patients with fractures of the upper end of the femur.

IMMOBILIZATION

Immobilization may be achieved by external or internal splintage.

External splintage

In order to achieve complete immobilization it is necessary to include the joint above and the joint below the fracture. In many instances, however, this may not be required, provided that the bone

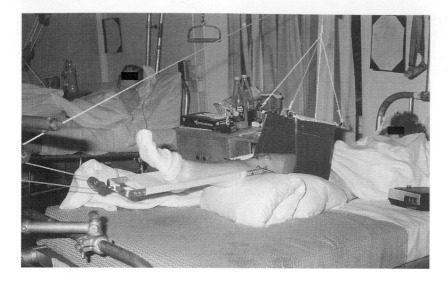

FIG. 4.10 Hamilton Russell balanced traction

ends can be locked in position; for example, in most fractures of the wrist and ankle in which the elbow or knee can be left free. There are several methods of external splintage:

- splintage, particularly by plaster of Paris;
- traction: fixed or balanced;
- external fixation devices.

The usual method of external splintage is by a plaster of Paris cast, in the application of which three practical points must be borne in mind. First, a skin-tight cast must never be employed because there is a risk of swelling; otherwise the circulation of the limb will be impaired. Second, care must be taken to prevent ridges or indentations as the plaster is applied; otherwise when they harden they may cause pressure sores. Third, the plaster should be applied smoothly, evenly and rapidly so that the whole cast sets in one piece, not in several layers, which may crack at a later date.

Traction is applied if deforming forces may threaten the stability of a reduction. It may be longitudinal, using a Thomas splint, and may be fixed or balanced, or it may be Hamilton Russell balanced traction (Fig. 4.10), Perkins split bed traction, or it may be calcaneum or distal tibial skeletal traction.

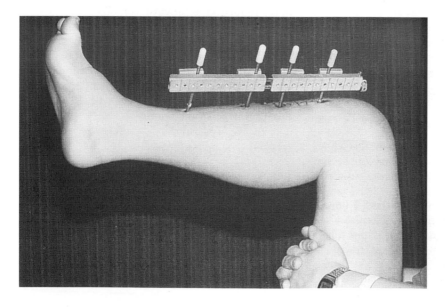

FIG. 4.11 External fixation of a fracture, single bar type

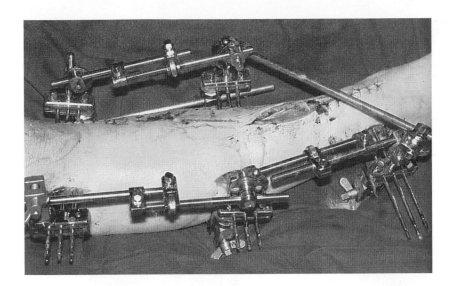

FIG. 4.12 External fixation using a frame

External fixation devices are also used for the treatment of fractures (Figs 4.11 and 4.12), particularly open and comminuted tibial fractures, their benefits being that the joints above and below are not immobilized and the soft tissue can be inspected.

Internal fixation

In open reduction of a fracture direct manipulation of the broken bone allows perfect restoration of position. This is followed by some form of internal or external fixation, which ideally should be strong enough to avoid the need for additional external support. The method employed will depend upon the nature and site of the fracture. Two basic forms of internal fixation are in use. First are those that obtain their hold by screws which traverse the bony cortex. Sometimes screws are used alone, as in ankle fractures (Fig. 4.13), otherwise they are used in conjunction with a plate. Second, fixation is obtained by the use of internal fixation traversing the medullary cavity of the bone. These take several forms, ranging from intramedullary nails that are locked at both ends to control rotation (Fig. 4.15), to various types of more flexible nails.

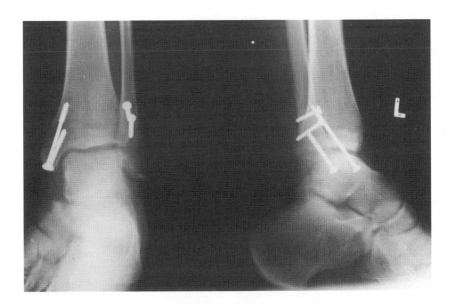

FIG. 4.13 Internal fixation of fractured medial malleolus using screws, A-P and lateral X-rays

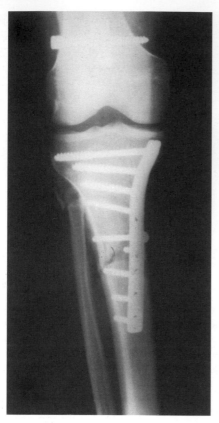

FIG. 4.14 Internal fixation of fractured tibial shaft using a plate and screws

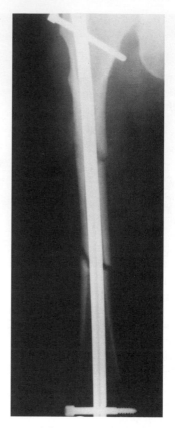

FIG. 4.15 Internal fixation of femoral shaft fracture using an intramedullary nail

REHABILITATION

Restoration of function is an essential part of the treatment of all injuries. In the majority of patients a full return to normal can be expected and the aim of rehabilitation is to achieve this as rapidly as possible. Less commonly, irreparable damage may have occurred at the time of injury, so a full return to normal function cannot be expected.

In most limb injuries, when full recovery can be expected, all that is required is encouragement to make the patient move all joints in the affected part that do not have to be immobilized. Then, as soon as splintage is removed, the injured limb should be used fairly actively until all the residual discomfort, stiffness and swelling have disappeared.

In fractures, the immobilization needed to permit bony union in good position accentuates stiffness caused by the associated soft-tissue damage. The joints below the site of injury are those mainly affected, because the muscles and tendons concerned with their movement will also have been damaged.

Methods of treatment will vary according to the severity of the injury and the mental attitude of the patient. In most patients, when the trauma was not very severe, encouragement to use the injured part (although painful at first) normally suffices. If the injury was more severe, a course of mobilizing exercises under physiotherapy supervision, coupled with local heat to overcome muscle spasm, should commence as soon as the period of immobilization is completed. These exercises are usually better carried out by a group of patients working together in a class, as thereby a mild spirit of competition may be introduced, which will help the more nervous individuals. Exercises done against increasing resistance, such as by lifting weights with the affected part, are very valuable at a later stage. Remedial games are also often helpful, particularly among younger adult patients, as thereby the exercises are made more enjoyable.

Occasionally, when injuries have been severe, and the patient's normal occupation involves hard physical work, a spell spent in a residential rehabilitation centre may be valuable, not only because such centres contain the best possible equipment and facilities, but also because treatment can be given to the patient continuously throughout the whole working day. In addition, an atmosphere is created that encourages maximal activity, and moreover, skilled assistance can be given to help the patient to carry out the specific activities that their normal occupation requires, and which they now find difficult.

In patients in whom some permanent disability is anticipated, rehabilitation has two aims: first, to minimize the functional effects of that disability and, second, to help the patient cope with both the social and physical problems which may arise as a result. The former is dealt with along the lines already described. The medical social worker can often assist in the social and financial problems that arise as a result of some permanent disability, and suitable employment may be found by registering the patient as disabled.

COMPLICATIONS

Malunion

A fracture may be united in a poor position either because the bone ends overlap, leading to shortening, or because the bone ends unite with an angular deformity or in a position of rotation in the longitudinal plane. The significance varies according to the bone involved. On the whole, malunion is of less importance in the upper limb than in the leg, in which shortening, unless compensated for by a raised shoe, will cause a limp, and also, as a result of altered stresses on the spinal column, may lead to various back problems. Angular deformities in the leg, particularly in the sagittal plane, are also important because the altered alignment in weight-bearing joints will lead to degenerative changes.

In the arm, minor deformities are important in fractures of the radial and ulnar shafts, as considerable restriction of rotation of the forearm may result. A valgus deformity of the elbow may be important; it may cause irritation of the ulnar nerve as it goes behind the medial epicondyle of the humerus.

An occasional cause of late deformities after injuries in childhood is premature epiphyseal fusion, due to a crushing injury of the epiphyseal cartilage. This is most commonly seen in the ankle, where forced adduction may cause crushing of the lower tibial epiphysis on its medial side, so that arrested growth, with normal growth in the lower fibular epiphysis, gradually produces a varus deformity of the ankle.

If there is a degree of malunion sufficient to cause early or late disability it must be treated by osteotomy – division of the bone at a suitable site.

Delayed and non-union

The rate of union in fractures is closely related to the local blood supply. At sites where the blood supply is abundant, union rarely presents a problem. At other sites, where the anatomical arrangement of the vessels is such that a fracture interrupts the blood supply to one fragment, union normally is slow, and perfect immobilization must be maintained until there is clinical and radiological evidence of union. Examples are fractures through the femoral neck, the waist of the scaphoid and the neck of the talus. In each case, if the blood supply to one fragment – the femoral head, the proximal pole of scaphoid, or the body of the talus – is completely cut off, avascular necrosis (osteonecrosis) will follow. This is first shown radiologically by apparent increase in bone density. In fact, this is due to relative osteoporosis in the surrounding bone which has a normal blood supply, resulting from hyperaemia caused by the injury, which in turn cannot affect the fragment as the latter is devoid of circulation. Later, the avascular portion of bone becomes brittle and, unless protected for a long period, collapses.

At other sites, the blood supply may be impaired by the severity of the local soft-tissue damage. Thus open fractures, especially those that result from severe violence, tend to take longer to mend than closed fractures at the same level. Fractures of the midshaft of the tibia are notoriously slow in uniting. This is partly because if the fracture is below the point of entry of the nutrient vessels, the endosteal blood supply to the lower fragment is cut off, and partly because the periosteum, being subcutaneous, is frequently damaged.

When union is taking longer than normal, but before there is definite sclerosis between the bone ends as seen radiologically, a state of delayed union is said to exist. Some such cases eventually do unite by bone, in others union never can occur.

Non-union is said to be present when, radiologically, there is an obvious gap between the bone ends, with sclerosis of the fragments (Fig. 4.17).

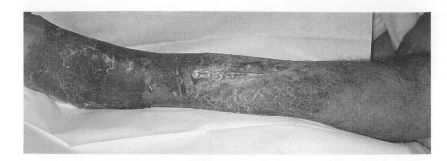

FIG. 4.16 Infected non-union of a fracture

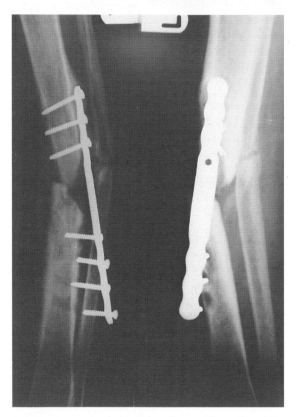

FIG. 4.17 Corresponding X-ray showing loosening of the plate and screws and visible fracture 9 months after initial treatment

The gap between the ends may be bridged by fibrous tissue, when fibrous union may be said to have taken place, or a false joint (pseudarthrosis) may form, the bone ends becoming lined by fibrocartilage. Clinically, some movement at the fracture site persists. In the case of fibrous union, this may be a mere jog with some discomfort. When a pseudarthrosis has formed there may be a considerable range of movement, which may be relatively painless.

If non-union is established, or appears to be inevitably developing, bone grafting should be employed.

Bone grafting

Phemister introduced the use of cancellous bone grafting to surgery. Cancellous bone is taken from the iliac crest and is transferred to the recipient site, which has been prepared for the graft. This commonly used procedure is an *autograft*. The fresh bone graft undergoes degeneration, proliferation and differentiation. The cancellous bone and its contained red marrow provide large numbers of osteogenic and potentially osteogenic cells and the graft actively contributes to osteogenesis. This grafted bone is then replaced by creeping substitution.

Sudeck's osteodystrophy

Sudeck's osteodystrophy is a late complication of an injury that may have been relatively trivial. There is stiffness and swelling of the limb, which in turn may be warm and painful. It is found particularly after a Colles' fracture or after a foot injury and may be due to overreaction of the sympathetic nervous system. The X-rays show marked osteoporotic changes in the bones. The treatment is to encourage active movement of the hand or foot, combined with adequate pain relief. Guanethidine blocks have proved useful, and transcutaneous nerve stimulation may be employed.

JOINT INJURIES

Types

Joint injuries may take four forms: a sprain, in which there is a tear of the capsular ligament without disturbance of the relationship of the opposing articular surfaces; a subluxation, in which, though displaced, the articular surfaces remain in contact; a dislocation, in which the articular surfaces are completely displaced from each other; and a fracture dislocation, in which, in order that the articular surfaces may become completely displaced from each other, a fracture of part of one of the bones must have taken place.

SPRAINS

Tears of the capsular lining of a joint may be of a trivial nature, or they may be severe, involving a complete disruption of one of the collateral ligaments in a joint such as the knee. In the latter case momentary subluxation will have taken place and, unless the ligamentous rent heals or is repaired, recurrent sprains from minor violence may follow.

SUBLUXATIONS

Partial displacement of the articular surfaces of a joint, with the bones still remaining in contact with each other, most commonly occurs in 'plane' joints such as the acromioclavicular. In these cases residual laxity usually persists.

DISLOCATIONS

For complete separation of the articular surfaces in a normal joint to be possible, the capsule of the joint must be completely torn through. This is, therefore, an injury resulting from considerable violence applied to the joint, and the soft-tissue damage may cause some residual stiffness through scarring. At certain sites where the cavity is shallow, residual capsular laxity may leave an unstable joint or, as in the shoulder, an unhealed rent may lead to recurrent dislocation. Pathological dislocations may occur if there is some inherent ligamentous laxity or abnormal muscle pull, such as in certain neurological disorders, leading to paralytic dislocations. Pathological dislocations may also occur if the joint lining has been destroyed by an infective process.

FRACTURE DISLOCATIONS

The fracture of the bony margin as it is dislocated may affect any joint, but it is most frequently seen in the more severe rotational injuries of the ankle.

Treatment of joint injuries

Treatment of joint injuries is similar in principle to that of fractures. In dislocations, fracture dislocations and subluxations, reduction is required first. This will be followed by a variable period of immobilization, after which the joint is actively mobilized.

REDUCTION

In dislocations and fracture dislocations, reduction normally requires an anaesthetic, whereas in subluxations, simple pressure applied in the reverse direction to the displacement may suffice – as in the acromioclavicular joint, for which strapping is employed to press the outer end of the clavicle downwards while the humeral shaft and shoulder are pressed upwards. Open reduction is required less frequently for true dislocations than in fracture dislocations. In fracture dislocations, particularly if there is an intra-articular fracture, operative reduction will be indicated; first, to ensure that a smooth articular surface has been restored, thereby avoiding the later development of osteoarthritis, and, second, to maintain accurate reduction of the bony fragment by internal fixation. Sometimes a flap of soft tissue may prevent manipulative reduction of the bony fragment. In true dislocations operative reduction will be necessary only on the uncommon occasions when the displaced bone becomes 'buttonholed' through a rent in the capsule and cannot be reduced by manipulative means.

IMMOBILIZATION

Unlike fractures, for which immobilization must be complete if malunion or non-union is to be prevented, only in fracture dislocations is perfect immobilization necessary. After dislocations, subluxations and sprains, immobilization is only necessary to prevent movement in the direction which caused the original injury, as in the shoulder, where the usual anterior dislocation is caused by external rotation, which is prevented by bandaging the arm, with the elbow flexed, to the side. Supportive immobilization is usually required for only 2–3 weeks.

MOBILIZATION

Cautious mobilization, avoiding strains in the direction that caused the capsular tear, should commence as soon as the initial reaction to the injury has begun to subside. The time will vary according to the natural stability of the affected joint and the degree of residual stiffness.

In all cases, movement must be active. Passive stretching of any injured part carries the risk of further damage and merely irritates the affected joint.

5 SKELETAL INJURIES OF THE SPINE AND PELVIS

CLINICAL CONSIDERATIONS

There are three important questions to be asked in vertebral fractures. The first question is whether pain will be temporary or permanent. Fractures of the spine will unite like any other bony injury and pain is usually temporary. A few individuals, however, do develop chronic back pain as a result of altered spinal mechanics. The physiological lumbar lordosis is important for the spine's strength and if this arch is lost as a result of a wedge fracture the spine can be permanently weakened. For the majority, however, the fractured spine can be compatible with a pain-free, normally functioning back.

The second question is whether as a result of fracture the spine is stable or unstable. Instability means that the spine is able to move in an excessive or erratic manner at the level of the fracture. This can then damage the spinal cord if the fracture is above L2 or the cauda equina in the lower lumbar region. A patient whose spine is unstable after a fracture or dislocation is at risk of neurological damage and must be treated by careful nursing or preferably by surgical fixation.

Stability can be fixed by the severity of the fracture. The spine can be considered as three columns: the anterior column being the anterior cortex of the vertebral bodies and the anterior discs, the middle column being the posterior cortex of the vertebral bodies and the posterior discs and the posterior column being the neural arch and posterior ligaments. Provided one of these columns is intact, the spine is probably stable. It is possible to have a burst fracture affecting the anterior and posterior cortex of the vertebral bodies with a stable spine because the neural arch is intact. It is not easy to identify the severity of the bony injury on plain X-ray and if instability is suspected, a CT scan is the imaging of choice.

It is unusual for a fracture of the thoracic spine to be unstable provided the ribs and sternum are intact. However, when a patient has a fractured sternum or fractured ribs in association with tenderness of the thoracic spine, an unstable spine fracture should be assumed until proved otherwise. Such a patient should be nursed with extreme care before imaging.

Any patient admitted with a neck injury or any patient admitted unconscious after trauma should be given a cervical collar and assumed to have an unstable neck injury until proved otherwise.

The third question is whether or not the fracture is associated with neurological symptoms or signs. There may be a complete spinal cord lesion from transection of the cord or contusion. This constitutes an emergency because early manual reduction of a dislocated neck with a contused cord can result in full neurological recovery. In the thoracic and lumbar spine, it is unusual for a complete neurological lesion to recover with surgical decompression. A partial neurological injury, however, can recover with prompt surgical decompression. Increasing neurological compromise can result from extradural bleeding or thrombosis after trauma.

FRACTURES OF THE THORACOLUMBAR SPINE

Fractures of the thoracolumbar spine may occur in three ways, depending upon the mechanism of injury: first, those due to direct blows on the back, leading to fractures of transverse processes or, more rarely, as a result of a direct blow on the midline, fractures of spinous processes; second, those due to vertical compression forces, which cause crush fractures of vertebral bodies; and third, those in which there is a combination of a compression force, with an anteroposterior shearing strain leading to a dislocation of one vertebra on another. In practice, therefore, the last type of injury follows when a forced flexion injury to the spine occurs in an individual who is moving forward at a speed, as in a motorcyclist thrown over their handlebars and landing on their head and shoulders. In this injury, the neurological contents of the spinal canal are almost inevitably damaged.

Fractures of transverse processes

Fractures of transverse processes follow direct blows, usually in the lumbar region, because in the thoracic spine the ribs are more liable to be fractured, and in the neck the mobility of the head is such that either the spine is undamaged or the force will have been so great as to cause a more severe injury.

The importance of fractures of transverse processes of the lumbar spine lies not in the bony injury, or the bruising of muscle that goes with it, but in the proximity of the abdominal viscera, which are often damaged at the same time. The organ most likely to be injured will be the kidney on the side that was struck.

TREATMENT

The actual fracture is unimportant and requires no specific treatment. To prevent adhesive formation in the muscle that has been damaged, and to help disperse the haematoma that inevitably forms, early mobilization by gentle exercises is encouraged. As the pain diminishes, the tempo of the exercises should be increased.

Because of the risk of renal or other intra-abdominal injury, all patients with fractures of the lumbar transverse processes should be admitted to hospital for a 24–48-hour period of observation, and their urine examined for fresh blood as a routine measure.

Fractures of the vertebral bodies

Fractures of the vertebral bodies occur when a vertical compression force is applied to the spinal column, such as when a heavy bulky object falls upon the patient's shoulders from above, or the patient falls from a height and lands on their feet. They may occur as

- a compression fracture, in which there is compression of the body; this is a flexion injury;
- a burst fracture, in which there is burst or collapse of the body, with splaying of laminae and widening of the interpeduncular space;
- a Chance fracture, which is also a flexion type injury causing disruption of the posterior column and a horizontal fracture through the vertebral body. This fracture is rare.

The majority of patients present with flexion/compression fractures (Figs 5.1 and 5.2). In all patients it is important to exclude injuries elsewhere. Other injuries caused by a fall from a height include fractures of the base of the skull and fractures of the calcaneum. Less commonly there may be a vertical fracture of the lower end of the tibia caused by the talus being driven upwards, and compression fractures of the condyles of the tibia or femur. Often these other injuries predominate, and unless the spine is checked, fractures may be overlooked. This applies particularly to patients

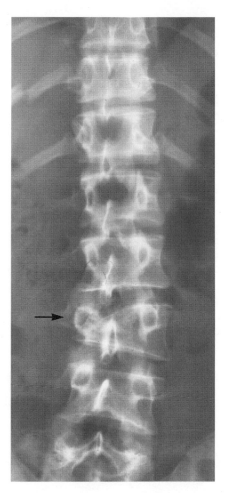

FIG. 5.1   Antero-posterior view of a flexion injury producing a fracture of the L3 vertebra

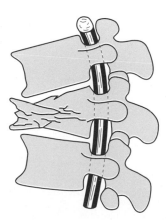

FIG. 5.2   Lateral view of a flexion compression fracture of a vertebral body

who are unconscious with fractures of the base of the skull.

Collapse of a vertebral body is also the most common type of pathological fracture. This is because they are filled with cancellous bone and blood-borne metastatic deposits from a neoplasm elsewhere are particularly liable to settle in a vertebral body, and any generalized skeletal decalcification will also involve vertebral bodies extensively. It is for the latter reason that vertebral collapse affecting several bones is common in elderly persons with senile osteoporosis.

On clinical examination, a fracture should be suspected if there is an area of local tenderness over one vertebral spine, which also feels a little more prominent than its neighbours. Irritation of the nerve root at the affected level also often causes referred pain in the region supplied by that nerve.

COMPLICATION

Paralytic ileus

Paralytic ileus is a state in which, owing to temporary suppression of autonomic nervous function, there is paralysis of the smooth muscle in the bowel. It is a condition that may follow any major injury, but is more common in injuries of the trunk, particularly when there is a retroperitoneal haematoma that may irritate the sympathetic trunk, such as may occur with any injury to the lumbar spine. There is rapid severe abdominal distension, with copious vomiting and a complete absence of normal bowel sounds. This leads to rapid dehydration and a serious risk of inhalation of stomach contents.

Treatment consists of immediate and continuous gastric suction by a nasogastric tube and intravenous fluid replacement, with nothing by mouth until there is evidence of return of normal bowel function, as shown by the passage of flatus per rectum, and the presence of bowel sounds on abdominal auscultation.

TREATMENT

Treatment will depend upon the age and general condition of the patient, the level of the lesion and the amount of bony damage present. In the frail and the elderly, management of the general condition will take priority over the local injury, and the possibility of some underlying pathological process requiring specific treatment – such as radiotherapy for a metastatic deposit – must be borne in mind.

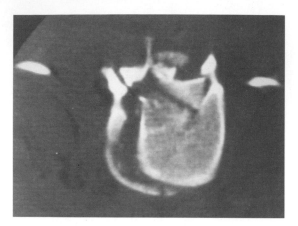

FIG. 5.3   CT scan showing a burst fracture

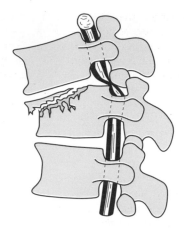

FIG. 5.4   Fracture dislocation of the spine, showing how the cord is damaged

Compression fractures of the thoracic spine are rarely serious as the ribcage provides some support. For the same reason, little active correction of any deformity is possible. Management, therefore, in the young, fit individual consists of an initial period of bedrest until the initial pain has subsided, which may be for a period of days. After this, exercises are commenced; when the patient becomes fully ambulant, their tempo is increased, and they may be better carried out in the competitive atmosphere of a 'back class'.

In the lumbar spine deformity is unlikely to occur, so, after a period of several days' recumbency to allow the initial reaction to subside, with extension exercises in bed, mobility and a period in the 'back class' follow. If later symptoms occur, these can be adequately controlled by the provision of a stout corset.

In flexion injuries and in burst fractures, the degree of posterior disruption should be assessed by CT scanning (Fig. 5.3). Surgery is indicated to stabilize the spine and to remove the retropulsed fragments. Anterior decompression and bone grafting are required, particularly when there is neurological involvement.

In the uncommon Chance fracture, the use of posterior compression rods with localized spinal fusion is recommended.

Fracture dislocation of the spine

Fracture dislocation of the spine is the most severe type of spinal injury, in which not only is a vertebral body fractured but the vertebra above is also displaced on that level below, usually in a forward direction (Figs 5.4 and 5.5). This causes narrowing and distortion of the spinal canal, such that, with the exception of the cervical spine, in which the

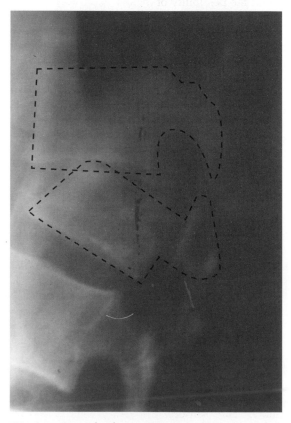

FIG. 5.5   X-ray of a fracture dislocation of the thoracolumbar spine

canal is larger than the cord, the neurological contents are also almost always severely injured. The nature and extent of nervous damage vary according to the level of injury, because the spinal cord in adults terminates at the lower border of the second lumbar vertebra, and below this level only the nerve roots contained in the cauda equina will be affected. Lesions above this level will involve both spinal cord and nerve roots. The significance of the level of the injury lies in the fact that, as nerve fibres contained in the roots have myelin sheaths, recovery is potentially possible, but the unmyelinated fibres in the cord cannot regenerate (for further details of the neurological aspect see *Management of established traumatic paraplegia* below). Management of fracture dislocations of the spine will be dominated by the neurological situation.

MANAGEMENT

First Aid

In all spinal injuries one must constantly bear in mind the possibility of an unstable spine, with the associated risk of incurring damage to the spinal cord as a result of injudicious handling of the patient. The greatest care must therefore be taken not to flex the patient's spine when they are being moved on to the stretcher, or from the stretcher on to a bed, during the radiological examination, or in any other manoeuvre. These patients need management in centres equipped to deal with the associated problems, and should be transferred there as soon as possible after the injury.

Without neurological signs

These injuries are unstable. However, fracture dislocations may reduce by laying the patient supine and may well go on to fuse spontaneously. Treatment is by lying flat on a firm mattress supported by boards with a pillow placed behind the fracture. The patient, however, needs to be turned regularly and at about 10 weeks the spine should be stable enough for the patient to be mobilized. Internal fixation is frequently practised in order to allow for early mobilization of the patient.

With neurological signs

It is essential to undertake a careful and precise neurological examination in all patients with spinal injuries. In patients with a local lesion, a full motor and sensory evaluation must be made because the slightest voluntary movement or aspect of sensation below the level of the cord

lesion is clear evidence of continuity of the cord. This is in contrast to total absence of motor power or sensation, which persists for more than 12 hours, is notable with active reflexes and means a complete cord compression. Radiological examination may then be completed with myelography and CT scanning.

TREATMENT

This can be considered under the following headings:

- nursing, to prevent pressure sores, contractures and urinary tract infection (see below);
- internal fixation, using distraction rods, cages, plates and pedicular screws in order to stabilize the spine, combined with bone grafting. This will not only help in mobilizing the patient but may also prevent further cord compression and spinal deformity;
- laminectomy: there is a very limited role for laminectomy after fracture dislocation of the spine. In progressive lesions the cord is best decompressed by an anterior approach. If a laminectomy is practised, it is absolutely essential to stabilize the spine by internal fixation because the spine will be rendered even more unstable by this procedure.

Management of established traumatic paraplegia

Immediately after injury there is complete suppression of all neurological activity in the cord below the site of injury. Then, after a variable interval, some reflex activity returns to the isolated distal segment of cord. This initial period of complete inactivity is known as spinal shock.

At first, therefore, not only is there complete loss of sensation below the level of cord transection – which will, of course, not alter with the passage of time – but also there is flaccid paralysis of all musculature. This includes the smooth muscle of the bladder and lower bowel, such that both distend passively. In the case of the bladder, when the intravesical pressure has built up sufficiently to overcome the passive resistance of the sphincters, dribbling overflow incontinence will follow. During this period, with a stagnating pool of urine in the bladder, chronic infection may occur.

After an interval, varying from 3 weeks to 3 months, the isolated segment of spinal cord below the lesion begins to recover reflex activity. Tone begins to return in the paralysed muscles, which change from being flaccid to spastic.

In the bladder, provided the muscle has not been allowed to become overdistended during the initial period of inactivity, and its lining has not become contracted owing to infection, when intravesical pressure reaches a certain level, reflex contraction takes place together with reflex relaxation of the sphincters. The result is that urine is passed with a normal stream, and the bladder emptied. This, however, takes place without either the knowledge or control of the patient, and is described as an automatic bladder. In the bowel a similar state occurs, so, provided the patient is neither constipated nor has loose stools, fairly regular evacuation will occur, such as happens after an interval with a colostomy.

In the lower limb, the return of muscle tone may enable the patient to be taught to stand, and even walk, with suitable orthoses. When this stage has been reached, the application of some stimulus that would normally cause pain provokes an automatic withdrawal reflex, or spasm. If violent, this may also cause emptying of the bladder and even evacuation of the rectum. Sometimes, because of either chronic urinary infection or pressure sores of the skin, these reflex spasms become exaggerated, being provoked by the slightest stimulus, thereby causing the patient a great deal of discomfort and seriously impeding efforts at rehabilitation.

COMPLICATIONS

There are three important complications of traumatic paraplegia: chronic urinary infection, pressure sores and contraction deformities. Pressure sores may occur because, owing to the absence of sensory stimuli, the patient will not alter the points of pressure as they lie or sit. In addition, during the initial stage of flaccid paralysis, owing to the absence of muscle tone, the peripheral circulation will not be very brisk, making the skin more delicate than normal. Sores occur over bony points such as the sacrum, greater trochanters, malleoli and heels. If not rapidly and adequately treated, full thickness skin loss down to the underlying bone quickly follows.

Later, when tone has returned, owing to unequal pull in opposing muscle groups, contraction deformities may develop unless care is taken to prevent them. Exaggeration of the normal withdrawal reflex that appears when muscle tone returns may cause severe spasms in the limbs, which may gravely interfere with efforts to rehabilitate the patient.

MANAGEMENT

Management of the traumatic paraplegic presents many complicated and specialized aspects, so, if possible, such patients are better transferred to a specialized spinal centre as soon as they can be. For practical purposes there are two phases: early, during the period of suppression of reflex activity, and later, when this has returned to the isolated segment of the cord.

Early

Prevention of pressure sores and control of the urogenital system dominates the early phase. Pressure sores can only be prevented by the regular and frequent alteration in position of the patient, with nursing treatment of all anaesthetic bony pressure points. The patient must therefore be turned every 2 hours by day and night, ideally from the moment of the accident. Established sores should be thoroughly cleaned and all dead tissues excised to encourage healing by granulation tissue. Occasionally, skin grafting may be required.

Management of the bladder in the early stage is aimed at control of distension, thereby preventing the vesical wall becoming stretched, and prevention of infection. Infection occurs because stagnant urine provides a good culture medium for organisms, which can reach the bladder fairly easily by ascending the urethra and passing through the relaxed sphincters. In practice both objectives may be achieved either by intermittent catheterization, conducted under the most perfect aseptic conditions, with regular bladder washouts using a mild non-irritant antiseptic lotion, or by employing an indwelling catheter, which may be made of non-irritant material and left on continuous drainage.

Late

In the later phase the principal aim in management turns to rehabilitation. As tone returns to muscles, it may be possible with suitable callipers and crutches to train the patient to walk after a fashion by swinging both legs through together – 'tripod gait'. Nevertheless, most patients will be mainly, if not entirely, dependent upon wheelchairs and time must be spent in teaching them how to make the best use of these.

When 'automatic' micturition becomes established, it is often possible to stimulate reflex bladder contraction by tickling the end of the penis, or some similar method. At first, to ensure that the bladder is completely empty, a catheter should be passed after voiding, but this procedure can soon be discarded. Bowel movement can, with suitable dietary care, be made fairly regular in much the same way as with a colostomy.

INJURIES OF THE CERVICAL SPINE

As the cervical spine is the most mobile part of the vertebral column, it differs in several ways from the spine below it, the main features being that the intervertebral articulations are placed more laterally than elsewhere and not so far behind the vertebral bodies, so that the nerve roots leave the spinal canal in an anterolateral direction. The bodies themselves are smaller in relation to the size of the vertebra as a whole, and therefore subluxations and dislocations of one vertebra upon another are more common than elsewhere. There is more room in the canal than in the thoracic region, so that the cord has a greater chance of escaping severe damage than lower down, though if it does occur and is not immediately fatal, all four limbs will be involved and the patient will therefore be quadriplegic.

Injuries to the cervical spine fall into two groups, those due to flexion and those due to extension, though rotatory forces also often play a part. Injuries of the atlantoaxial region will be considered separately.

Flexion injuries

Flexion injuries may take three forms. First, there are those in which the posterior ligament complex is intact but the body of the vertebra may form a wedge. This is not a serious injury, though it may cause irritation of a nerve root leading to pain in the arm or side of the neck, depending upon the level. It may lead to early disc degeneration at this site, resulting in cervical spondylosis later.

Second, there may be flexion and rotation injuries, in which there will be frank dislocation of the intervertebral joints, which may be unilateral or bilateral (Fig. 5.6), with or without a fracture of the vertebra. Dislocation, particularly if unilateral, often results in locking of the facet joints. Severe

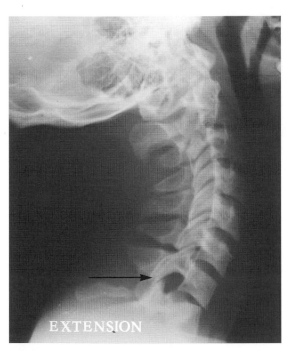

FIG. 5.6 Bilateral fracture dislocations of the cervical spine of C7 on T

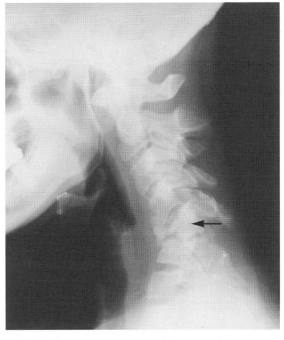

FIG. 5.7 Compression fracture of the cervical spine

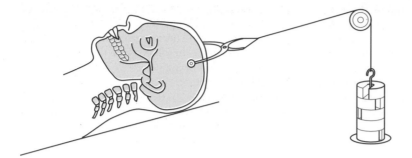

FIG. 5.8   Skull traction

irritation of the nerve root emerging at the affected level is almost inevitable, and damage to the spinal cord may also be present in this type of injury.

Third, a burst fracture of the vertebral body may occur. This is usually stable, but cord impingement results in neurological loss.

TREATMENT

Minor injuries merely require the use of a supporting collar for 6–8 weeks, followed by a period of exercises to regain mobility.

More severe injuries require very careful handling from the outset. For this reason all patients attending hospital with neck injuries must not be moved until the extent of the damage is known, and the greatest of care must be taken during the initial radiological examination. The possibility of associ-

ated injury to the cervical spine must be borne in mind whenever a patient is brought to hospital unconscious from a head injury. Dislocations of intervertebral joints should be treated by traction using skull callipers inserted under local anaesthesia so that the patient is not inadvertently moved (Fig. 5.8). By this means the facets may usually be disengaged, as considerable weight (up to 20 kg) may be applied to the skull without causing discomfort. If after a few hours radiographs show the dislocation to be reduced, traction is maintained for a further 6 weeks, or a halo–body device is

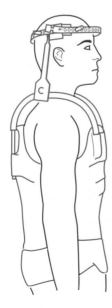

FIG. 5.9   A halo–body fixation system

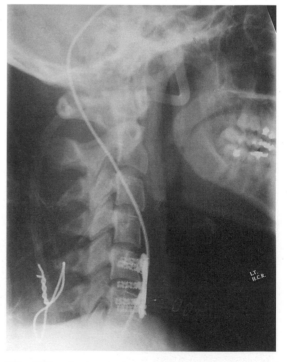

FIG. 5.10   Anterior and posterior fixation of dislocated spine

fitted, which consists of a jacket extending down the trunk to the iliac crests and a ring round the forehead, over the eyebrows (Fig. 5.9); it, too, is worn for about 6 weeks. If there is no fracture, only a ligamentous injury, the cervical spine is unstable and surgery is essential. An anterior and posterior cervical fusion is performed (Fig. 5.10), leaving the patient in skull traction or the halo–body system. An alternative means of maintaining the traction is to use a Minerva plaster cast.

Occasionally reduction may be difficult, in which case, with skull traction still in place, open reduction is performed with the patient lying prone. At the same time the position is stabilized by wiring the spinous processes together, with cancellous bone graft taken from the iliac crest.

Extension injuries

Extension injuries occur when the head is violently driven backwards. They are therefore very common in road accidents, in which, sometimes, when the trunk strikes the back of the car seat the head is then thrown forwards again – the so-called whiplash injury. Extension injuries often show no radiological abnormality on the X-rays, the anterior and posterior longitudinal ligaments being torn. Occasionally, possibly owing to momentary pressure from the ligamentum flavum and lamina posteriorly, severe cord damage occurs (Fig. 5.11). Extension injuries should be suspected in patients with evidence of injury to the face suggesting that the head has been knocked backwards, and can be demonstrated radiologically by flexion/extension

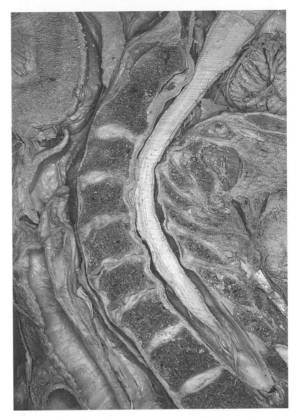

FIG. 5.11   Side view of the anatomical structures related to the cervical spine

views of the cervical spine carried out under medical supervision.

(a)

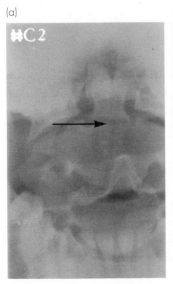

(b)

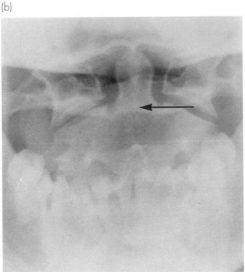

FIG. 5.12   Atlantoaxial injuries: (a) fracture of the odontoid process; (b) 1 year later, fracture healed

TREATMENT

Treatment consists of supporting the head in a firm collar or cervical brace, if the neck is stable. However, if the ligaments are torn, posterior cervical fusion, which may be combined with anterior fusion, is necessary. If the cord is compressed, it is decompressed anteriorly at the same time.

Atlantoaxial injuries

Three forms of atlantoaxial injury commonly occur. First, there is displacement of the atlas on the axis with fracture of the odontoid process (Fig. 5.12), an injury from which the patient usually survives. Second, there is displacement with dislocation of the odontoid process backwards, which is almost invariably fatal owing to sudden pressure on the vital centres below the foramen magnum. This is the injury produced by judicial hanging (hangman's fracture). (Fig. 5.13.) Third, a vertical blow from driving the head downwards may split the atlas in a lateral direction (Jefferson's fracture).

TREATMENT

Fractures of the atlantoaxial complex are serious injuries, because the neck is no longer stable. Reduction is essential, first to relieve the pressure on the spinal cord and second to obtain the best anatomical condition for stabilization.

Reduction is usually achieved by skull traction, and the fracture is immobilized by fusion of the vertebrae, either by the posterior route and incorporating the occiput in the fusion mass, or by the transpharyngeal approach.

INJURIES OF THE PELVIS

Injuries to the pelvis are of three main types: fractures of the pelvic ring; isolated fractures of either the pubic rami or the ilium, and fractures of the acetabulum.

Pelvic ring

Pelvic ring fractures may occur in three forms: the anterior portion of the ring may be disrupted if all four pubic rami are broken, the loose portion being driven backwards; one side of the pubic symphysis may be fractured and the anterior sacroiliac joint ruptured, producing an 'open book' fracture; and one side of the pelvic ring may be fractured and not only roll outwards but may also be displaced upwards (Malgaigne's fracture). (Figs 5.14–5.16)

As with all bony injuries of the trunk, the possibility of visceral damage must be constantly borne in mind. This applies particularly in pelvic injuries because the rectum, bladder and urethra are contained within the pelvic cavity, and the membranous urethra is especially vulnerable as it passes through the pelvic diaphragm. A distended bladder is also very liable to be ruptured by a blow hard enough to disrupt the pubic bones.

FRACTURES OF ALL FOUR PUBIC RAMI

Detachment of the whole anterior segment of the pubis follows a severe blow on the front of the pelvis.

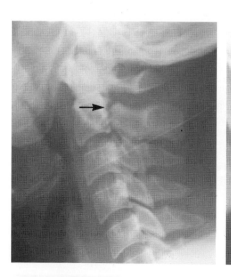
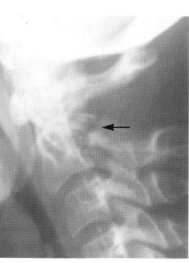

FIG. 5.13 Hangman's fracture of C2

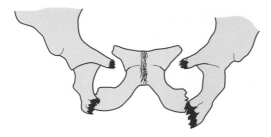

FIG. 5.14   Fractures of the pubic rami

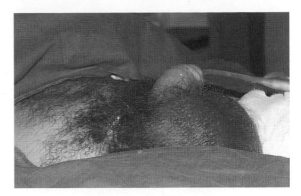

FIG. 5.17   Massive perineal haematoma after pelvic fracture, associated with rupture of the urethra

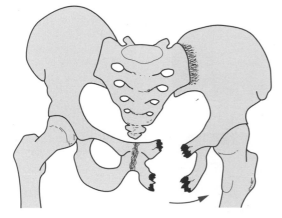

FIG. 5.15   Fracture of the pelvis with lateral displacement

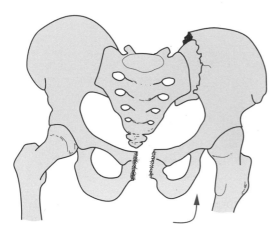

FIG. 5.16   Fracture of the pelvis with lateral and upward displacement

Such injuries usually result from road accidents, or sometimes from a fall from a height, when the patient lands prone, striking this region on some hard object. The significance of injuries of this nature lies in the grave risk of associated damage to the bladder or urethra (Fig. 5.17). The bony injury is important only if the fracture line extends into the hip joint, or, in women of child-bearing age, when residual displacement may obstruct normal delivery.

Treatment

Treatment is mainly symptomatic. An initial period of rest is necessary until the floating fragment begins to become stabilized, because otherwise the opposing pull of the abdominal muscles above, the hip adductors and intrapelvic muscles below, causes considerable discomfort. The pelvis is frequently X-rayed to detect any movement in the fragments. As soon as possible, active movements of the lower limbs are begun, the patient remaining in bed for 4–6 weeks after injury.

'OPEN BOOK' FRACTURE AND MALGAIGNE'S FRACTURE

In these injuries the pelvic ring is broken in two places, anteriorly through the pubic rami or pubic symphysis and posteriorly through the ilium, ala of the sacrum or the sacroiliac joint. The force required to produce the disruption of the pelvic ring is enormous and can occur when a patient is partially run over in, for example, a road traffic accident.

Treatment

Treatment is aimed at closing the gap in front of the pelvis. An external fixation bar with pins in the iliac crest is used to close the diastasis in the 'open book' fracture, as the posterior sacroiliac ligament is intact and the compression applied by a transverse bar hinges on this ligament.

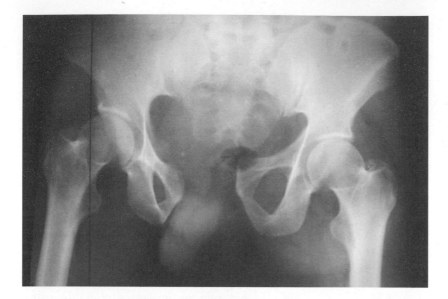

FIG. 5.18 Malgaigne's fracture dislocation of the pelvis

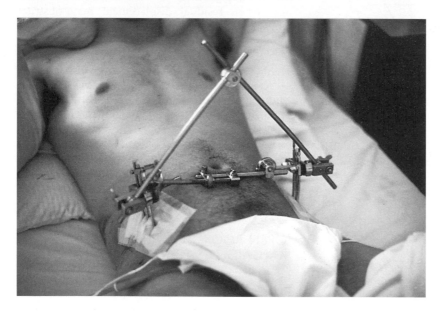

FIG. 5.19   'A' frame for stabilizing pelvic fracture

However, in the shear fracture of the Malgaigne injury, the sacroiliac ligaments are completely disrupted and the pelvis is totally unstable. (Fig. 5.18.) Control can be achieved by using a trapezoid fixation frame (Fig. 5.19), and it may be necessary to fix the sacroiliac joint internally at the same time.

Isolated fractures

Isolated fractures follow direct blows and occur rather more readily in the osteoporotic bone of the elderly.

Fractures of the ilium alone, although less common than fractures of the pubic rami, usually result from greater trauma and therefore cause more constitutional upset to the patient. Fractures of the pubic rami on one side only are of little significance unless they extend into the acetabulum (see below).

TREATMENT

After more serious intrapelvic damage has been excluded, these injuries should be treated in the

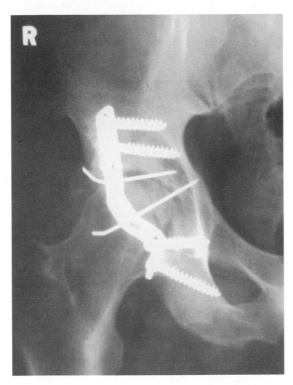

FIG. 5.20   Internal fixation of an acetabular fracture

same way as severe bruising, that is by early mobilization. Weight bearing can be resumed within a few days.

Acetabular fractures

The acetabulum may be fractured in a variety of different ways, and the Letournel–Judet classification lists ten different types. Essentially, though, the fractures may involve either the anterior wall or the posterior wall, or result in a central fracture dislocation of the acetabulum. CT scanning has demonstrated the extent of these fractures, which affect the stability of the hip joint, and damage to the articular cartilage, leading to early osteoarthri-

tis. At the same time the blood supply to the femoral head may be impaired, resulting in avascular necrosis (osteonecrosis).

TREATMENT

After careful identification of the extent of the fracture, early surgery is essential to restore the joint surface to as near normal as possible and hence prevent osteoarthritis (Fig. 5.20). The acetabulum can be approached by the anterior or the posterior route, depending on the fracture, which is then reduced and stabilized by means of plates.

COMPLICATIONS OF PELVIC INJURIES

Injury to the main iliac vessels

The internal iliac artery is the main vessel involved in injuries to the pelvis. There is a wide cross-circulation between the four main branches, obturator, superior and inferior gluteal and internal pudendal. Massive blood loss can occur and large transfusions of up to 8 litres may be necessary.

Angiography is performed and intravascular tamponade is produced using gel-foam to block the bleeding vessels.

Injury to the sciatic nerve

The sciatic nerve may rarely be involved in a traction injury (axonotmesis) in severe pelvic injuries, in which there is disruption to the pelvic ring especially when involving the ala of the sacrum. Muscle weakness occurs in the buttock, hamstrings and calf muscles. The prognosis is variable, recovery being good in milder cases and poor in severe cases.

EXAMPLES

Spine

A 20-year-old woman was involved in a road traffic accident. She was not wearing a seat belt and, although in the back seat of the car, was thrown half out of the car injuring her neck.

She was fully conscious and was taken by ambulance to the Accident and Emergency Department and after ABC assessment immediately had a skeletal survey. Neurological evaluation revealed Medical Research Council (MRC) grading of power 3 and 4 in the upper and lower limbs. X-rays revealed a dislocation of C5 and C6.

Questions
- What is the immediate management?
- Is this injury stable?
- Is surgery necessary?

Answers
- Arrange for cervical calipers to be applied and the dislocation reduced.
- No, this is an unstable injury and may progress to cord damage.
- Yes, anterior and posterior stabilization is necessary as all the soft tissues, ligaments, discs and joints have been disrupted.

Pelvis

A 30-year-old man is involved in a road traffic accident and is admitted to the Accident and Emergency department in a state of shock. On arrival he is conscious and breathing but has a BP of 80/20 mmHg and a pulse of 160 min.

He is acutely tender in his abdomen. The skeletal survey shows a fractured pelvis with disruption to the sacroiliac joint. Peritoneal lavage reveals blood-stained fluid.

Questions
- What is the immediate management?
- How can the blood loss be controlled?
- Where is the bleeding taking place?

Answers
- Stabilize the pelvis by sandbags immediately and then arrange for external pelvic fixation to be applied.
- Arterial embolization, after stabilizing the pelvis, is invaluable.
- Into the retroperitoneal space.

6 UPPER LIMB – SHOULDER, ARM AND ELBOW INJURIES

FRACTURES OF THE CLAVICLE

Fractures of the clavicle occur very commonly throughout life, being seen most frequently in children and young adults. The majority of fractures are situated in the middle third of the bone, and are due to a fall on the point of the shoulder. Sometimes fractures of the outer end follow direct blows.

Complications are very uncommon. Rarely, the subclavian vessels are trapped as they pass between the clavicle and the first rib.

Treatment

Fractures of the clavicle almost invariably unite rapidly, despite the fact that true splintage is almost impossible. However, malunion is common, although this is rarely accompanied by loss of function. The mass of new bone is usually palpable at the site of the united fracture. In theory, the only way of attempting to avoid this complication when for cosmetic reasons it is thought desirable, would be to nurse the patient flat in bed and allow the shoulders to fall back over a sandbag placed vertically between the scapulæ. However, this is never practised and usually a sling is all that is necessary.

A figure-of-eight bandage can be used, but needs regular adjusting to prevent displacement and compression on the axillary nerves and vessels.

DISLOCATION OF THE STERNOCLAVICULAR JOINT

Dislocation of the sternoclavicular joint is an uncommon injury, resulting from a fall on the shoulder forcing the inner end of the clavicle forwards. Rarely, it is displaced backwards where it may injure the vessels of the neck or damage the trachea.

In the true dislocation, reduction is obtained by direct pressure on the bone end, while the shoulder is drawn outwards. Reduction is usually simple to obtain, but maintenance is not so easy, although stability can be achieved by internal fixation of the clavicle to the manubrium. However, recurrent displacement and subluxation are common, but rarely cause any disability. In the occasional patient with repeated pain and subluxation a further operation may be required, and the bone is then anchored by the use of either a fascia lata strip or the tendon of the subclavius muscle.

INJURIES TO THE ACROMIOCLAVICULAR JOINT

Acromioclavicular joint injuries result from a blow on the shoulder, forcing it downwards. The joint may be completely dislocated or merely subluxed. In the latter the strong coracoclavicular ligament remains intact, whereas in dislocations this must be torn through to allow full displacement. Clinically, apart from obvious marked prominence of the outer end of the clavicle, when the coracoclavicular ligament has been torn, there will be tenderness and bruising over the coracoid process and the acromioclavicular joint.

Treatment

Treatment varies according to whether the joint is subluxed or dislocated.

Subluxations require only that the joint is protected, by supporting the arm in a triangular bandage sling for about 10 days.

Dislocations are more difficult to treat, as it is necessary to provide downward pressure over the outer end of the clavicle, at the same time raising the shoulder joint. A simple method consists of passing non-stretch zinc oxide strapping over the clavicle, down the upper arm anteriorly, under the flexed elbow, and then up behind to cross the clavicle again, felt pads being used to protect the bony points. This strapping should be retained for 3 weeks. Sometimes reduction is prevented by the outer end of the clavicle becoming trapped above the trapezius muscle. Then operative reduction may be necessary, which can be secured by an intramedullary pin or screw passed through the acromion and down the clavicle.

FRACTURES OF THE SCAPULA

Fractures of the scapula, affecting either the neck or the body of the bone, follow a direct blow on the scapular region. The bony injury is unimportant, and treatment therefore consists of early mobilization using a sling for protection until the acute pain has subsided.

DISLOCATION OF THE SHOULDER

In order to permit a really wide range of movement, the glenoid cavity is shallow, and the shoulder joint depends for stability upon the surrounding soft tissues. Movements at the shoulder girdle are both glenohumeral and scapulothoracic. Dislocation of the shoulder is therefore a very common injury, usually resulting from a fall on the hand with the arm abducted. The head of the humerus most commonly is forced out of the glenoid cavity inferiorly and then moves up to lie anteriorly because, as the body is moving forwards, the shoulder is externally rotated at the same time – this is anterior dislocation of the shoulder. Sometimes the head is driven directly forwards

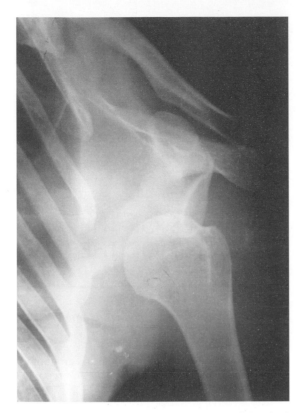

FIG. 6.1   *Appearance of anterior dislocation of the shoulder*

when the cartilaginous labrum glenoidale is torn from its anterior attachment. This leaves a potential cavity into which the head can repeatedly slip if primary healing fails to take place – this is known as recurrent dislocation. More rarely, the humeral head is displaced behind the glenoid – posterior dislocation. It is absolutely essential to take both anteroposterior and axillary X-rays of all injuries to the shoulder joint, to define the direction of the dislocation.

Anterior dislocation (Fig. 6.1)

The clinical picture of anterior dislocation is characteristic. There is flattening of the normal shoulder contour, because the humeral head is absent from the glenoid and, below the deltoid, the arm is held in about 30° of abduction. Radiologically, the head usually lies below the coracoid process (subcoracoid position). Occasionally it remains below the empty glenoid cavity (subglenoid position).

COMPLICATIONS

The axillary nerve, as it passes round the neck of the humerus, may be injured with paralysis of the deltoid muscle, which is shown by the inability to abduct the arm in association with an area of numbness over the skin of the lateral border of the deltoid. Rarely, when severe violence causes the injury, the brachial plexus, in part or as a whole, may be damaged, as may the axillary vessels. The greater tuberosity is sometimes fractured at the same time (group VI fracture, see below) which may delay full return of function for a while. On occasions there is an associated fracture through the surgical neck of the humerus, leaving the head lying free in front of the glenoid.

TREATMENT

Kocher's method of reduction is normally employed. Under general anaesthesia the arm is fully externally rotated, then, in this position, adducted across the body, and finally, still adducted, it is swung into internal rotation. Alternatively, the Hippocratic method may be used. In this the operator's 'unbooted foot' is placed in the patient's axilla, and, with traction on the hand, the humeral head is gently lowered back into the glenoid fossa. X-rays are then taken to confirm the reduction.

After reduction the arm is supported by a sling and bandaged to the side for 3 weeks, thus preventing external rotation, allowing the capsular tear to heal and diminishing the risk of recurrent dislocation. After this, a period of exercises to restore movement is usually required.

An axillary nerve injury is usually a lesion in continuity, and invariably recovers.

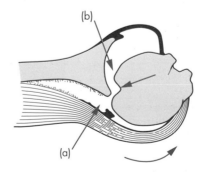

FIG. 6.2   *Causes of recurrent dislocation of the shoulder: (a) rent in the glenoid labrum; (b) notch in the head of the humerus*

Recurrent dislocation (Fig. 6.2)

Recurrent dislocation is due to the presence of an unhealed rent in the anterior humeral attachment of the labrum glenoidale, leaving a pocket into which the humeral head can slip when the arm is externally rotated and abducted. Associated with this, a notch may develop in the head posteriorly where it strikes the margin of the glenoid as it dislocates (Hill–Sachs lesion). This notch renders the head unstable.

TREATMENT

Treatment is surgical, by repair of the rent in the anterior attachment of the labrum and deliberately restricting the range of external rotation by taking a tuck in the subscapularis tendon and anterior part of the joint capsule. Postoperative treatment consists of keeping the arm firmly bound to the side for 6 weeks.

Posterior dislocation (Fig. 6.3)

Posterior dislocation is comparatively uncommon and is due to an internal rotation-abduction force. It occurs in epileptics. It can be overlooked if only

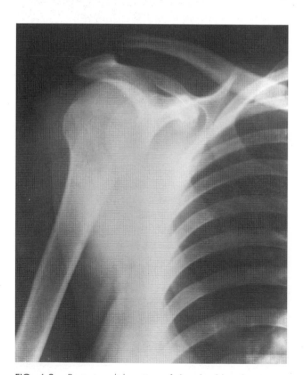

FIG. 6.3 Posterior dislocation of the shoulder showing a 'light bulb' sign

anteroposterior X-rays are taken of the shoulder joint because the head of the humerus, although lying behind the glenoid, may not be displaced medially. Therefore, axillary views must also be taken to demonstrate the relationship of the humeral head to the glenoid.

Reduction is obtained by adducting the arm across the trunk, followed by external rotation. If recurrent dislocation occurs, this is best prevented by deepening the posterior glenoid margin by inserting a bone block.

FRACTURES OF THE UPPER END OF THE HUMERUS

Fractures of the upper end of the humerus are common, and follow a fall on the outstretched hand. Neer has classified these injuries according to the number of fragments and the amount of displacement seen on the X-ray.

Group I – undisplaced fractures

Group I includes all undisplaced fractures, regardless of the number of fractures, and fractures in which there is no displacement or angulation greater than 45°.

Treatment is by early immobilization after a short period in a collar and cuff.

Group II – fracture through the anatomical neck

Fracture through the anatomical neck is rare and may escape detection. Osteonecrosis may develop. A hemiarthroplasty may be inserted in this group.

Group III – fracture through the surgical neck

Group III includes all displaced fractures of the surgical neck of the humerus, in which the displacement is more than 1 cm or there is more than 45° of angulation of the fragments. But the rotator cuff remains intact and the head is in neutral.

- Group IIIA: the head is impacted and angulated more than 45°;
- Group IIIB: the fracture of the surface neck is separated, with more than 1 cm of displacement;
- Group IIIC: the fracture of the surgical neck is comminuted and displaced.

All these fractures may require internal fixation (Fig. 6.4), but can be treated conservatively with the risk of malunion, non-union or avascular necrosis.

Group IV – fracture of the greater tuberosity

In group IV the greater tuberosity is fractured with more than 1 cm of displacement. These fractures imply a rupture of the rotator cuff. The two-part fracture may be associated with a dislocation of the humeral head. The three-part fracture is associated with a separation through the surgical neck of the humerus and is combined with displacement because of the pull of the subscapularis and retraction of the humeral shaft by the pectoralis major. The result is that the humeral head turns to face posteriorly.

Open reduction and internal fixation are essential.

Group V – fracture of the lesser tuberosity

Group V consists of fractures of the lesser tuberosity of the humerus, into which the subscapularis muscle is inserted. The two-part fracture occurs as an isolated fracture and can be treated conservatively. The three-part fracture, however, involves displacement of the surgical neck and the humeral head rotates. Open reduction and internal fixation are required. The four-part fracture involves both tuberosities and the surgical neck. The blood supply to the humeral head is lost and therefore it is necessary to replace the bone with a hemiarthroplasty.

Group VI – fracture dislocation (Fig. 6.5)

A fracture of the greater tuberosity commonly occurs in association with anterior dislocation of the head of the humerus. If the rotator cuff remains intact, closed reduction usually leads to accurate

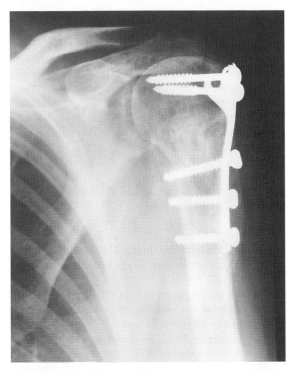

FIG. 6.4   Internal fixation of fractured humerus, (group III)

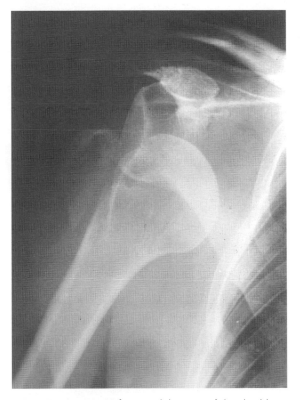

FIG. 6.5   A group VI fracture dislocation of the shoulder

replacement of the tuberosity. This is also invariably so for two- and three-part fractures. However, if there is a four-part fracture dislocation, the head is separated from its blood supply. This severe fracture may be associated with damage to the axillary vessels or the brachial plexus. Closed reduction needs to be performed with care, preferably by the hippocratic method, and internal fixation or a hemiarthroplasty may be necessary (Fig. 6.6).

Group VII – articular fractures

In group VII, part of the articular surface is crushed against the glenoid. The result will be a defect in the articular surface with fragments extruding into the joint.

Conservative treatment will usually suffice, although, if there are fragments involving more than 20 per cent of the articular surface, internal fixation of the fragments should be performed if possible or they should be removed. With more than 50 per cent of the surface damaged, dislocation is inevitable and a hemiarthroplasty must be performed.

Fractures in children

In children, greenstick fractures of the surgical neck are undisplaced and may be treated conservatively.

Epiphyseal injuries may be reduced by a closed means, but may require internal fixation with a pin. Open reduction is not normally necessary.

SOFT-TISSUE INJURIES OF THE SHOULDER

Because the shoulder is largely dependent upon surrounding soft parts for its stability, these are, naturally, subject to injury. Musculotendinous structures intimately related to the joint are, first, the flat muscles arising from the scapula and inserted into the tuberosities on the humeral head – the subscapularis, supraspinatus, infraspinatus and teres minor, which together form the 'rotator cuff' – and, second, the tendon of the long head of the biceps brachii crossing over the head of the humerus within the joint, to enter the bicipital groove between the greater and lesser tuberosities on its way to join the short head of the biceps in the arm.

Injuries of the rotator cuff

Some tearing of the musculotendinous fibres of the rotator cuff must occur when a normal shoulder is dislocated, but this is rarely important. If, however, in a fall the abducted arm is forcefully brought to

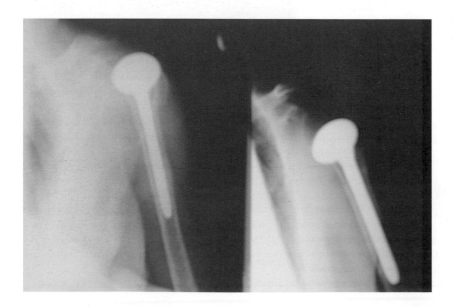

FIG. 6.6   Hemiarthroplasty for fracture dislocation (group VI)

the side, there may be an extensive tear of the rotator cuff and capsule of the shoulder. Usually this involves mainly the supraspinatus tendon, though other parts of the cuff may also be torn, depending upon the direction of the fall.

Clinically, there will be marked tenderness over the humeral head and complete inability to initiate abduction. Soon after injury, however, before reaction has caused general stiffness in the joint, it may be possible to demonstrate that if abduction is initiated passively, the patient can then continue to raise their arm actively, using the deltoid muscle. In these cases, also, as the abducted arm is lowered, sudden pain will be experienced, causing the arm to drop to the side. This occurs when the torn tendon impinges upon the undersurface of the acromion.

TREATMENT

In the elderly, preservation of movement is the most important aspect of treatment, so, as soon as the initial reaction has subsided, mobilizing exercises are started. Occasionally, direct operative repair of extensive tears is required.

Rupture of the long head of the biceps

Rupture of the long head of the biceps is an injury of elderly patients, and is associated with attrition of the tendon of the long head as it passes through the bicipital groove, which may be somewhat roughened.

Frequently, this occurs almost spontaneously, so no actual moment of rupture can be recalled, the patient becoming aware of pain in the shoulder, with tenderness over the bicipital groove, and a characteristic bulging of the biceps muscle belly when the elbow is flexed against resistance. Usually, however, there is a specific moment when sudden sharp pain is experienced as the patient is lifting some heavy object.

TREATMENT

In the large majority of cases no active treatment is indicated. The patient is instructed to continue using their arm as normally as possible, and to ignore the bulge in the arm as the muscle belly contracts. Very rarely in younger persons, the torn lower end of the tendon may be reattached to the bicipital groove, though no attempts should be made to repair the tendon itself.

FRACTURES OF THE HUMERAL SHAFT

Fractures of the humeral shaft (Fig. 6.7) occur at all levels, and may result from direct or indirect violence, the former having a transverse or comminuted fracture line, and the latter oblique. These fractures occur at all ages, but they are rather less common than fractures of the shafts of the other long bones. Possibly this is because the wide range of movement in the shoulder joint absorbs some of the violence of an injury.

Pathological fractures, though, are common in the humerus. In children, they may occur through a solitary bone cyst, the upper shaft of the humerus being the commonest site for this condition. In adults, the humerus is a common site for metastatic deposits, particularly from neoplasms of the breast or bronchus. Often, a pathological fracture is the first sign of abnormality in the bone, and, in the case of bronchial carcinoma, may also be the presenting symptom of the disease as a whole.

Complications

The radial nerve, being closely related to the bone as it lies in the spiral groove, is often injured in

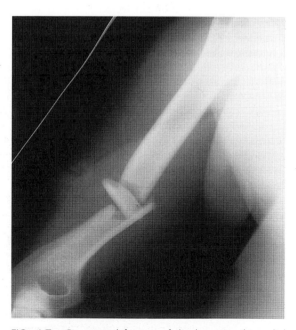

FIG. 6.7 Comminuted fracture of the humerus; the radial nerve is at risk from this fracture

fractures of the humeral shaft. This may be merely bruising – 'neurapraxia' – in which full recovery occurs spontaneously after an interval of 2–4 weeks. Alternatively, however, more permanent damage is done to the nerve on axonotmesis or neurotmesis.

Non-union can present a very great problem when it occurs, partly because of the difficulty of providing really adequate immobilization of the bone.

Treatment

In uncomplicated fractures of the humeral shaft, treatment does not usually provide a problem. Reduction is relatively simple, and minor degrees of overlap or angulation are of less significance in the humerus than in any other long bone. With the patient sitting, leaning slightly to the injured side, and with the wrist supported so that the elbow is flexed at 90°, the fracture automatically realigns itself. While in this position a plaster of Paris slab is applied extending from the axilla, down the inner side of the arm, beneath the elbow and up the outer side, to end lying over the shoulder in the region of the acromioclavicular joint. This 'U' plaster slab is secured by a crepe bandage, applied before it has set. The wrist is then supported in a collar-and-cuff sling. Anaesthesia is not required. Immobilization is continued for 6–8 weeks, after which mobilization is commenced, with the arm protected by a triangular sling for a further 2–3 weeks.

When there is difficulty in obtaining adequate reduction, or if there are multiple injuries elsewhere, rendering early mobility desirable, and in patho-

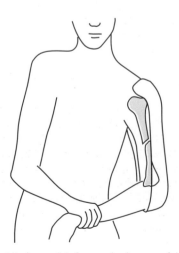

FIG. 6.8 'U' plaster slab fixation for fracture of the humeral shaft

logical fractures through a neoplastic deposit, internal fixation should be used. The best method is by a locked intramedullary nail inserted from above and driven across the fracture site; the proximal and distal ends of the nail are locked with a screw to prevent rotation. This may be preceded or followed by radiotherapy in neoplastic lesions.

Treatment of complications

INJURY TO THE RADIAL NERVE

The integrity of the radial nerve must be tested in all fractures of the humeral shaft. In a neurapraxia, full recovery is almost certain, but it is not always possible to tell which lesion is in continuity and which is from a divided nerve when there is a closed injury.

A good index of radial nerve recovery is the brachioradialis muscle, which is visible when the elbow is flexed against resistance. If there is no sign of recovery after 12 weeks, the nerve could be explored. The radial nerve is largely motor in function and therefore results of direct suture are usually good. However, if it is not possible to repair the nerve or the suture fails, good function can be obtained by tendon transfers. The radial nerve extends the wrist, thumb and fingers, therefore

- flexor carpi ulnaris is transferred to extensor digitorum, to extend the fingers;
- palmaris longus, if present, is inserted into extensor pollicis longus to extend the thumb;
- pronator teres is inserted into extensor carpi radialis brevis or longus to extend the wrist.

NON-UNION

Non-union occurs when the blood supply to the humerus has been impaired, and therefore is commonly associated with severe local trauma. If, after a reasonable interval, union has failed to take place, the fracture should be grafted. A locked intramedullary nail is used to provide internal fixation, and cancellous iliac bone graft should be employed as the graft.

INJURIES OF THE ELBOW

The range of elbow movement in flexion and extension is shown in Chapter 1. It must be appreciated that, although residual stiffness in the elbow is serious, loss of flexion is a much greater disability than loss of extension. Therefore, not only must the elbow never be splinted in extension, but also, when mobilization is begun, flexion is the more important movement to restore. Furthermore, the weight of the forearm tends to extend the joint passively at the expense of regaining flexion; so the elbow must be supported in a sling until a reasonable range of movement has returned.

Passive movements are to be avoided, as they merely irritate the joint and so increase the stiffness. Sometimes myositis ossificans may be provoked by such means.

The close proximity of the main vessels and nerves must always be borne in mind when dealing with major injuries, and the state of these should be checked regularly.

Fractures of the lower end of the humerus

The lower end of the humerus may be fractured in several ways, depending upon the direction of force. In a fall on the outstretched hand, the lower end may be driven backwards – a posterior supracondylar fracture of the humerus. This is a very common injury of childhood whereas in an adult a similar force would dislocate the elbow joint. Falls in which the point of the elbow is struck from behind may cause an anterior supracondylar fracture of the humerus. In a fall directly upon the flexed elbow, the olecranon may split the lower end of the humerus vertically, causing a Y-shaped fracture. If a severe lateral angulatory force is applied to the elbow, the lateral humeral epicondyle may be displaced upwards. Occasionally the medial humeral epicondyle may be avulsed, an injury of later childhood occurring before this epiphysis joins the main bone.

Supracondylar fracture of the humerus

As stated above, supracondylar fracture of the humerus with posterior displacement is a very common injury of childhood, caused by a fall upon the outstretched hand. The lower end of the humerus is displaced backwards. All degrees may occur, from undisplaced cracks to complete separation of the lower fragment. If displacement is severe, considerable soft tissue damage may be done.

COMPLICATIONS

The brachial artery may be injured by impinging upon the sharp lower end of the main fragment. The vessel is not often torn through but the damage to its wall causes it to go into severe spasm, which, if not relieved rapidly, will cause permanent ischaemic changes in the forearm and hand, with infarction of muscle, leading to the condition known as Volkmann's ischaemic contracture (already described). It is important to appreciate that injury to the brachial artery may occur during injudicious attempts at reduction of the fracture.

The median nerve may also be injured when it is stretched over the lower end of the main fragment, and occasionally severe damage is done in this way.

The ulnar nerve may be damaged by traction between the point where it passes through the medial intermuscular septum (above the fracture site) and where it is anchored in its groove below the medial epicondyle of the humerus. Irritation may also occur if the fracture unites with a valgus deformity; this causes late development of weakness in the intrinsic muscles of the hand and numbness of the ring and little fingers – a complication known as delayed ulnar neuritis.

Myositis ossificans, as already mentioned, may follow attempts to mobilize the stiff elbow at a later stage.

TREATMENT

Manipulative reduction is employed, but, because of the risk of injury to the brachial vessels, it should be conducted under full general anaesthesia, with X-ray control.

Procedure

There are two principal deformities to correct, posterior and lateral displacement. To do this the elbow is gently extended and strong longitudinal traction is applied; the lateral displacement is corrected at this stage. Then the surgeon flexes the elbow with one hand and at the same time, while maintaining continuous traction in the long axis of the forearm, guides with the other hand the distal fragment onto the proximal end of the humerus, correcting the posterior displacement. After reduction, the fracture can be maintained in good position merely by keeping the elbow flexed, thus tightening the posterior humeral periosteum, which, though stripped off the bone, was not torn through. However, if

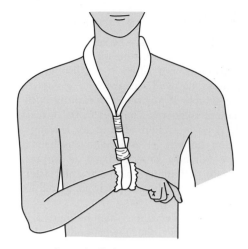

FIG. 6.9   Collar-and-cuff sling

swelling is considerable, full flexion may impair the circulation, so the procedure may have to be deferred for 2 or 3 days, and after reduction a very careful watch must be kept on the radial pulse for at least 24 hours. A collar-and-cuff sling worn under the clothes so that it cannot be removed, provides sufficient immobilization. (Fig. 6.9.)

TREATMENT OF COMPLICATIONS

Vascular

Circulatory impairment is shown by an absent pulse, pain on extending the fingers when the wrist is dorsiflexed, absent capillary return on pressure to the finger nails and blue or white fingers. It is accompanied by paraesthesia.

It is imperative to restore the blood flow as soon as possible. Once the decision has been made, no time should be wasted. The patient is taken to theatre, an extensive incision is made through the deep fascia to expose the artery, and warm saline packs are applied to the wound. If this is not effective the damaged segment of artery should be excised, the clot in the distal segment removed and continuity restored by a primary anastomosis or by the use of a graft.

Neurological

The median or ulnar nerve may be damaged, but in most cases recovery occurs within a few weeks. However, if after a few months there is no sign of recovery, the nerves should be explored under a bloodless field. The ischaemic nerve is excised and reconstructed by a nerve graft.

A useful sign of median nerve damage is the pointing index finger sign, and is particularly helpful when examining a child.

Delayed ulnar neuritis
If evidence of late ulnar nerve irritation appears, the nerve should be dissected free from its bed in the groove behind the medial epicondyle and transplanted to lie in front of the humerus.

Myositis ossificans

If the recovery of movement ceases, X-rays should be taken; any evidence of the development of myositis ossificans is an indication for active exercises.

Anterior displacement

Anterior displacement is a much less common injury than supracondylar fracture of the humerus with posterior displacement, and it is also an injury of adults rather than children. It results from a backward fall onto the point of the elbow, thereby driving the smaller fragment forwards, along with the forearm. Complications, other than residual joint stiffness, are uncommon.

TREATMENT

The reduced fracture is stable in extension, but in view of the risk of stiffness this position is impracticable and usually some residual deformity must be accepted. The elbow is rested at first in a collar and cuff; exercises are started as soon as the pain has settled. In young adults an open reduction can be performed to obtain an anatomical reduction.

Y-shaped fractures of the lower end of the humerus

Y-shaped fractures are not very common. They occur in adults, and are due to a powerful blow striking the lower end of the humerus, splitting it longitudinally. Displacement may be severe, and in younger adults open reduction with internal fixation may be required.

Fractures of the lateral humeral condyle (Fig. 6.10)

Fractures of the lateral humeral condyle are due to lateral angulatory forces applied to the extended

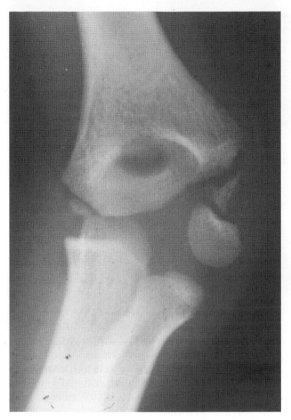

FIG. 6.10   Fracture of the lateral humeral condyle

elbow. They are seen in adults and children, but are more common in the latter. In children the true extent of injury may not be appreciated from X-rays because of the amount of epiphyseal cartilage present.

COMPLICATIONS

Unless an almost perfect reduction is obtained, a residual valgus deformity will follow. As a result, delayed ulnar neuritis may occur. (Fig. 6.11.)

NON-UNION

This is fairly common and may lead to later development of a valgus deformity.

TREATMENT

In order to ensure close bony apposition, open reduction is indicated. The detached condyle is secured by an internal fixation.

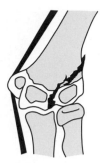

FIG. 6.11   Fracture separation of the epiphysis for the lateral humeral condyle, showing how the ulnar nerve may be stretched

Fracture of the capitulum

In adults, the capitular portion of the lateral epicondyle may be fractured, the loose fragment being displaced upwards. As the fragment may be almost free in the joint, with only a small soft-tissue attachment, avascular necrosis often occurs.

Open operation is the best method of treatment. If there is a reasonable soft tissue attachment, the capitulum may be reattached by subperiosteal sutures reinforced by a screw.

Avulsion of the epiphysis of the medial condyle (Fig. 6.12)

In severe lateral angulatory strains of the elbow, particularly when there is also powerful contraction of the wrist flexors attached to the medial

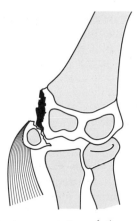

FIG. 6.12   Fracture separation of the epiphysis of the medial condyle

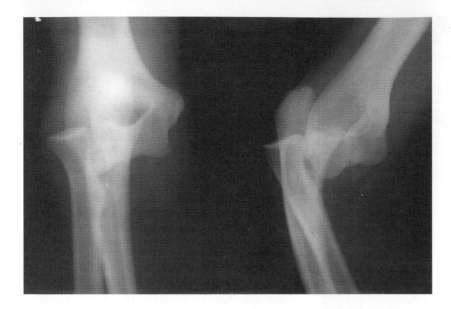

FIG. 6.13 Dislocation of the elbow joint

condyle, this fragment may be avulsed. This can only occur in later childhood, when the epiphysis for the epicondyle is well developed but not yet attached to the humerus itself. This injury in effect represents a tear of the medial joint capsule, and it is often associated with dislocation of the elbow, when the condyle becomes lodged between the joint surfaces, blocking reduction.

Fibrous union is the rule after avulsion of the medial condyle, but, as the articular surfaces of the elbow joint are unaffected, this is of no significance.

COMPLICATIONS

Delayed ulnar neuritis or immediate damage to the ulnar nerve are common, because the nerve is so closely related to the bone at this point. Delayed neuritis at this site is due to the nerve becoming strangled by scar tissue as it lies in its groove.

TREATMENT

Avulsion of the condyle indicates severe capsular damage to the elbow joint. A period of rest in a collar and cuff for 2–3 weeks is therefore required, followed by gentle active mobilization.

If the condyle is trapped between the articular surfaces of the humerus and ulna, open reduction is indicated and the ulnar nerve can be transplanted at the same time to prevent the onset of delayed neuritis.

Dislocation of the elbow

Dislocation of the elbow (Fig. 6.13) is a common injury occurring throughout adult life, and is due to a fall on the outstretched hand with the elbow a little flexed. In a child a similar fall would cause a supracondylar fracture. The elbow is normally a stable hinge joint, so, in order to produce a dislocation, extensive tearing of the joint capsule must take place, sometimes with avulsion of bony fragments (such as the medial epicondyle already described). Sometimes the radial head is fractured at the same time as the dislocation. Displacement is either backwards or laterally, and sometimes is a combination of both.

COMPLICATIONS

Nerve injuries

Nerves related to the elbow joint are occasionally damaged, particularly the ulnar nerve because of its close relationship with the humerus. In most cases the injury is slight, and full recovery follows.

Myositis ossificans

Myositis ossificans may occur later on, affecting the brachialis muscle. The ossification extends from the coronoid process into the brachialis muscle, thus limiting flexion.

Recurrent dislocation

Recurrent dislocation follows on rare occasions, if the coronoid process has been fractured.

Treatment

Manipulative reduction is usually simple. It is accomplished by gentle traction on the semiflexed joint, the flexion being cautiously increased, while direct pressure is exerted over bony points to overcome the displacement. Open reduction is required only in cases in which a loose bony fragment causes a block to manipulative reduction. After reduction, the joint is rested in a collar and cuff. At about 2 weeks active mobilization is encouraged. Full movement takes several months to return, and slight residual stiffness is common.

Fractures of the olecranon

Fracture of the olecranon (Fig. 6.14) usually results from sudden contraction of the triceps as the elbow is forcibly flexed, the olecranon thereby being snapped over the lower end of the humerus. Because of the pull of the triceps, some separation of the loose fragment invariably occurs. Occasionally the olecranon is fractured by a direct blow on the point of the elbow, when there is comminution without separation of the fragments because the periosteum is intact.

TREATMENT

Because of the pull of the triceps, apposition of the fragments could be achieved only by splinting the elbow in full extension, which would certainly leave severe permanent limitation of flexion. For this reason, operative treatment is the rule (Fig. 6.15). When there is a single fragment, internal fixation using wires gives good results. If there is comminution the fragments can be excised and the triceps tendon reattached to the stump of ulna,

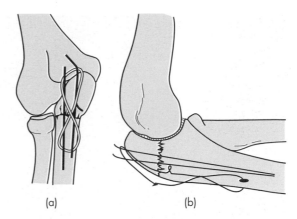

FIG. 6.15 Fracture of the olecranon: (a) anteroposterior view, treated by internal fixation with wires; (b) lateral view, showing wires in the olecranon

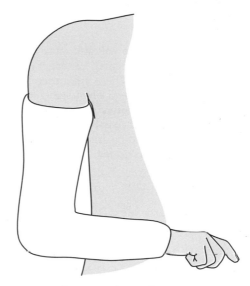

FIG. 6.16 Axilla-to-wrist plaster of Paris cast

however if at all possible the fragments should be reduced and will then need to be internally fixed.

Postoperatively a plaster of Paris cast from axilla to wrist is applied and retained for about 4 weeks, after which gentle active mobilization is commenced.

Fractures of the head of the radius (Fig. 6.17)

Radial head fracture is caused by a fall on the hand that drives the radial head against the capitulum. It is important to appreciate that a blow of sufficient

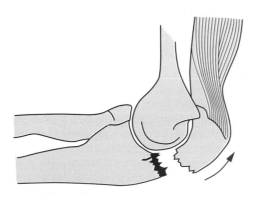

FIG. 6.14 Fracture of the olecranon

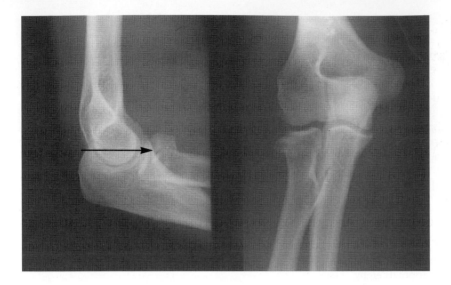

FIG. 6.17 Fracture of the head of the radius

severity to break the bone will also cause considerable damage to the articular cartilage on both surfaces. Radiologically, there may merely be a vertical crack in the bone, or one fragment may be considerably displaced outwards and downwards, or the whole radial head may be comminuted. The head of the radius may be fractured at the same time as the elbow is dislocated.

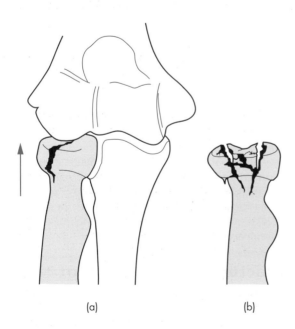

(a)   (b)

FIG. 6.18   Fractures of the head of the radius: (a) vertical crack; (b) comminuted

TREATMENT

When displacement is slight, treatment should be conservative, the arm being protected in a collar-and-cuff sling for 2 or 3 weeks, gentle active flexion in this being permitted. This is followed by increasing active movement, with the arm in a triangular sling worn outside the clothes until a reasonable range of movement has been regained. If the displacement is minimal the fracture can be reduced and held by a single screw.

If displacement is severe, the head of the radius may need to be excised. Fractures of the head of the radius complicating dislocation of the elbow are often comminuted, and require excision, but in these cases it is better to wait several weeks until the reaction to the original trauma has subsided before operating on the injured joint and encouraging dislocation.

Fractures of the neck of the radius (Fig. 6.19)

Fractures of the neck of the radius are injuries of childhood, the fracture being of a greenstick nature. Slight displacement can be accepted, but an attempt should be made to correct angulation greater than about 30°. Often this can be done by direct pressure with the thumbs, but if much swelling is present it may be better to expose the annular ligament surgically and apply direct pressure on the bone.

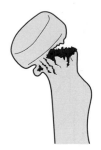

FIG. 6.19   Fracture of the neck of the radius

'Pulled elbow'

'Pulled elbow' is an injury of young children and is due to a dislocation of the radial head out of its annular ligament as a result of the infant being lifted up by the hand. Treatment consists of flexing the elbow and supinating the forearm under anaesthesia.

Rupture of the biceps insertion

Rarely, if there is sudden, forcible extension of an actively flexing elbow, the insertion of the biceps may be avulsed from the neck of the radius. This is demonstrated clinically by loss of active flexion and marked bruising in the cubital fossa. Treatment is by operative repair.

EXAMPLES

Shoulder

An 80-year-old woman falls down on the pavement injuring her right shoulder. In the Accident and Emergency Department she is found to have a four-part fracture of her right humerus.

Questions
■ What is the treatment?
■ What is the prognosis?

Answers
■ The options available are non-operative and operative.
■ This patient is 80 years old but is otherwise fit and healthy and it is her dominant arm. She lives alone and values her independence.
■ Hence a hemiarthroplasty is a reasonable line of management.
■ If treated operatively the prognosis is reasonable, in that pain and restoration of function can be achieved. However, if this fracture is treated conservatively with pain relief and immobilization, problems of non-union and shoulder stiffness could occur, which would affect her overall function.

Elbow

A 12-year-old boy falls out of a tree injuring his left elbow. He is seen in the Accident and Emergency Department with a swollen left elbow and tingling in his hand.

X-rays demonstrate a supracondylar fracture of the left humerus.

Immediate treatment is to reduce the fracture under general anaesthetic and the postoperative X-rays show the fracture has been reduced.

However, the patient still complains of tingling in his hand.

Questions
■ Why has he got tingling in his hand?
■ What treatment is advocated?

Answers
■ He has tingling because the blood supply to the median nerve is compromised because of a compartment syndrome.
■ This syndrome is associated with supracondylar fractures and is brought about by swelling of the muscles within tight compartments.
■ The clinical presentation is tingling in the hand; poor capillary filling in the hand; pain in the forearm on passive extension of the hand; and absence of peripheral pulses, a late manifestation.
■ The treatment is to arrange for the forearm fascial planes to be decompressed immediately in order to overcome the effect of the swelling on both the neurovascular structures and prevent muscle ischaemia.

7 UPPER LIMB – FOREARM, WRIST AND HAND INJURIES

FOREARM

In considering fractures of forearm bones it is necessary to appreciate that preservation of rotation at the wrist is very important, and this must be borne in mind during reduction and subsequent treatment. The elbow is basically the humeroulnar joint, with supination and pronation occurring at the humeroradial joint, whereas the wrist is the radiocarpal joint. If, therefore, one bone only is fractured and displaced, there will be dislocation of the more mobile end of the other. With fractures of the ulnar shaft the head of the radius is dislocated, and with fractures of the radial shaft the lower end of the ulna is displaced.

Fractures of radial and ulnar shafts

Fractures of radial and ulnar shafts may follow direct or indirect violence. In those due to direct violence, both bones will be broken at about the same level, and the fracture will be either comminuted or transverse. In these injuries there may also be considerable soft-tissue damage, with injury to the median, ulnar or posterior interosseous nerves. In addition, if severe swelling is present, this may interfere with arterial circulation to the muscles, such that Volkmann's ischaemic contracture may occur.

Radial and ulnar shaft fractures due to indirect violence are rather more common in children. In these, the ulnar fracture is spiral, but the radial fracture is at a different level and often transverse, because in the forceful twist it is snapped directly across the ulna. In children the radial fracture may be of greenstick type.

COMPLICATIONS

Apart from the soft-tissue complications already mentioned, non-union of forearm fractures, especially those due to direct violence, is fairly

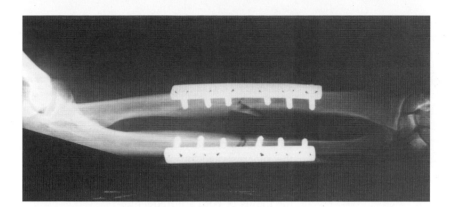

FIG. 7.1 Internal fixation of fractures of the radius and ulna

common. Occasionally, usually where there has been an open fracture with low grade infection, cross-union, in which a bridge of bone joins the radius to the ulna, may occur. This is serious, because it completely prevents any rotation movement of the forearm.

TREATMENT

Fractures of both radius and ulna

Perfect reduction must be obtained, particularly when there is displacement. Closed reduction can be achieved; however, open reduction is required in order to reduce the fractures accurately and to prevent angulation of the radius or ulna. This angulation occurs after closed reduction plaster is applied, for, as the swelling in response to the injuries diminishes, the fractures displace within the loose plaster. Therefore open reduction is followed by internal fixation with a plate to both forearm bones. (Fig. 7.1.)

Fractures of the ulna

An undisplaced fracture of the ulna caused by a direct blow can be treated in an above-elbow plaster. However, a displaced fracture of the ulnar shaft must be associated with a dislocation of the radial head – a Monteggia fracture dislocation (see below).

Fractures of the radius

Fractures of the radial shaft usually occur in the distal third because the proximal two-thirds are well covered by muscle. An isolated displaced fracture of the radius will not occur without a dislocation of the distal radioulnar joint. This is Galeazzi's fracture dislocation (see below).

Fracture of the ulna with dislocation of the radial head (Monteggia) (Fig. 7.2)

Displacement may be either forward bowing of the ulnar shaft, with anterior dislocation of the radial head, or backward, with posterior displacement of the radial head. The former, which is more common, results from a forced pronation twist,

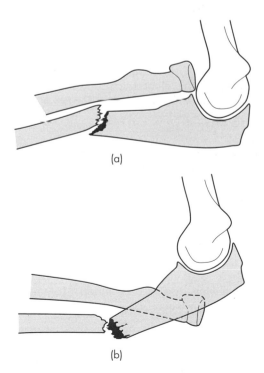

(a)

(b)

FIG. 7.2 Monteggia fracture of the ulna shaft, with dislocation of the radial head: (a) forward; (b) backward

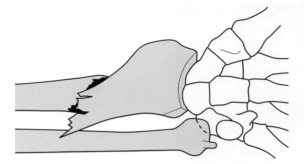

FIG. 7.3 Galeazzi fracture of the radial shaft with dislocation of the lower end of the ulna

which extends the elbow at the same time. The less common backwardly displaced type is due to a flexion–supination force. In children the ulnar fracture may be of greenstick type, in which case its significance may not be appreciated, and in consequence the displacement of the radial head may be overlooked.

TREATMENT

In the more common type, with forward dislocation of the head of the radius, manipulative reduction should be employed in children. This consists of flexing the elbow and fully supinating the forearm. In adults, when there is either an anterior or a posterior dislocation of the radial head, open reduction of the ulnar fracture is required, after which the radial head reduces. The ulnar fracture is held with a plate.

Fracture of the radius with dislocation of the lower end of the ulna (Galeazzi) (Fig. 7.3)

The Galeazzi fracture, which is the reverse of the Monteggia type of fracture, consists of a displaced fracture of the lower half of the radial shaft, with dislocation of the lower end of the ulna. It also follows a rotational strain, and the ulnar head is almost always displaced posteriorly. It is not seen in children, in whom greenstick fractures of both bones occur.

TREATMENT

Unless perfect reduction of the radial fracture is maintained, residual displacement at the inferior radioulnar joint will follow. Open reduction, with internal fixation of the radius by a plate, is therefore indicated.

Lower end of radius and ulna

Fractures of the lower end of the radius due to falls on the hand are very common in all ages. In adults, the ulnar styloid process may be avulsed by its attachment to the fibrocartilaginous disc. In children, greenstick fractures near the lower end of the ulna, the radius or both are frequent.

ADULTS

In adults two forms of displacement may occur, depending upon the direction of the injury force. In falls with the hand outstretched, there is backward displacement of the lower end of the radius. When the wrist is flexed, there is forward displacement.

Fracture of the lower radius with posterior displacement (Colles' fracture) (Fig. 7.4)

Fracture of the lower end of the radius with posterior displacement of the distal fragment was first described in 1814 by Abraham Colles, an Irish surgeon who was Professor of Anatomy, Physiology and Surgery at the Royal College of Surgeons in Ireland. He described this fracture without the aid of X-rays.

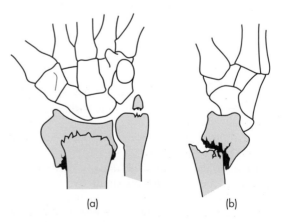

(a)   (b)

FIG. 7.4 Colles' fracture: (a) anteroposterior view; (b) lateral view

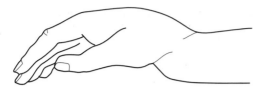

FIG. 7.5   The clinical appearance of a Colles' fracture

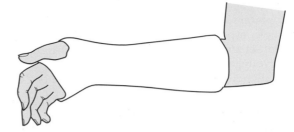

FIG. 7.6   Colles-type below-elbow plaster of Paris cast

A Colles' fracture occurs commonly throughout adult life, but particularly in the elderly, and is probably related to the increased incidence of osteoporosis in this age group. As, at the moment of impact, the patient is usually moving forwards, supination is also a factor in producing the characteristic appearance.

Deformity of the lower end of the radius is three-fold: displacement backwards, tilt backwards and tilt in a radial direction (Fig 7.5). Depending upon the degree of violence, some comminution may be present, particularly posteriorly. The ulna styloid is also usually avulsed. Clinically, the displacement causes what is described as a 'dinner-fork' deformity.

COMPLICATIONS

Complications may involve:

- Bone: malunion, a common end result, due to the displacement of the fracture during union. It may cause a problem, however, because of shortening of the radius at the wrist joint, resulting in the loss of supination and pronation.
- Joint: stiffness and loss of function can occur at the wrist joint, and the shoulder joint may become stiff through immobility.
- Nerve: the median nerve may be compressed during the healing of the fracture, producing a carpal tunnel syndrome.
- Tendons: the extensor pollicis longus tendon may rupture, particularly in patients with minimally displaced distal radial fractures. This is because the blood supply to the tendon is impaired from the fracture haematoma as it lies within the tight extensor compartment.
- Sudeck's osteodystrophy can occur, resulting in a stiff, painful, swollen hand and wrist with erythema of the skin.

TREATMENT

When there is significant displacement, manipulative reduction under general or regional anaesthesia is required. This is achieved by disimpacting the fracture by firm longitudinal traction and reducing it by direct pressure on the displaced lower fragment with the operator's thumbs, as the same time rotating the carpus into a position of pronation and ulnar deviation. After reduction, a 15 cm wide plaster of Paris slab is applied over the dorsum of the wrist, and moulded round its radial side to retain the ulnar deviation of the hand. A check X-ray is then taken. As swelling may occur, for the first 1 or 2 days the slab is secured by a crepe bandage and the cast is completed later. It should extend from the metacarpal heads posteriorly, and the proximal palmar crease anteriorly, to just below the elbow, and is retained for 5 or 6 weeks.

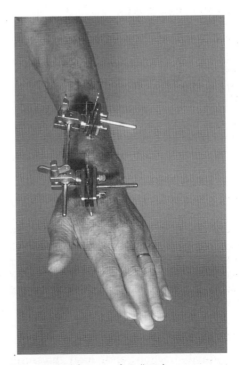

FIG. 7.7   External fixation of Colles' fracture

As the majority of patients are elderly, it is important to encourage early use of the limb as a whole, especially of the fingers and the shoulder joint; otherwise, stiffness may be a problem later. In younger patients, in order to maintain joint length and reduce stiffness an external fixator can be employed. (Fig. 7.7.)

TREATMENT OF COMPLICATIONS

- Malunion, with loss of supination and pronation, is best left for a period of time. If loss of movement persists, the distal end of the ulna can be excised to improve rotation.
- Stiffness of joints: active physiotherapy is commenced from the beginning to prevent this complication.
- Carpal tunnel syndrome usually resolves spontaneously, but division of the flexor retinaculum is required if median nerve compression persists.
- Rupture of the extensor pollicis longus tendon requires repair. The extensor indicis to the index finger, which runs on the ulnar border of the extensor tendon, is sacrificed and its proximal part is sutured to the distal portion of the ruptured extensor pollicis longus tendon.
- The treatment of Sudeck's osteodystrophy in the stage of painful dystrophy is by splintage in the position of function, combined with active use of the rest of the limb. As soon as the painful episode has resolved, active functional exercises are carried out under supervision of the physiotherapist. It may take the patient 6 months or more to recover.

   Iuanethidine, a ganalion blocker, can be used to treat resistant cases.

Fracture of the lower radius with anterior displacement (Smith's fracture)

Smith's fracture, which may also be described as a 'reversed Colles' fracture', follows a forcible flexion injury to the wrist. It is uncommon and occurs in younger adults, sometimes resulting from accidents on bicycles or motorcycles, because of the position of the hands on the handlebars. Like a Colles' fracture, this is not associated with any articular injury and is a fracture of the lower part of the radius.

TREATMENT

Longitudinal traction and local pressure can reduce the anterior displacement and correct the angulation. However, the problem is to maintain this position and so above-elbow plaster with the forearm supinated will be required. Because these fractures tend to occur in younger people and the disability after unsatisfactory reduction is much greater, open reduction and internal fixation with a T-plate are necessary.

Fracture of the lower end of the radius (Barton's fracture)

Barton's fracture should not be confused with Colles' or Smith's fractures because first, it involves the articular surface of the lower end of the radius, and second, it is associated with radiocarpal instability. This fracture is not uncommon and is caused by a fall on an outstretched hand. The damaged articular surface is frequently comminuted.

TREATMENT

As these fractures occur in a younger age group than Colles' fracture and because the articular surface is damaged, accurate reduction is essential. This is achieved either by open reduction and internal fixation with a T-plate or by closed reduction and external fixation.

Fracture of the radial styloid

The radial styloid alone may be fractured by a fall that forces the hand in a radial direction. Displacement is not usually significant. Treatment consists of a below-elbow plaster, worn for 3 or 4 weeks.

CHILDREN

Fractures of the lower ends of the radius and ulna in children are very common, usually resulting from falls on the outstretched hand or blows that dorsiflex the wrist. They may take two forms: a fracture separation of the epiphysis or a fracture of the distal radius.

Fracture separation of the lower radial epiphysis

In this injury there is backward displacement of the radial epiphysis, to which is attached a triangular fragment of variable size from the metaphysis – a Salter–Harris type II injury. There is also,

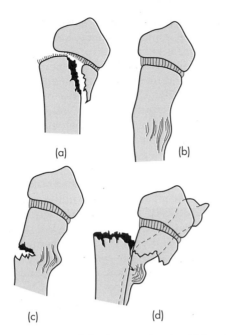

FIG. 7.8 Fractures of the lower radius in childhood: (a) fracture separation of the lower radial epiphysis; (b) 'buckle' fracture of the lower radius; (c) greenstick fracture of the lower radius; (d) fracture with overlap of the radius, with greenstick fracture of the ulna

often, a greenstick fracture of the distal end of the ulna.

TREATMENT

Because of the natural tendency for the deformities to correct with growth, very minor displacement can be accepted. When reduction is required, it is carried out by the same manoeuvre as that employed with a Colles' fracture. Immobilization, by a below-elbow plaster, is required for 3 weeks, with the wrist fully plantar flexed to hold the reduction.

Greenstick fractures of the lower end of the radius and ulna

Greenstick fractures of the lower end of the radius and ulna are very common (Fig. 7.8c), particularly to a minor degree in younger children. In this case, the radius alone is affected, usually about 2–3 cm proximal to the epiphysis. There is no actual break in bony continuity, the dorsal surface of the radius being merely buckled. In more severe injuries there is an appreciable angular deformity with a break in continuity on the anterior surface of the bone. Both bones are often involved in these cases.

TREATMENT

In 'buckle' fractures of the lower radius, protection only is required for 2 or 3 weeks by a below-elbow plaster. It is probable that many of these injuries are never referred for medical opinion, yet uneventful recovery always takes place.

In fractures in which there is more marked displacement, with angular deformity that is visible clinically, manipulative reduction is required. In carrying this out, it is important to appreciate that unless the fracture is completed, by snapping through the angulated posterior radial cortex when the wrist is palmar flexed, the normal resilience in children's bones will cause the deformity to reappear as soon as the operator's pressure is relaxed. Over reduction is almost impossible because of the tough dorsal periosteum. After reduction, 3 weeks' immobilization in a plaster cast is required.

Fracture of the lower end of the radius with overlap

Fracture at the lower end of the radius with overlap (Fig. 7.8d) follow more severe falls. There is usually an associated greenstick fracture of the lower end of the ulna, though sometimes there is a complete fracture in this bone also.

TREATMENT

It is necessary, first, to overcome the overlap of the fractured bone ends. Therefore, before any attempt is made to correct the dorsal displacement, longitudinal pressure down the shaft of the radius is exerted by the operator's thumbs. Often cautious, slight increase in dorsal angulation may assist in 'hitching' the bone ends, after which the deformity is corrected by palmar flexion. In these cases, immobilization in an above-elbow cast for 3–4 weeks is required.

CARPUS

The wrist is the radiocarpal joint. Significant injuries involving carpal bones, therefore, are usually restricted to the scaphoid and lunate.

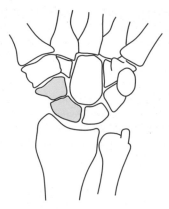

FIG. 7.9   Fracture of the waist of the scaphoid

Fracture of the waist of the scaphoid (Figs 7.9 and 7.10)

Fracture of the waist of the scaphoid results from forcible radial deviation of the carpus, usually due to a fall on the outstretched hand. The waist of the scaphoid is broken by being pinched between the radial styloid and capitate bone. If violence is considerable, some displacement occurs, and there may be an associated fracture of the tip of the radial styloid, but often there is merely a hairline crack that is difficult to detect radiologically. For this reason, the clinical features of a fractured scaphoid are important. There will be tenderness and some swelling in the 'anatomical snuffbox' bounded by the tendons of the extensor pollicis longus, abductor pollicis longus, extensor pollicis brevis and the radial styloid, and any attempt to move the hand in a radial direction will aggravate the pain. Fractures of the waist of the scaphoid are often more easily visualized on X-ray if oblique views are taken in addition to routine anteroposterior and lateral projections. Furthermore, if the clinical features in any way suggest a fractured scaphoid, the wrist should be immobilized, and fresh films taken 2 weeks later, when the absorption at the fracture line will make it more easily visible radiographically.

COMPLICATIONS

Most of the blood supply to the scaphoid enters at its distal end. Fractures through its waist, therefore, may cut off the circulation to the proximal fragment. Because of this anatomical arrangement, delayed union, non-union and avascular necrosis (osteonecrosis) may occur. Avascular necrosis may be diagnosed 6–8 weeks after the occurrence of the injury, when X-ray will show apparent increase in density of the proximal fragment. This in fact is because, having no blood supply, it cannot share in the osteoporosis that follows a fracture. Later there is softening of the avascular fragment, such that it collapses, the shape is distorted and osteoarthritis of the wrist follows.

TREATMENT

Because of the poor blood supply to the proximal fragment, immobilization must be complete. A plaster cast is used, immobilizing the wrist and including the metacarpophalangeal joint of the thumb (Fig. 7.11). To allow use of the hand in the cast, it should be applied in the 'position of function', with the wrist slightly dorsiflexed and slightly adducted, and the first metacarpal in some degree of opposition. Immobilization must continue until union has occurred, usually about 6 weeks in all. To prevent stiffness, the patient should be encouraged to use their hand as normally as possible in the plaster.

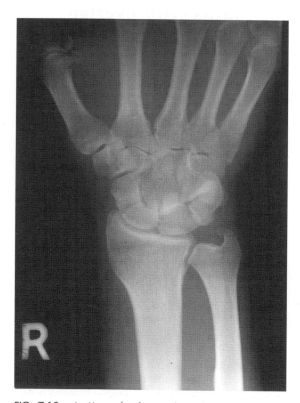

FIG. 7.10   An X-ray of a fractured scaphoid

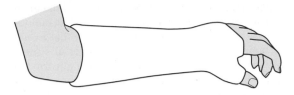

FIG. 7.11   Scaphoid plaster of Paris

TREATMENT OF DELAYED UNION AND NON-UNION

Early surgical intervention is indicated if a fracture shows evidence of displacement during treatment or cystic changes are detected. Internal fixation of the fracture with a compression screw is performed. Bone grafting may be undertaken for any large cysts that have formed.

In established non-union of the scaphoid it is not usually necessary to operate unless there are clear signs of pain from the fractured scaphoid.

Fracture of the tuberosity of the scaphoid (Fig. 7.12)

Fracture of the tuberosity of the scaphoid is an injury that results from a direct blow on the thenar eminence. As there is normal blood supply to this segment of the bone, and the main articular surfaces are not involved, treatment need by symptomatic only. Often, supportive strapping for 2 weeks is sufficient.

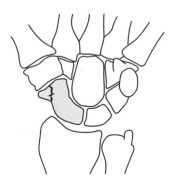

FIG. 7.12   Fracture of the tuberosity of the scaphoid

Dislocations of the carpus

DISLOCATION OF THE LUNATE (Fig. 7.13)

If there is an injury to the carpus that involves forced dorsiflexion, occasionally the joint between

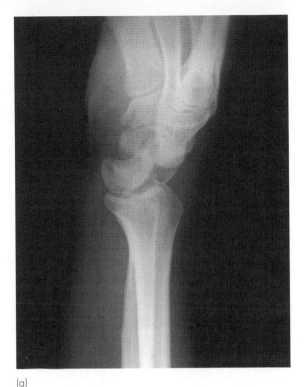

(a)

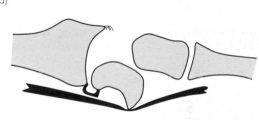

(b)

FIG. 7.13   (a) An X-ray showing dislocation of the lunate; (b) dislocation of the lunate, showing how the median nerve may be damaged

the capitate and lunate becomes dislocated. Then, as the wrist returns to the neutral position, the lunate becomes displaced forwards. Pressure on the median nerve by the dislocated lunate causes paraesthesia in the thumb, index and middle fingers.

Complication

Apart from median nerve compression, avascular necrosis (osteonecrosis) in the displaced lunate commonly occurs, as the widespread capsular stripping will interfere with its blood supply.

Treatment

Manipulative reduction consisting of traction on the wrist, which is then palmar flexed slowly, together with direct pressure on the lunate, usually succeeds. Open reduction is necessary if there is damage to the median nerve, when closed methods have failed or when the dislocation is more than 2 weeks old. Excision of the lunate may be necessary if osteonecrosis develops and the space can be filled with a Silastic implant.

Other carpal dislocations occur, which fortunately are not very common but are due to considerable violence. They are seen in fit young adults, for, in children or older people, fractures will result from this degree of violence.

TRUE DISLOCATIONS OF THE RADIOCARPAL JOINT

True dislocations of the radiocarpal joint are the least common; usually a carpal bone remains articulating with the radius.

PERILUNAR DISLOCATION OF THE CARPUS

In perilunar dislocation of the carpus, the lunate remains in place, and the carpus is dislocated round it.

TRANS-SCAPHOID PERILUNAR FRACTURE DISLOCATION

In trans-scaphoid perilunar dislocations, not only does the lunate remain in contact with the radius, but also there is a fracture of the scaphoid, the proximal pole remaining attached to the radius and the distal pole being displaced with the carpus.

Treatment

In all these carpal dislocations, reduction is rarely difficult, but in trans-scaphoid perilunar dislocations – which are the least uncommon – osteonecrosis of the scaphoid fragment almost invariably follows.

SPRAINED WRIST

The term 'sprained wrist' is used to describe an injury in which the wrist is palmar flexed, thereby tearing the posterior capsule and probably injuring the triangular fibrocartilage of the inferior radioulnar joint. A diagnosis of sprain should not be made without careful X-ray examination that includes anteroposterior, lateral and right and left oblique views of the wrist. An X-ray may show that a flake of bone has been avulsed from the dorsal surface of the triquetral and is associated with a tearing of a ligament. Arthrography and arthroscopy help to evaluate these lesions.

Treatment is symptomatic, and early mobilization is encouraged to prevent a stiff wrist.

HAND

The hand is perhaps the most unique part of a human being. Phylogenetically it is very close to the basic primitive mammalian pattern, yet, because of the high tactile sensation it possesses, and the wide range of movement possible in the digits, it has been suggested that, second to the human cerebral cortex, it is our most useful organ! The nomenclature of the hand is shown in Fig. 7.14. Movements of the digits are concerned with either grasp or pinching. In the former, the fingers surround an object in one direction, with the thumb surrounding it in the opposite way, and considerable power may be exerted. In the latter, the tip of the thumb is brought into contact with that of the index and

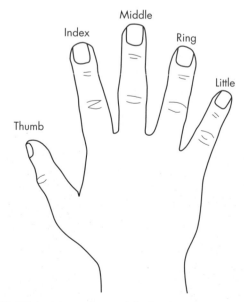

FIG. 7.14   Nomenclature of the hand

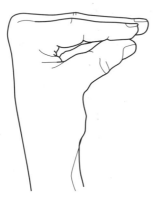

FIG. 7.15 Position for immobilizing the hand

It is also important in the treatment of all hand injuries to encourage active mobilization in all joints that do not specifically require to be immobilized. In all injuries, swelling should be discouraged, and if present, measures taken to reduce it. This applies particularly to the hand for two reasons: first, because the resulting pain will prevent active movements by the patient, and second, the presence of either blood or oedema fluid in the tissue planes is liable to cause adhesions that in the hand would interfere with the free gliding of tendons.

Individual hand injuries will be dealt with in two parts – those involving bones and joints, and those affecting the soft tissues – but it must be emphasized that, more than elsewhere in the body, the management of bony and soft tissue injuries go together.

middle fingers. This is the position employed in doing finer work.

In considering the management of hand injuries, therefore, the preservation of movement is of great importance, and if any residual stiffness is anticipated the part must be held in the position functionally most useful. The fingers should only be immobilized with the metacarpal phalangeal as flexed as far as possible, and the interphalangeal joint as extended as far as is possible. This is in order to maintain tension in the collateral ligaments. The thumb should be placed with its metacarpal in 'opposition', that is, rotated through 90° to the plane in which the finger metacarpals lie, and abducted. The wrist itself should ideally be held slightly dorsiflexed and also in ulnar deviation (Fig. 7.15).

SKELETAL HAND INJURIES

Skeletal injuries can be grouped into those of the metacarpus and those of the phalanges.

Injuries of the metacarpus

FRACTURES OF THE BASE OF THE FIRST METACARPAL

Fractures of the base of the first metacarpal are common and result from a longitudinal thrust down the metacarpal shaft. Two forms occur: a vertical fracture line through the base, with dislocation of the

(a) (b)

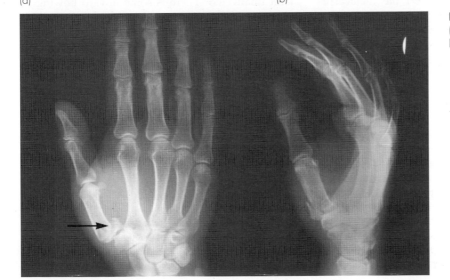

FIG. 7.16 A Bennett's fracture; (a) anteroposterior view; (b) lateral view

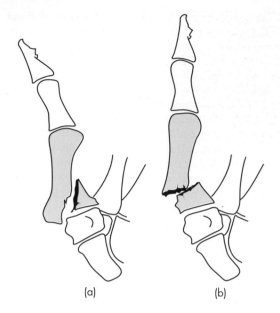

FIG. 7.17   Fractures of the base of the first metacarpal: (a) Bennett's fracture dislocation; (b) fracture through the base of the metacarpal shaft

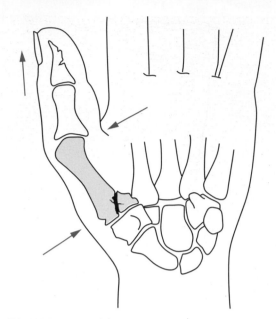

FIG. 7.18   Lines of force employed in the reduction of a Bennett's fracture

joint between the metacarpal and trapezium, and a fracture with a transverse line, involving the metacarpal alone.

FRACTURE DISLOCATION (BENNETT'S FRACTURE) (Figs 7.16 and 7.17a)

Bennett's fracture is seen most frequently in young men, often due to injuries at sport. A large fragment of the base is sheared off the metacarpal shaft, which is adducted and displaced proximally.

Treatment

If osteoarthritis in the joint at the base of the first metacarpal is to be avoided in later life, perfect reduction is essential. Closed reduction is usually possible. Traction is exerted in the line of the thumb, which is then abducted while pressure is applied over the base of the bone (Fig. 7.18). A scaphoid type of plaster cast is then applied in this position, being carefully moulded at the base of the metacarpal, and includes the interphalangeal joint. In order to maintain the metacarpal in full abduction, the metacarpophalangeal joint must be immobilized in an extended position. The cast is maintained for 4 weeks, during which time frequent X-rays through the plaster are required to ensure that re-displacement does not occur. If

any difficulty is experienced with maintenance of the position, fixation with a Kirschner wire is indicated.

FRACTURE THROUGH THE PROXIMAL PART OF THE FIRST METACARPAL (Fig. 7.17b)

In fractures through the proximal part of the first metacarpal the fracture line is transverse, and the joint unaffected. There is some inward bowing in most cases. In children there may be a fracture separation of the epiphysis of the metacarpal, which, in the case of the first, is situated at its base.

Treatment

As no joint is involved, perfect reduction is not vital. If displacement is marked, the fracture may be reduced in the same way as a Bennett's fracture. Immobilization is by a scaphoid type of plaster cast maintained for 3–4 weeks.

FRACTURES OF THE BASES OF THE SECOND TO FIFTH METACARPALS

Fractures of the bases of the second to fifth metacarpals follow direct blows on the dorsum of the hand, and may take all forms from minor cracks to comminuted fracture dislocations of the

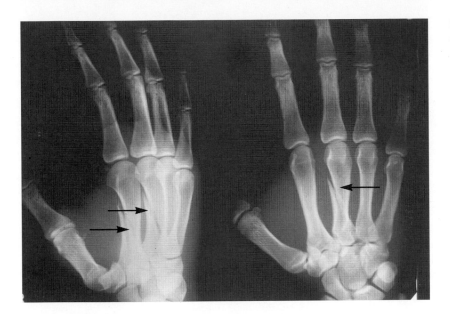

FIG. 7.19 Fractures of the second and third metacarpals

carpometacarpal joints. Reduction, if required, is rarely difficult, and is followed by immobilization in a boxing glove dressing. If indicated, internal fixation with Kirschner wires, followed by mobilization of the hand, may be undertaken.

FRACTURES OF THE METACARPAL SHAFTS (Fig. 7.19)

Fractures of the metacarpal shafts may be either oblique or transverse, depending upon the direction of force that caused the injury.

Oblique fractures lead to some shortening of the metacarpal shaft, but alignment is not often significantly disturbed. Transverse fractures are more liable to an angular deformity, and there may also be overlap of the fragments.

Treatment

Uneventful union invariably occurs in oblique fractures; therefore early mobilization is encouraged, to prevent joint stiffness. Transverse fractures do require reduction if displaced. If there is overlap of the fragments, open reduction and internal fixation using transverse Kirschner wires is often useful as external splintage may thereby be avoided, allowing greater mobility of the hand from the outset.

FRACTURES OF THE METACARPAL NECKS

Fractures of the metacarpal necks (Fig. 7.20) are common injuries resulting from a blow on the

metacarpal head. In children this leads to a fracture separation of the epiphysis from the head. It occurs most commonly in the fifth metacarpal, known as a boxer's fracture, followed by the fourth and second, being least common in the first. The smaller fragment is displaced forward.

Treatment

Manipulative reduction is achieved by flexing the finger fully at both the metacarpophalangeal and proximal interphalangeal joints, when pressure along the line of the proximal phalanx will push the displaced metacarpal head back into place.

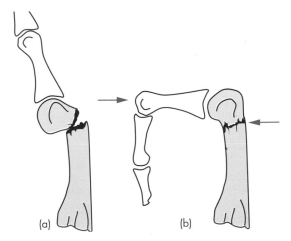

FIG. 7.20 Fracture of the metacarpal neck showing: (a) displacement; (b) method of reduction

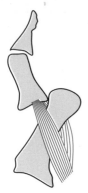

FIG. 7.21   Dislocation of metacarpo-phalangeal joint of the thumb

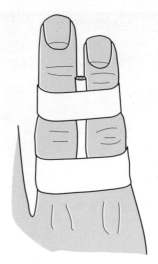

FIG. 7.22   Method of strapping an injured finger to its neighbour

After reduction, the finger is immobilized with the metacarpophalangeal joint flexed and the inter-phalangeal joints extended, held on an aluminium splint, for 2 or 3 weeks, and then gently mobilized.

DISLOCATION OF THE METACARPOPHALANGEAL JOINTS

In dislocation of the metacarpophalangeal joints (Fig. 7.21), the proximal phalanx is normally dis-placed backwards in relation to the metacarpal head. It is most common in the thumb, followed by the index finger. Occasionally, particularly in the thumb, the dislocation is associated with a vertical split in the volar plate, which then becomes buttonholed round the metacarpal neck, forming a block to reduction.

Treatment

Manipulative reduction is achieved by first hyper-extending the proximal phalanx, and then, by direct pressure at its base, lowering it over the metacarpal head. If traction is applied, reduction may be prevented by the metacarpal head being gripped between the flexor tendons or, in the case of the thumb, the long flexor and the thenar muscles. If the volar plate has buttonholed, open reduction is necessary.

SPRAINS OF THE METACARPOPHALANGEAL JOINTS

Side to side movement at the metacarpophalangeal joints is prevented by the collateral ligaments, so that if a digit is subjected to a sideways stress, the ligament may be torn through, thus allowing the joint to become subluxed. This occurs most commonly in the thumb, followed by the little and index fingers. In the thumb, a flake of bone may

be avulsed from the base of the proximal phalanx by the collateral ligament, and when this occurs, unless the fragment becomes reattached, residual laxity remains. This is most frequently seen on the ulnar side.

Treatment

In the thumb, supportive strapping for 10–14 days suffices in minor injuries (Fig. 7.22). If a bony flake has been avulsed, immobilization in a scaphoid type of plaster cast is required for 3 or 4 weeks, or surgical repair is necessary. In fingers, the affected digit should be strapped to its healthy neighbour, thereby permitting flexion and extension but restricting lateral movement.

Digital injuries

FRACTURES OF THE PHALANGES

Phalanges may be damaged either by direct violence from a blow or a crushing force, in which case soft-tissue damage may well have occurred at the same time, or by indirect violence.

Fractures due to direct violence are usually transverse, at midshaft level, and, owing to the combined pull of the flexor and extensor tendons, displacement consists of forward angulation, in which case the bone ends will impinge upon the flexor tendons in their sheath (Fig. 7.23).

Fractures due to indirect violence may be oblique, with some lateral displacement, or one of

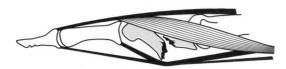

FIG. 7.23   Fracture of midshaft phalanx, showing relationship to the flexor tendons

the articular condyles at the distal end may be sheared off.

In children, fracture dislocation of the epiphysis at the base occurs.

Treatment

If there has been forward angulation, reduction is achieved by traction and flexion of the finger. If interference with the gliding of the flexion tendons in their sheath is to be avoided, perfect reduction is essential. Occasionally an intramedullary wire is employed to provide internal fixation.

After reduction, the finger is splinted in a position of extension at the interphalangeal and flexion at the metacarpophalangeal joints. An aluminium finger splint provides a simple means of doing this.

FRACTURES OF THE DISTAL PHALANX

The end of the distal phalanx may be crushed as a result of a direct blow. The fracture here can be ignored, and the injury regarded as involving soft tissues only. A subungual haematoma is often present and requires evacuation if the nail is to be preserved.

In children, fracture separation of the epiphysis may occur, and if displacement is severe, reduction may be required. The nail in this case must be removed to obtain reduction; if the nail is avulsed from its bed but is still covered by skin this prevents reduction. However, after the nail has been removed the fracture reduces on its own. A

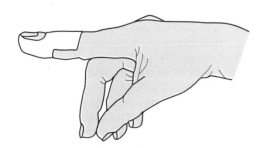

FIG. 7.24   Mallet finger splint

flake of bone may be avulsed from the base by the extensor tendon; this injury is treated for 6 weeks as if there is a tendon rupture, on a 'mallet finger' splint in which there is hyperextension of the distal interphalangeal joint and complete freedom of movement of the proximal interphalangeal joint (Fig. 7.24).

DISLOCATION OF INTERPHALANGEAL JOINTS

Dislocations of the interphalangeal joints may be in the anteroposterior or lateral planes. In the former, reduction by traction will be required, after which the position is stable. However, disruption of the extensor mechanism may occur, leading to a 'boutonnière' deformity. In the latter, spontaneous reduction often takes place, but, because the collateral ligament on one side has been completely disrupted, recovery may be prolonged.

Treatment

After reduction, the finger is supported by strapping it to an unaffected neighbour for 2–3 weeks. Active movement is encouraged.

SOFT-TISSUE INJURIES

Skin

In skin injuries of the hand, two points require to be considered – first, the siting of the scar and, second, replacement of skin loss.

SCARS

In accidental lacerations, the direction of the cut is entirely fortuitous, and the important consideration is to obtain rapid, uneventful healing with minimal reaction. When surgical procedures of any kind are performed in the hand, however, the line of incision must be carefully planned, so that at no point is a natural crease line crossed directly by the cut.

REPLACEMENT OF SKIN LOSS

Skin may be lost in three ways. First, an area may be cleanly sliced off by something sharp, such as a knife or piece of broken glass. Second, loss may be by a combination of crushing and shearing forces, which both lacerates and devitalizes the skin. Finally, if the hand is caught in the moving parts of some machine, skin may be torn off; this is known as 'degloving'. In a finger, the skin may be avulsed in this way if a ring is accidentally violently pulled off.

In replacement of skin, at any part of the hand which is commonly subject to direct pressure, a full thickness graft must be employed.

Nerves

It is important to appreciate that sensory loss in the hand, particularly the fingertips, is extremely disabling because it impedes function and, by removing a protective mechanism, makes further injury more likely to occur. For this reason, divided digital nerves should be repaired whenever possible with the use of magnification or the operating microscope. Occasionally, partial sensation to the tip of the thumb or index finger may be restored by moving an island of skin, together with its neurovascular bundle, from some less vital site, such as the ulnar side of the ring finger.

Tendon injuries

In the hand itself, the flexor tendons differ greatly from the extensor tendons in nature and method of operation, so the two groups will be considered separately.

FLEXOR TENDON INJURIES

Flexor tendons to the fingers and thumb have wide excursions. In order to work efficiently, they must be able to glide freely; yet, whatever position the digit may occupy, they must not alter their relationship to surrounding structures. Where, therefore, they may have to move round corners, they pass through synovial sheaths, lubricated with synovial fluid, and these in turn are anchored by fibrous tissue.

In the fingers the synovial sheaths, in which the flexor tendons run, end opposite the distal interphalangeal joint. In the index, middle and ring fingers, the sheath commences proximally opposite the heads of the metacarpals, whereas in the little finger it is continuous with the general synovial sheath in which all the finger flexors run at the level of the wrist joint. In the thumb the flexor pollicis longus tendon runs on its own, and its sheath extends from the wrist to the interphalangeal joint (Fig. 7.25).

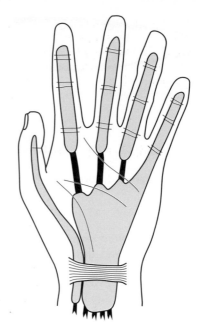

FIG. 7.25 The anatomy of the flexor synovial tendon sheaths in the hand

The flexor tendons in their synovial sheath at the wrist are held in place by the tough flexor retinaculum stretching from the scaphoid to the pisiform. In the fingers there is a fibrous sheath running the length of the synovial sheath. This is firmly attached to the sides of the shafts of the proximal and middle phalanges and their opposite joints. In the thumb the fibrous sheath commences at the metacarpal head, extending only to the interphalangeal joint.

There are two sets of flexor tendons to each finger. The flexor digitorum profundus tendons run through to be inserted into the bases of the distal phalanges, arising from their muscle belly, which lies deep in the forearm. The tendons of flexor digitorum superficialis lie more superficially and, over the proximal phalanges, each one splits so that the two parts pass on either side of the profundus tendon, which lies beneath, to be inserted into the borders of the middle phalanx.

Arising from the profundus tendons in the hand are the small lumbrical muscles, which pass in the interdigital cleft, where each joins the tendon of one of the interossei to be attached to the extensor expansion on the dorsum of the proximal phalanx. This makes it possible to flex the metacarpophalangeal joint while active extension of the interphalangeal joints is maintained. The two ulnar lumbricals and all the interossei are supplied by the deep branch of the ulnar nerve, so an injury to this nerve permits hyperextension of the metacarpophalangeal joints with loss of active extension at the interphalangeal joints. The resulting deformity is known as a 'claw-hand'.

Treatment

Two factors govern the treatment of flexor tendon injuries. First, because of their wide excursion and free movement, where there is complete division wide retraction of the proximal end inevitably occurs, such that an extensive exposure may be necessary at the time of surgical repair. Second, if normal function is to be restored, there must be no adhesion formation within the synovial sheath, which would prevent their free gliding movement. The method of repair, therefore, will depend upon the competence of the surgeon, the level of injury and also the extent of trauma to surrounding structures that occurred at the time of division. A severe crushing injury, particularly if it has also caused a concomitant fracture at the same level, may entirely preclude a successful result from direct tendon repair, and some alternative, less satisfactory, form of treatment may have to be adopted.

Clean incisions of the tendons will be considered first.

In the palm

At the level of the palm direct repair of the tendon is usually possible, using the Kessler method of suture, which is strong and yet minimizes further scar formation at the actual site of the division (Fig. 7.26).

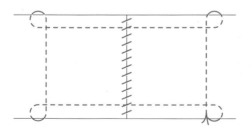

FIG. 7.26   A Kessler suture of a tendon

In the finger

In the finger, as the division is in the synovial sheath, direct tendon repair can produce poor results because of adhesion formation between the sheath and suture line. However, with meticulous technique repair is possible, particularly if the tendon is sutured using a Kessler technique and then mobilized with Kleinert traction. If failure is encountered after primary repair, or if the patient's injury is treated late, tendon grafting may be employed.

After primary or secondary repair, Kleinert traction is used for 4 weeks to permit the suture lines to heal, after which active mobilization is started.

The timing of the flexor tendon repair is important in order to minimize scar formation. If the wound is contaminated, or there has been crushing in the original injury, operation should be postponed until all tissue reaction has settled down and a full range of passive movement has been regained.

If the flexor digitorum profundus alone has been divided opposite the middle phalanx, satisfactory repair can be obtained by excising the short distal stump of tendon and bringing the proximal end directly up to the base of the distal phalanx. This procedure is known as tendon advancement.

If there has been extensive soft-tissue damage as well as flexor tendon division, the prospects of a successful tendon repair by any means are not good. In this case it may be better to accept a finger that is stiff in the position of function, by arthrodesing the interphalangeal joints in the semi-flexed position. Occasionally, when there has been extensive damage to one finger alone, especially if sensation has also been impaired, best results will be obtained by amputation, usually through the metacarpophalangeal joint.

In the wrist

In the wrist all the finger flexor tendons run in one synovial sheath, with the median nerve in close proximity. Any laceration at the wrist that divides these tendons is very likely to divide the nerve as well. Surgical repair is a complicated procedure, and to begin with all the flexor digitorum profundus and superficialis tendons are repaired. The median nerve can be repaired at the same time. However, it is possible to leave the nerve repair until later when the tendons are functioning.

EXTENSOR TENDON INJURIES

Only at the level of the wrist do the extensor tendons run in synovial sheaths. In the fingers, the extensor apparatus ceases to be a true 'tendon' and is better described as the 'extensor aponeurosis'. For this reason, the problems of retraction of the severed ends, and free gliding of the tendons, which are so important in the repair of flexor tendons, do not exist.

Treatment

Direct suture of the divided tendon ends, followed by a suitable splint to maintain the tendon in a relaxed position for 3 weeks, gives good results.

Individual extensor tendon injuries

Extensor pollicis longus

As has been mentioned as a complication of a Colles' fracture, the extensor pollicis longus tendon may rupture as it passes over the dorsum of the wrist within the extensor retinaculum. The ruptured tendon is repaired by transplanting the proximal tendon of extensor indicis into the dorsal end of the ruptured extensor pollicis longus.

Proximal interphalangeal joint (boutonnière deformity) (Fig 7.27a)

At the proximal interphalangeal joint the extensor apparatus is in three slips: a central slip, which is inserted into the base of the middle phalanx, and two side slips (into which are inserted the tendons of the intrinsic muscles), which unite together to be inserted into the base of the distal phalanx.

Injury at this level will divide the central slip alone, so the proximal interphalangeal joint will assume a flexed position, whereas the two side slips become displaced forwards and hyperextend the distal phalanx. The resulting appearance is known as a 'boutonnière deformity'.

Treatment Initially the proximal joint is splinted in extension; then the finger is placed in a dynamic splint. Later, if the deformity persists, rather than attempt repair to the central slip, which would be difficult, reasonably good results are obtained if the two lateral slips are sutured together longitudinally over the interphalangeal joint.

Distal interphalangeal joint ('mallet finger')

Mallet finger (Fig. 7.27) is a very common closed injury, in which the extensor is avulsed from its

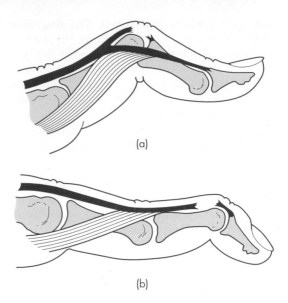

(a)

(b)

FIG. 7.27   Finger extensor expansion injuries: (a) proximal interphalangeal joint ('boutonnière' deformity); (b) distal interphalangeal joint ('mallet finger' deformity)

attachment to the base of the distal phalanx. Occasionally a small fragment of bone is pulled off with the extensor. The cause is usually forceful flexion of the actively extruded finger, as when it is stubbed against some fixed object.

The appearance is characteristic, the distal interphalangeal joint being flexed, whereas the proximal joint tends to assume a hyperextended position.

Treatment The finger should be splinted with the distal interphalangeal joint hyperextended and the proximal joint mobile, thus allowing the torn ends to come together (Fig. 7.24). This position is maintained for about 6 weeks. The splint may be made of plaster of Paris, or a strip of aluminium lined with felt or a plastic material.

In a few cases some residual lag may remain but, as functional disability is slight and the risk of leaving permanent stiffness if surgical repair is attempted is great, the deformity should be accepted.

EXAMPLES

Wrist

A 25-year-old man falls, injuring his right wrist. He is seen in the Accident and Emergency Department with a painful wrist and inability to use his right hand because of the pain.

X-rays demonstrate a fracture at the waist of the right scaphoid.

Questions
- What is the treatment?
- What is the outcome?

Answers
- The treatment is to immobilize the fracture in a scaphoid plaster in order to allow fracture union to occur.
- As this fracture is through the waist of the scaphoid it is probable that the blood supply to the proximal pole of the scaphoid is disrupted.
- If this occurs there is a real risk of osteonecrosis developing with eventual collapse of the scaphoid and the onset of a painful osteoarthritis in a young man.
- The fracture needs to be immobilized for a minimum of 8 weeks followed by bone grafting and internal fixation if evidence of non-union occurs.

Hand

A 20-year-old man sustains an injury to his non-dominant hand in a fight. In the Accident and Emergency Department the hand is swollen and painful and X-rays reveal an angulated fracture of the fifth metacarpal neck.

Questions
- What is the treatment?
- What is the outcome?

Answers
- The treatment is to reduce the angulation, usually under local anaesthetic, and then to immobilize the fracture with the metacarpal phalangeal joint flexed. This position prevents joint contracture.
- The outcome is excellent, even if there is some shortening. The fracture heals quickly and active movement is encouraged as soon as possible, usually after 4 weeks.

8 LOWER LIMB – HIP AND FEMORAL INJURIES

DISLOCATION OF THE HIP

Traumatic dislocation of a normal hip can only follow considerable violence because, unlike the glenoid in the shoulder, the acetabulum is a deep cavity into which the femoral head fits snugly. The head of the femur may be displaced either forwards (anterior dislocation) or backwards (posterior dislocation); the latter is considerably more common. In addition, a direct thrust along the line of the femoral neck occasionally shatters the acetabulum, so the femoral head is displaced into the pelvic cavity. This amounts to a fracture dislocation of the hip, and is often described as a 'central dislocation'.

Posterior dislocation of the hip (Fig. 8.1)

The head of the femur can be driven backwards out of the acetabulum if a longitudinal thrust is applied along the shaft of the femur when the hip is flexed and also slightly adducted. It is therefore an injury commonly due to road accidents. The

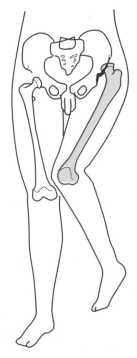

FIG. 8.1   The clinical appearance of posterior dislocation of the hip

clinical appearance is characteristic; the affected leg is internally rotated, adducted and shortened.

Two important complications may occur.

IMMEDIATE COMPLICATIONS

The sciatic nerve may be stretched as it runs round the back of the femoral neck. Damage varies from mild neurapraxia to a severe traction injury (axonotmesis) causing total paralysis. Usually, however, damage is not severe, the lateral popliteal division of the nerve being most vulnerable, causing foot drop and numbness over the outside of the calf.

LATE COMPLICATIONS

The rent that occurs in the capsule of the joint, coupled with the inevitable complete avulsion of the ligamentum teres from the acetabulum, may cut off the blood supply to the femoral head, leading to osteonecrosis. This will cause an apparent increase in density of the femoral head on X-ray, and can also be demonstrated by decreased uptake on the bone scan. If osteonecrosis occurs, then later on the head will collapse, and severe osteoarthritic changes will follow.

TREATMENT

Manipulative reduction is usually successful. The anaesthetized patient is laid on their back, with an assistant anchoring the pelvis by pressure on the iliac crests. The operator flexes the hip to 90° so that the displaced femoral head comes to lie directly behind the acetabulum, then, by traction combined with slight adduction of the hip, the dislocation is reduced.

After-treatment consists of maintaining the leg in traction for about 4 weeks to permit healing of the capsular tear, after which weight bearing is permitted. X-rays, along with regular bone scans, should be taken at monthly intervals for the first 3 or 4 months, so that osteonecrosis of the femoral head may be detected early, before collapse has occurred.

Occasionally, manipulative reduction fails if there is a loose fragment, or, if the posterior lip of the acetabulum has been fractured, redisplacement occurs. In such cases, open reduction using a posterior approach is necessary. The loose fragment is removed, and the lip of the acetabulum, if fractured, may be held in place by screws.

TREATMENT OF COMPLICATIONS

Usually the sciatic nerve is not damaged in a dislocation of the hip.

However, if there is a fracture dislocation involving the acetabulum, the sciatic nerve may be trapped between bone fragments. In this case an operation may be necessary in order to free the nerve and to screw the acetabular fragment back into place.

Osteonecrosis is treated in its early stages by the rigid avoidance of weight bearing until radiographs show that the bony texture of the femoral head has returned to normal. In practice this may take many months, and if this management fails and femoral head collapse continues then, as the patients with traumatic dislocation of the hip are usually young fit adults, surgical treatment is necessary. Total hip replacement is probably the treatment of choice; alternative treatments include arthrodesis, femoral osteotomy and bone grafting of the femoral head, which is effective only in the early stages of osteonecrosis.

Anterior dislocation of the hip

Anterior dislocation of the hip is rare and results from an injury that forcibly abducts the extended hip, causing the femoral head to lie below and in front of the acetabulum. The leg assumes a characteristic position of abduction and external rotation. Complications are less common than in posterior dislocation of the hip.

TREATMENT

Reduction is effected by a combination of adduction, internal rotation and flexion of the hip. This is followed by about 3 weeks' traction to allow repair of the soft-tissue damage.

'Central' dislocation of the hip

'Central' dislocation of the hip is due to direct violence, which drives the femoral head through the floor of the acetabulum. The articular surfaces of both are therefore extensively damaged. There may be intrapelvic haemorrhage, leading to profound shock, which will require treatment.

TREATMENT

If the central displacement is marked and there is gross comminution of the acetabulum, with extensive articular damage, treatment is difficult. Conservative treatment consists of applying longitudinal traction for about 6 weeks. Mobility of the hip may be encouraged by use of weighted slings to support the thigh (Hamilton–Russel traction). Surgical treatment involves reconstruction of the destroyed acetabulum with the aid of internal fixation. If painful osteoarthritis occurs later on, total joint replacement may be necessary.

FRACTURES OF THE UPPER END OF THE FEMUR

Because of the angle formed between the neck and shaft of the femur, fractures of the upper end are very common. They usually result from an indirect twisting force, and are most often seen in the elderly, in whom senile osteoporotic changes are present. It is clear that every patient who has sustained an injury to the hip, whether direct or indirect, must be X-rayed.

The fractures may be grouped according to the level at which they occur:

- subcapital fractures: in which the neck joins the head;
- intertrochanteric fractures: often comminuted, occur through the trochanters;
- subtrochanteric fractures: these are least common, are in fact fractures that occur transversely through the upper femoral shaft.

In addition, occasionally, the lesser trochanter may be avulsed by a sudden pull by the psoas muscle inserted into it, and the tip of the greater trochanter may be cracked by a direct blow over it.

Fractures of the femoral neck are common and carry a mortality of around 20 per cent in the first year.

There are certain notable risk factors:

- age: risk doubles over age of 50 years
- sex: risk is 2–3 times greater in women than men
- race: risk is 2–3 times greater in Caucasians than Negroes

- social: urban dwelling
                    alcohol
- medical history: previous hip fracture
                    senile dementia.

Subcapital fractures of the femoral neck

Subcapital fractures of the femoral neck are common in elderly women, probably due to senile osteoporosis, which tends to be more marked in postmenopausal women. The fracture may present in two ways – it may be impacted, when the neck is driven into the head of the femur, or unimpacted, when the head is free to move within the hip joint and has no remaining soft tissue attached. Garden has classified these injuries into four types or grades.

GRADE I (Fig. 8.2)

In Grade I injuries, the head of femur is in an abducted position, so that it rests on the top of the neck where, as a result of muscle pull, the head and neck become impacted together.

Clinically, there may be little beyond pain in the hip after an injury to suggest a fracture. In the elderly the injury may be a seemingly trivial fall. There is no shortening or rotational deformity and active movement may be possible.

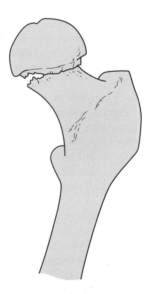

FIG. 8.2   Impacted abduction fracture of the femoral neck

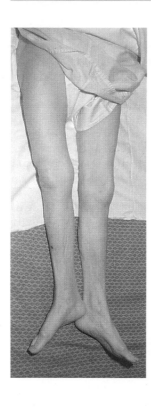

FIG. 8.3 The clinical appearance of displaced fracture of the neck of the right femur

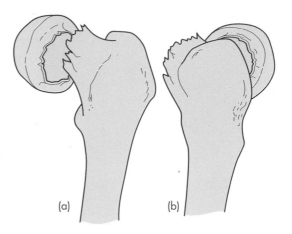

FIG. 8.4 Unimpacted fracture of the femoral neck: (a) anteposterior view; (b) lateral view

GRADE II

In Grade II injuries, the fracture is undisplaced on anteroposterior and lateral radiographs. Soft tissue may still be attached, providing some blood supply.

GRADE III

In Grade III injuries, the femur is adducted at the fracture site, but the head is separated from the neck. The patient is usually unable to stand or move the affected limb and complains of severe pain in the hip. On examination, the injured leg lies with the foot externally rotated. Despite point contact between the bones, soft-tissue disruption is severe. (Fig. 8.3.)

GRADE IV (Figs 8.4 and 8.5)

There is gross rotation of both fragments with complete loss of contact between the fractures in Grade IV injuries.

TREATMENT

The treatment of subcapital fractures is operative, unless the general condition of the patient does not permit surgery. The patient needs to be mobilized

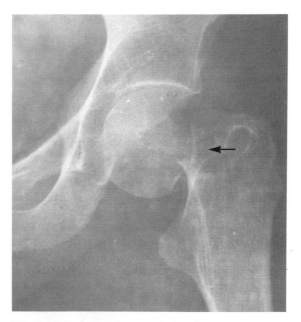

FIG. 8.5 Subcapital fracture (displaced)

as soon as possible. It has been shown that bedrest and conservative management leads to broncho-pneumonia, pressure sores, pulmonary embolus, urinary tract infection, muscle wasting, institutional dependence and death.

The impacted stable grade II fracture has a tendency to displace, but does not need reduction. Internal fixation is carried out using either multiple cannulated cross screws or compression screws and plates (Fig. 8.6).

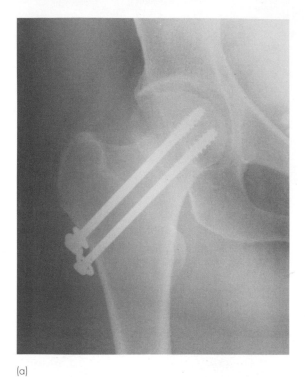

(a)

In grade II and III and in young people with a grade IV fracture every effort is made to reduce the fracture and fix it internally.

Grade IV patients, particularly if they are elderly, are best treated by excision of the fractured femoral head, replacing it with a hemiarthroplasty (Austin–Moore prosthesis) (Fig. 8.7). In fit elderly patients with grade IV fractures it is reasonable to proceed immediately to a total hip replacement in order to ensure long-term pain-free activity. Hemiarthroplasty tends to lead to residual shortening of the leg and erosive changes in the acetabulum with loosening of the component in the more active individual. However, it remains a very useful, quick and relatively complication-free procedure for the elderly patient.

Intertrochanteric fractures of the femur

Intertrochanteric fractures of the femur, like subcapital fractures, are very common injuries in

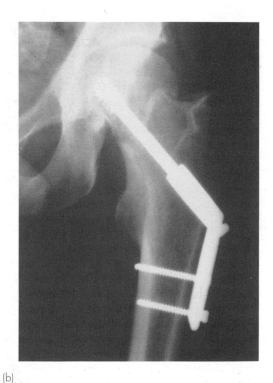

(b)

FIG. 8.6   (a) Cannulated screws inserted for a grade II undisplaced fracture, (b) compression screws and plate inserted after reduction of a grade II fracture

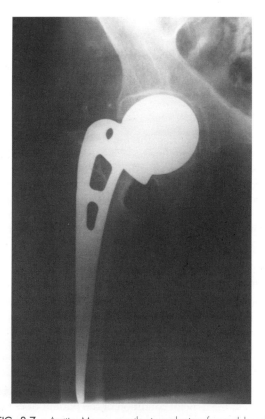

FIG. 8.7   Austin–Moore prosthesis replacing femoral head

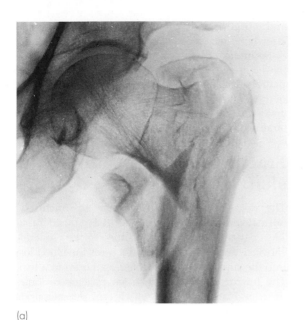

(a)

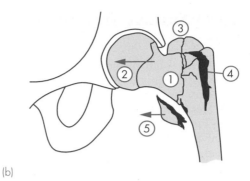

(b)

FIG. 8.8   (a) Intertrochanteric fracture of the upper end of the femur; (b) diagram of the intertrochanteric fracture showing the many fragments of the fracture

elderly people. At this level, however, they occur with equal frequency in men and women. They are often comminuted, and the lesser trochanter is frequently avulsed and pulled upwards by the iliopsoas muscle, which is inserted into it.

TREATMENT

Union of these fractures rarely presents a problem, so simple traction on the injured leg allows the fracture to unite in a reasonably satisfactory position. In contrast to fractures through the femoral neck, in which non-union is frequent, the problem in intertrochanteric fractures is malunion, producing coxa vara and external rotation deformity. However, the patient who sustains such an injury is almost always elderly, and the risks of immobility that this entails are considerable. These risks include pneumonia, pressure sores, urinary tract infection (possibly from an indwelling catheter) and pulmonary embolism. For this reason internal fixation using a compression screw and plate is to be preferred in virtually every patient, (Fig. 8.9) as the patient can be mobilized freely in bed immediately, and, if a secure hold on both main fragments has been obtained, ambulation may commence within a few days of operation.

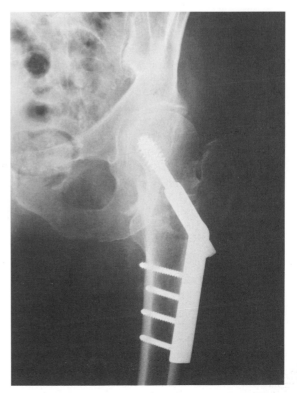

FIG. 8.9   Intertrochanteric fracture of the femoral neck treated by compression screw and plate

Subtrochanteric fractures of the femur

Fractures at the subtrochanteric level are really through the upper femoral shaft. They are comparatively uncommon unless the bone at this site is abnormal. Metastatic carcinomatous deposits are common in the upper end of the femur, leading to pathological fractures. The bone at this site may also be weakened through the changes of Paget's disease (see Chapter 17).

TREATMENT

The aim of treatment is to provide stability with a compression screw and plate or a modern reconstruction device. If the fracture is pathological the defect in the bone can be filled with bone cement. If a neoplastic deposit is present a primary source should be sought and usually a course of radiotherapy is administered.

Isolated fractures of the trochanter

Occasionally, the tip of the greater trochanter is cracked as a result of a direct blow, or avulsed by the pull of a muscle. Protecting the limb by avoiding weight-bearing for a few weeks until the reaction to the trauma has settled down is usually all that is required.

The lesser trochanter may also be avulsed by the pull of the psoas muscle. In itself this is of no importance, but sometimes it occurs because the bone at this level is weakened through pathological change, particularly a secondary neoplastic deposit. This possibility must therefore always be borne in mind, and if necessary a biopsy should be taken. In adolescents, avulsion of the lesser trochanter can occur, particularly during exercise. Treatment is bedrest, with the hip in flexion by supporting the thigh on a pillow.

FRACTURES OF THE SHAFT OF THE FEMUR

Fractures of the shaft of the femur are common severe injuries, which may occur at any level. Usually they are due to considerable direct violence, and are therefore often associated with injuries elsewhere, and frequently result from road accidents.

Secondary carcinomatous deposits are common in the femur, particularly in its upper shaft, so pathological fractures can occur. Oblique fractures of the femoral shaft also frequently occur in infants and young children due to indirect rotational strains on the bone.

Fractures of the femoral shaft in adults

The degree of trauma necessary to fracture a normal femoral shaft in an adult is considerable. The patient therefore is liable to be severely shocked, and even in closed fractures the blood loss into the surrounding tissues may amount to a litre. The fracture line may be transverse or comminuted, and displacement, which will depend upon the direction of the causative force, may be severe.

COMPLICATIONS

- The fat embolus syndrome is believed to be more common in fractures of the femoral shaft than in other bones.
- Because the bone is surrounded by muscle, injuries to the femoral vessels or sciatic nerve are not very common.
- Residual stiffness of the knee because of scarring in the quadriceps muscle anchoring it to bone at the level of the fracture may be a problem.
- Non-union of the bone sometimes occurs, especially in open fractures.

TREATMENT

Treatment may be conservative or operative, and is governed by the general condition of the patient, the level of the fracture and the presence of injuries elsewhere. The role of internal fixation in multiple injuries has already been discussed.

CONSERVATIVE TREATMENT

Temporary traction can be applied using adhesive strapping attached to weights slung over the end of the bed or attached to a Thomas' splint and may be either 'fixed' or 'balanced' (Fig. 8.10). In 'fixed' traction a pin is placed through the bone and cord attached to the pin. The cord is then attached directly to the end of the splint, and is secured to the splint by strapping. In 'balanced' traction

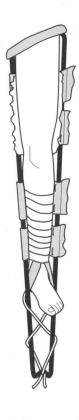

FIG. 8.10 Thomas' splint using 'fixed' skin traction

alike as more internal fixation of fractures is being carried out. The addition of a hinged attachment at the knee (Pearson) allows knee flexion to be practised without interrupting traction. In practice, fixed traction is employed mainly in the early stages, particularly if the patient has to be moved.

When the fracture is clinically and radiologically united, which in a normal adult takes about 12 weeks, traction is dismantled. The patient is nowadays more likely to be placed in a cast brace, hinged at the knee and made out of a light-weight cast material, at about 8 weeks after fracture. Weight-bearing is then encouraged.

OPERATIVE TREATMENT

The femoral shaft is one of the fracture sites most suitable for internal fixation, using a 'locked' intramedullary nail (Fig. 8.12). Malunion and non-union have been virtually abolished by such treatment and hospital stay can be reduced to a few days. The absolute indications for internal fixation of femoral shaft fractures include a flexed and abducted short proximal fragment, multiple injuries and pathological fractures. The nail is usually inserted over a guide wire that has been passed through the fracture from the proximal end of the bone under radiographic control. The fracture site is therefore left unopened, which preserves the blood supply to the bone fragments and reduces the risks of infection. Cross-screws proximally and distally 'lock' the nail and bone fragments together allowing early weight-bearing.

weights are not only attached directly to the limb, but are also used to suspend the splint allowing the patient to be nursed more easily and to avoid prolonged pressure from the ring of the splint on the groin (Fig. 8.11). These skills are unfortunately being rapidly lost by medical and nursing staff

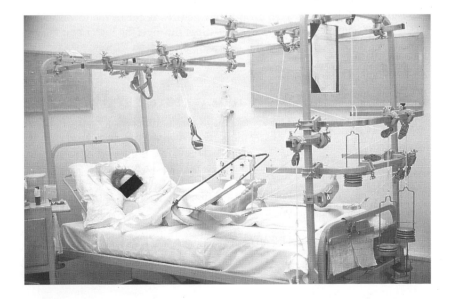

FIG. 8.11 Thomas' splint using balanced skeletal traction with a knee hinge

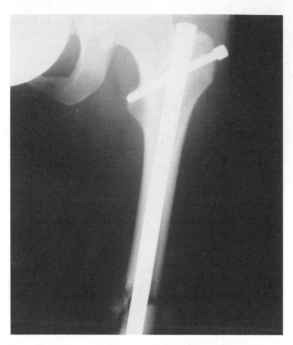

FIG. 8.12 Internal fixation of femoral shaft fracture using an intramedullary nail, with a proximal locking screw to prevent rotation

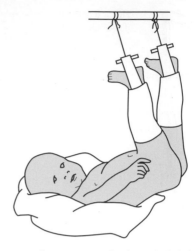

FIG. 8.13 'Gallows traction' for femoral shaft fractures in early childhood

In infants and children under 3 years of age 'gallows traction' provides a simple and effective method of management (Fig. 8.13), but may, rarely, result in a sciatic or lateral popliteal nerve palsy. This should be looked for regularly and the traction dismantled if it occurs.

Fractures of the femoral shaft in infancy and childhood

Unlike femoral shaft fractures in adults, those occurring in children are often due to indirect rotatory twisting strains, having oblique fracture lines. A baby's femur is also sometimes fractured during a difficult delivery, especially in breech presentations with extended legs. If there is overlap, the infant must be treated by suspension from a 'gallows' splint, which allows traction by the child's own weight, with the hips flexed to a right angle, which is normal in the infant. Uncorrected overlap leads to permanent shortening, whereas angular deformity becomes spontaneously corrected with growth.

TREATMENT

Rapid union is the rule and, as residual joint stiffness is very uncommon in children, 3–4 weeks of 'fixed' traction on a Thomas' splint is all that is required.

FRACTURES OF THE LOWER END OF THE FEMUR

Two groups of fractures occur in the lower end of the femur: fractures through the lower end (supracondylar fractures) and fractures of femoral condyles.

Supracondylar fractures

The lower end of the femur has no muscle attachments anteriorly, whereas the two heads of the gastrocnemius have their origin posteriorly. As a result, in supracondylar fractures there is a characteristic flexion deformity of the lower fragment. Because of this the medial or lateral popliteal nerves of the femoral vessels may also be injured (Fig. 8.14).

TREATMENT

Reduction can be maintained only if the flexing force of the muscles is relaxed by holding the joint

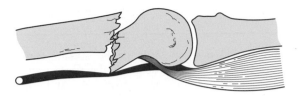

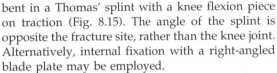

FIG. 8.14 Supracondylar femoral fracture, showing how the femoral artery may be damaged

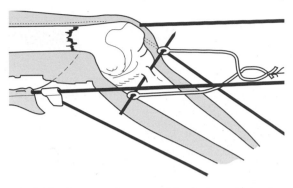

FIG. 8.15 Diagram of supracondylar fracture with traction

bent in a Thomas' splint with a knee flexion piece on traction (Fig. 8.15). The angle of the splint is opposite the fracture site, rather than the knee joint. Alternatively, internal fixation with a right-angled blade plate may be employed.

In children a fracture separation of the lower femoral epiphysis may occur, with displacement similar to that seen in supracondylar fractures in adults. As there is no risk of stiffness developing, reduction may be maintained by holding the knee flexed to a right angle in a plaster of Paris cast. Unstable reductions are held by percutaneously inserted wires.

Fractures of the femoral condyles

Fractures of the femoral condyles are comparatively uncommon. They may take two forms: either one condyle alone may be fractured, as a result of a sideways blow just above the knee, or both condyles may be fractured in a 'Y' pattern, due to a direct blow on the femoral condyles when the knee is fully flexed.

TREATMENT

Treatment is difficult because with an intra-articular injury early mobilization is desirable but maintenance of the reduction to prevent residual angular deformity and loss of joint surface contact is very important. Fortunately, union of the fracture rarely presents a problem.

The simplest way of treating these fractures is by manual compression, followed by traction for about 3–4 weeks. Perkins' split-bed traction is particularly helpful (Fig. 8.16). Full weight-bearing should not be permitted for several weeks. This method can be employed when there is severe comminution osteoporosis and no articular incongruity.

In the majority of patients, however, internal fixation with plates and screws is necessary to reduce the fractured articular surfaces accurately and allow early mobilization.

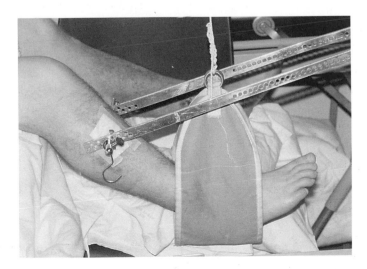

FIG. 8.16 A patient with Perkins' type traction

EXAMPLES

Hip fractures

A 70-year-old woman falls down on the street. She lives on her own in a ground floor flat and is independent in that she does her own shopping and is visited regularly by her relatives. In the Accident and Emergency Department she is found to be healthy apart from being a diabetic; her diabetes is controlled by diet alone. X-rays reveal a displaced intertrochanteric fracture of her right femoral neck.

Questions
- What is the treatment?
- What are the complications of this injury?
- What is the outcome?

Answers
- The patient needs admission to hospital for closed reduction and internal fixation of her fracture. This should be done the next day, on the trauma list.
- Wound infection, deep vein thrombosis (DVT) and pulmonary embolus are all risks that affect patients with these fractures. Indeed there is an overall 12 per cent mortality associated with femoral neck fractures within the first 3 months.
- After the fracture has been reduced and stabilized, it is important that the patient is mobilized as quickly as possible, that is 1–2 days after surgery, and that if at all possible she is returned to her own environment relatively quickly.
- This will need the help of the nursing staff, physiotherapists, occupational therapists, social workers, orthopaedic geriatricians and the patient's own general practitioner.
- Fractured neck of femurs are common and the fracture should be treated as only one part of the rehabilitation process, which is directed at getting the patient back into the community.

Femoral fractures

A 20-year-old man is involved in a road traffic accident.

His only injury is a displaced fracture of the midshaft of his left femur.

Questions
- What is the treatment?
- What complications can occur?

Answers
- Admission to hospital and the fracture is stabilized on either traction or a splint.
- As soon as possible the patient is taken to theatre and under image intensification the fracture is reduced and stabilized by means of an interlocking intramedullary nail.
- The complications that occur are infection, malunion, non-union, joint stiffness and possible fat embolus syndrome. However, most of these complications can be avoided by early management of the fracture which includes stabilization of the fracture and early mobilization of the patient.

9 LOWER LIMB – KNEE INJURIES

The knee is the largest joint in the body and, because the femur and tibia are also the longest bones, it is subjected to very powerful forces in all directions. During active flexion, forces many times the body weight are transmitted by the surrounding tendons, muscles and ligaments in addition to the forces transmitted by the bones themselves. Anatomically, the knee is classified as a 'hinge joint', but in fact the upper end of the tibia consists of two very shallow saucer-like depressions, and the femoral condyles are elliptical in shape so that on flexion the femur rolls back across the tibia. On extension the knee also tightens its ligaments by internal rotation of the tibia. This property is important from the functional aspect, as, when standing with the knees straight, it becomes possible to relax the thigh musculature. Any loss of full extension thus imposes a strain upon the patient when standing.

Of the muscles that assist in providing stability, the quadriceps is the most important because active extension is essential for standing and walking. Therefore, after any significant knee injury active quadriceps exercises must be insti-

tuted. A sizeable effusion may also inhibit movement and should be aspirated to reduce tension with the joint capsule. Aspiration also provides a useful guide to the nature and severity of the injury. If the fluid is clear yellow, this indicates that there has been no actual tearing of the joint lining at the time of injury, whereas if it is blood-stained this can only be the result of an intracapsular injury or a fracture involving the articular surfaces. In particular, rupture of cruciate ligaments should be considered and anteroposterior stability tested. Fat globules in the aspirate indicate an articular fracture.

Temporary splintage by means of a well padded bandage (Robert Jones) (Fig. 9.1) or a canvas splint or plaster cylinder, should only be carried out until facilities are available to obtain a definitive diagnosis by means of arthrogram, Magnetic Resonance Imagery (MRI) or arthroscopy. A plaster of Paris cylinder may be useful once ligamentous injury has been diagnosed (Fig. 9.2). However, instability should always be assessed by an experienced surgeon in order to select those patients requiring operative stabilization.

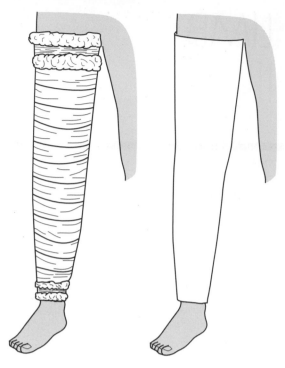

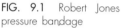

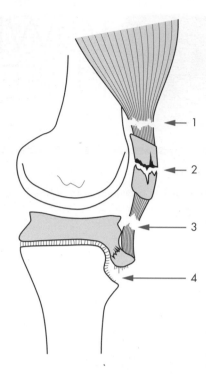

FIG. 9.1 Robert Jones pressure bandage

FIG. 9.2 Plaster of Paris cylinder

FIG. 9.3 Injuries to the extensor apparatus: (1) rupture of quadriceps insertion; (2) fracture of the patella; (3) rupture of the ligamentum patellae; (4) avulsion of the tibial tubercle

INJURIES TO THE EXTENSOR APPARATUS

With the exception of injuries to the patella due to direct blows, the extensor apparatus is liable to damage when the knee is forcefully flexed at a moment when the quadriceps muscle is actively contracting. The injuries occur in five ways, to some extent depending upon the age of the patient. (Fig. 9.3.)

Rupture of the quadriceps insertion

Rupture of the quadriceps insertion usually occurs in middle-aged individuals, in whom the muscles are beginning to lose some of their elasticity. Clinically, there is a sudden pain above the patella and the patient is unable actively to extend the knee. At first, a gap may be felt above the patella, but this soon becomes filled by haematoma.

TREATMENT

The correct treatment is to reattach the muscle to its tendon by surgical repair. This is not necessary if there is incomplete division and the patient can actively extend their leg. A plaster cylinder is applied for 4 weeks, after which it is removed and early mobilization encouraged.

Fractures of the patella

Fractures of the patella take two forms. If there has been a direct blow, the patella breaks into several pieces, but, because the quadriceps expansion remains intact, separation of the fragments is uncommon. This type is known as a *stellate* fracture, and may occur at any age. Radiologically this should not be confused with a bipartite patella, in which the bone has developed from the two centres of ossification.

In the second type, the patella is fractured transversely by indirect violence and is cracked across the femoral condyles by a sudden contracture of the quadriceps muscle. In most *transverse* fractures,

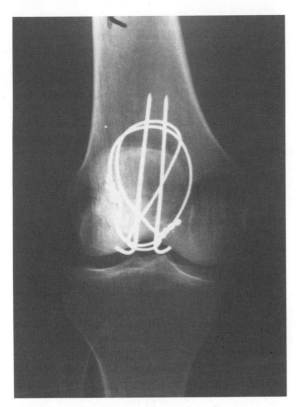

FIG. 9.4   Internal fixation of fractured patella

the quadriceps expansion is also torn on either side, with consequent wide separation of the fragments.

TREATMENT

In some stellate fractures, when the articular surface is still congruent, conservative management is possible with immobilization in a plaster cylinder for 4–6 weeks. Aspiration of the haemarthrosis may be performed under sterile conditions for comfort. In severely comminuted fractures, however, the patella should be excised, the fragments of bone being dissected from the aponeurosis, interfering as little as possible with the quadriceps mechanism so that mobilization of the knee may be commenced 2 or 3 weeks after operation.

In transverse fractures, it may be possible to repair the patella by a combination of longitudinal and circumferential wires, which form a 'tension band' mechanism. The principle of a 'tension band' is that flexion of the knee increases the tension in the wires, thereby compressing the bone fragments together and encouraging union (Fig. 9.4). The quadriceps expansion must be repaired at the same time. If, however, there is any comminution at the fracture line, patellectomy should be carried out, with careful repair of the quadriceps mechanism. This is because any significant irregularity of the articular surface will inevitably lead to later osteoarthritis. Transverse fractures require about 6 weeks' postoperative splintage in a plaster of Paris cylinder during which ambulation should be encouraged.

Rupture of the ligamentum patellae

Like rupture of the quadriceps insertion, rupture of the ligamentum patellae usually occurs in middle-aged individuals. There is tenderness and a palpable gap below the patella, with loss of active extension. Occasionally, in younger individuals, a small fragment of the lower pole of the patella is also avulsed.

TREATMENT

Treatment is surgical, by repair of the ligament. If the lower pole of the patella has been avulsed, this is excised and the tendon sutured to the main portion, which is drilled so that the sutures may be firmly attached. Reinforcement of the repair with a wire suture around the patella is usually carried out. Postoperatively, 6 weeks' splintage is required.

Avulsion of the tibial tubercle

Avulsion of the tibial tubercle is an uncommon injury of late childhood, in which the tongue-like extension of the upper tibial epiphysis to which the ligamentum patellae is attached becomes pulled upwards. Significant displacement is rare.

Dislocation of the patella

The patella may be displaced laterally to differing degrees. An incomplete dislocation, called a subluxation, most commonly reduces itself as the knee is extended. Occasionally, however, assistance is required to reduce a dislocation.

This is an injury that may result from a direct blow from the medial side but is usually caused by a sudden contraction of the quadriceps mechanism

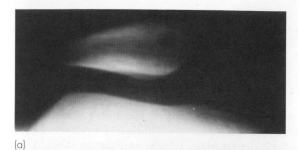

(a)

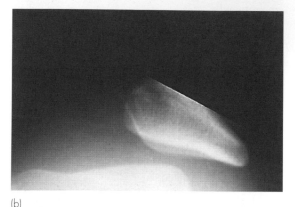

(b)

FIG. 9.5 (a) The patella in normal position; (b) lateral dislocation of the patella

with the knee in valgus and slightly flexed position. Tibial external rotation may also play a part. Congenital anomalies such as a small, high patella, general ligamentous laxity (hypermobility syndrome), a deficient lateral femoral condyle and genuvalgum may predispose a patient to such dislocation. The condition is commoner in young girls. Repeated incidents of the knee 'giving way', with momentary 'locking' of the joint stretches the medial joint capsule and patellar retinacular ligaments. Pain and tenderness is therefore mainly on the medial aspect of the patella. If the patella is pushed laterally as the knee is gently flexed, the patient becomes typically apprehensive, as they feel dislocation is liable to be precipitated. This is called a positive 'patellar apprehension test'. However, the most important consequence of a dislocation is the injury to the vastus medialis muscle, which then fails to contract and compounds the instability.

TREATMENT

After a first episode, a trial of conservative treatment is usually carried out, which involves splinting in extension for 3 weeks. An intensive course of exercises is then prescribed to strengthen the vastus medialis muscle, with most effort concentrated on lifting the leg with the foot externally rotated. This selectively builds up the vastus medialis muscle.

When recurrent dislocation of the patella occurs, operation is indicated. An arthroscopic lateral release of the lateral patellar retinacular ligaments may be tried in the first instance. However, in the presence of severe malalignment or deformity, realignment of the extensor apparatus may be necessary, including transposition of the tibial tubercle to a more medial and distal position.

INJURIES TO BONE AND ARTICULAR SURFACE

Femoral and tibial condylar fractures

Compression and angulatory strains on the knee can result in injuries to the bones. Supracondylar and condylar fractures of the femur have already been discussed (Chapter 8). Fracture of a single condyle is often due to a direct blow to one or other side of the knee. This is known as a 'bumper fracture'. The condyle as a whole may be split, crushed or have a central portion driven downwards with meniscus becoming wedged between the fragments.

TREATMENT

The same principles of management apply in the tibia as in the femur. Undisplaced fractures in the elderly may be treated conservatively. However, in a younger patient in whom articular irregularities and malalignment occur, open reduction and internal fixation of the fractures must be carried out. In order to support early mobilization and weight-bearing, 'buttress plating' with multiple cross-screws may be necessary. If both condyles are involved plating must be performed medially and laterally. When bone stock is deficient, bone grafting is carried out.

Osteochondral fracture

Various compression forces can damage the articular surface of any part of the joint. Splitting and damage to the articular cartilage can coexist with damage to the underlying subchondral bone. This is best seen on MRI images, which show 'bruising' or internal fracturing of the cancellous bone beneath the articular surface. The relationship between pain and such findings is still poorly understood. Treatment is conservative and consists of partial weight-bearing on crutches for several weeks. Articular damage, however, does not heal other than by weak fibrocartilage formation.

Osteochondritis dissecans

Osteochondritis dissecans (see Chapter 12) is one variant of osteochondral fracture that is common in young men and involves the gradual separation of a piece of articular cartilage and a small amount of cancellous bone from the weight-bearing portion of the femoral condyle. Treatment consists of attempting to fix the fragment back using screws or pins after first abrading the base of the defect. This is carried out in order to encourage increased blood supply to the area.

Articular degeneration

The commonest presentation of a knee problem in the middle-aged and elderly patient today is that of severe articular degeneration. This can either be primary osteoarthritis or osteoarthritis secondary to acute or chronic trauma. In this situation arthroscopic examination can determine the extent and severity of the changes. The outer-bridge classification is useful in which

- Grade 1 changes mean softening of the articular cartilage;
- Grade 2 means fibrillation appearing as fronds elevated from the surface;
- Grade 3 means partial thickness cartilage loss and fissuring;
- Grade 4 means exposed bone.

Remarkably, patient symptoms do not always correlate with the degree of damage. Indeed, the relationship between articular damage, patients' symptoms and bone changes remains poorly understood.

In inflammatory arthritis, a gradual 'secondary' atrophy of the articular surfaces and menisci occurs, although traumatic damage to articular surfaces can also occur simultaneously.

Arthroscopic lavage, removal of loose bodies and cartilage shaving can temporarily reduce the amount of inflammation within a joint for up to 6

months. More aggressive attempts to remove osteophytes and carry out extensive drilling procedures can make patients worse. In certain situations, however, localized drilling procedures can remove obstacles to motion, reduce pain and encourage healing of small articular defects.

LIGAMENTOUS INJURIES

Ligamentous injuries tend to occur in younger adults with good bone density. The two main types of ligament tear are the collateral ligament tear and the cruciate ligament tear. However, they often occur in combination.

Collateral ligament injury

The medial and lateral collateral ligaments provide mainly mediolateral stability and testing for injury and instability involves valgus and varus stressing, respectively. However, in extension the collateral ligaments tighten and this provides the basis for the 'Lachman test' in which an 'anterior drawer test' manoeuvre tests for stability of the knee in extension. This is usually only important in the presence of a coexisting anterior cruciate ligament tear.

- Grade 1 tear is only a sprain, which can have strapping applied and then be mobilized almost immediately.
- Grade 2 is a more severe sprain for which immobilization is recommended for 3 weeks in a slightly flexed cylinder cast.
- Grade 3 implies significant disruption and opening of the joint on stressing but which can still be managed conservatively because of some residual stability in extension. Immobilization may be for up to 6 weeks.
- Grade 4 implies significant opening of the joint in both extension and flexion, implying that no fibres of the ligament remain intact. Examination under anaesthesia can be required to assess such severe injuries. Operative repair and immobilization for up to 2 months is required. Often the menisci are torn from the ligament and require reattachment if possible. Cast braces can also be used to allow early protected knee flexion.

Occasionally a few fibres of the medial ligament are torn from its femoral attachment. These may raise a small flap of periosteum such that some calcification may occur, and be visible radiologically adjacent to, but distinct from, the upper part of the adductor tubercle. This condition, known as 'Pellegrini–Stieda syndrome', may cause persistent pain at the upper attachment of the medial ligament, made worse by lateral rotation or attempted full extension. Treatment consists of immobilization. If pain persists, a local injection of hydrocortisone suspension may be employed.

Cruciate ligament injury

Injuries to the cruciate ligaments are usually caused by excessive force in the anteroposterior plane. Force thrusting the tibia anteriorly in flexion will rupture the anterior cruciate ligament. Posterior force applied to the tibia, often in hyperextension, may rupture the posterior cruciate. However, the anterior cruciate ligament is also responsible for direction and some rotational movement of the tibia on the femur, and, therefore, so-called anterolateral tibial rotation may injure the anterior cruciate.

Grading of injury is important and is best carried out by anterior drawer testing with the knee flexed. Once again this is best performed under anaesthesia.

- Grade 1 means that the tibia moves forward no more than 5 mm more than the intact side;
- Grade 2 is up to 10 mm of difference;
- Grade 3 is up to 15 mm of difference;
- Grade 4 greater than 15 mm of difference.

Grade 1 and 2 are most likely to be managed with intensive physiotherapy and possibly bracing alone. Grade 3 and 4 are most likely to require reconstruction. Such decisions are often based upon patient requirements and symptoms rather than the absolute grade of injury. For example, a building worker with a Grade 2 instability in extension would not require reconstructive surgery. The so-called 'pivot shift testing' in which a clunking sensation is obvious during extension of the knee with a valgus stress applied under anaesthesia can be used to identify rotational instability.

Arthroscopic examination is essential not only to grade the instability but also to identify the common, associated injuries of meniscal tear and articular damage. Initial treatment is, however, usually along conservative lines and isolated ruptures are easily missed. An effusion is aspirated and the presence of blood is highly suggestive of a cruciate rupture. Quadriceps exercises are instituted. Some residual anteroposterior laxity in the joint will often persist, but good quadriceps muscles can, in the majority of individuals, compensate for this.

Immediate direct repair of the cruciate ligaments themselves has been shown to be unrewarding. Late repair using artificial fibres, however, has been advocated in the past but has more recently been shown to be useful only in older age groups of patients with lower demands. The two principal methods of reconstruction in use today involve precise drilling of tunnels in the bones to locate the origin and insertion of the ligaments and the use of patellar tendon attached to bone or multiple hamstring tendons to recreate the ligament. Various methods are then used to hold the grafts in the tunnels or surrounding soft tissues. Results are now good as the need for very strong grafts and prolonged protection during the 12 month healing phase has been realized.

Combined ligamentous and bony injuries

In cases in which combinations of rotation, compression and angulation occur, ligaments, capsule (including collateral ligaments) and bone may be injured simultaneously. Treatment consists of bony and ligamentous repair in combination. Late reconstruction of cruciate ligaments may be necessary. Avulsion of the tibial spine indicates a cruciate ligament injury and therefore open reduction and screw fixation should be carried out.

Dislocation of the knee

Dislocation of the knee is a very severe injury, which is fortunately rare, resulting from a violent shearing force applied to the knee. Because the popliteal vessels are anchored by deep fascia, these are often damaged, as are the main nerve trunks. Reduction by manipulation usually succeeds but surgical intervention will probably be required to stabilize the knee.

MENISCAL INJURY

Rotational and compressive forces applied to the knee are liable to cause injury to the menisci. The latter are the remains of the complete cartilaginous discs that in fetal life separate the articular surfaces of the femur and tibia. The medial meniscus is attached to the medial collateral ligament, so that it does not move with the femoral condyle. On the lateral side, the meniscus has no attachment to the lateral ligament and it also has a hiatus for the popliteus muscle posteriorly. Both menisci are, however, vulnerable to injury.

Types of tear

Throughout childhood, blood vessels in the middle of the menisci retreat outwards towards the capsule, leaving a horizontal plane of cleavage that may be vulnerable to injury. Similarly, a tear at the circumference may lead to an unstable 'bucket handle segment' becoming jammed in the joint leading to a 'locked knee'. The true 'locked knee' in this situation usually has only a 10–20° block to full extension. A radial split may also give rise to mechanical symptoms. Splits that extend out to the capsule are often painful and also give rise to cysts in which gelatinous debris collects outside the knee capsule causing a painful swelling (Fig. 9.6).

Effusion, joint-line tenderness and pain on compressing the appropriate compartment are the usual positive physical signs. Often, if the knee is flexed and then slowly extended while at the same time it is abducted and externally rotated, a characteristic 'click' may be heard or felt as the torn portion momentarily catches between the femoral and tibial condyles. This is known as McMurray's sign.

In middle age, the menisci become brittle and widespread breakdown can occur. In the elderly, the menisci become soft and degenerate. All these types of tear give rise to combinations of pain, swelling, effusion and mechanical symptoms, including locking and giving way. They also are all capable of causing damage to the adjacent weight-bearing articular surfaces.

Diagnosis may be confirmed by arthrography (Fig. 9.7) or preferably by an MRI scan. More commonly, when the diagnosis is less in doubt, arthroscopic examination provides the simultaneous opportunity to identify and treat the lesion precisely.

Treatment of meniscal injury

Treatment is usually that of arthroscopic resection. In younger patients attempts are usually made to preserve a sizeable 'remnant' in order to assist

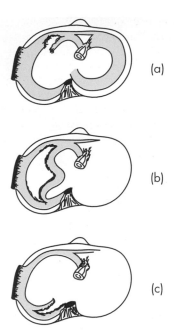

FIG. 9.6 Tears of the medial meniscus: (a) anterior horn tear; (b) 'bucket handle' central tear; (c) posterior horn tear

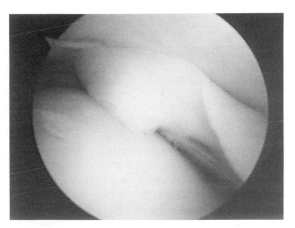

FIG. 9.7 Torn medial meniscus seen through the arthroscope

stability and spread loads over the joint surface. Certain types of tear are nowadays repaired using absorbable intra-articular sutures. In middle age, however, the remnants are more likely to continue breaking up and a more radical resection is required. Extracapsular cysts are decompressed

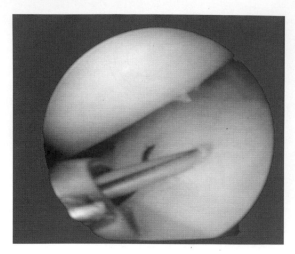

FIG. 9.8   Arthroscopic powered meniscal debridement

arthroscopically and strapping is applied until fibrosis seals the defect.

Meniscal degeneration

Senile meniscal degeneration may be accompanied by crystal formation within the substance of the meniscus in a condition called 'chondrocalcinosis'. As the meniscus breaks up, large quantities of inflammatory material are released into the joint, causing pain, swelling and articular damage. Radical meniscal resection and general debridement is then required (Fig. 9.8).

SYNOVIAL PATHOLOGY

Local synovial lesions

Thickened fibrotic synovial folds (plicae/shelves), which can be congenital in origin but may also be acquired by acute or chronic trauma, can cause severe pain, swelling and mechanical symptoms within the anterior compartment of the knee. In severe cases, patellofemoral joint impingement and abrasion of articular surfaces may occur. Treatment is by localized arthroscopic synovial resection.

Generalized synovitis

In rheumatoid, seronegative and psoariatic chronic synovitis that has not responded to medical treatment total arthroscopic synovectomy can provide relief from severe inflammation for up to about 5 years. Prevention of articular degeneration after with surgery is much more difficult to prove, as often significant articular damage has occurred long before surgery.

EXAMPLES

Knee injuries

A 70-year-old woman sustains an injury to her left knee when she falls onto the pavement. When seen in the Accident and Emergency Department she is found to have a supracondylar fracture of her left femur, which is T-shaped and hence involves the joint surface.

Questions
- What is the treatment?
- What is the outcome?

Answers
- These fractures are real problems in management, that is, the elderly woman may well have osteoporotic bone. This makes it difficult to fix the bones internally. However, the more conservative means of traction and mobilization in traction mean the patient needs to be in hospital for some time, and this affects her ability to return to her own environment.
- If possible, open reduction and internal fixation is advocated.
- Alternatively, replacement arthroplasty may be more appropriate.
- The outcome is dependent on getting good fixation and stabilization of the fracture as soon as possible. Thirty per cent of elderly patients with this type of fracture end up with complications of treatment, which may result in amputation and death.

A 25-year-old footballer injured his right knee while playing.

He is seen immediately in the Accident and Emergency Department with a swollen right knee that is painful and cannot be moved. It is unstable to examination.

Questions
- What is the diagnosis?
- What is the management?

Answers
- If the knee is unstable, especially in either a medial or lateral direction, it suggests that the main ligaments of the knee joint have been ruptured.
- If the knee is unstable in an anterior or posterior direction it suggests that the cruciate ligaments may have been ruptured.
- If the effusion in the knee joint is bloodstained it suggests that there has been soft tissue or bony damage.
- Therefore the possible diagnosis of this patient's injured knee are: torn medial or lateral ligament; torn anterior or posterior cruciate ligament; torn or detached menisci; intra-articular fracture; or any combination of these.
- Hence it is important to be able to examine the knee carefully; this is best carried out under an anaesthetic. The joint can be examined by means of an arthroscope, the blood washed out and the true injury assessed, after which the damaged structures can be repaired.

10 LOWER LIMB – INJURIES OF THE TIBIA AND FIBULA

Fractures of the tibia and fibula may result from direct or indirect violence. Because the tibia has a large subcutaneous surface, it is one of the bones in which open fractures readily occur. In addition, the tibial shaft, particularly in its lower half, has a blood supply that is vulnerable to injury. The configuration of the fracture also frequently renders the fragments quite unstable. Combinations of circumstances therefore occur that predispose to delayed union, malunion and non-union.

FRACTURES OF TIBIA AND FIBULA (Fig. 10.1)

Direct blows tend to cause transverse fractures whereas rotational forces cause spiral fractures of the tibia and fibula. Longitudinal compression and bending forces cause butterfly fragments and comminution to occur. However, the bony injury itself is only important in terms of the potential stability of the fracture. A more significant consequence of the trauma is the degree of soft-tissue damage, which, except in severely compound fractures, usually remains unseen beneath the skin.

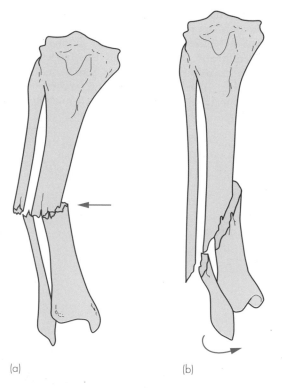

(a)   (b)

FIG. 10.1   Fracture of the midshaft tibia and fibula: (a) due to direct violence; (b) due to indirect violence

So-called high-energy fractures, for example a motor cycle injury, are most at risk in this respect.

The human body, however, does have the callus formation mechanism to attempt to heal even the most comminuted of fractures, and indeed a significant proportion of these will heal perfectly well with careful conservative management involving careful traction or prolonged immobilization. However, in the days before internal fixation non-union rates of over 10 per cent were not uncommon and many patients spent up to 8 or 9 months in plaster. Also, prolonged hospitalization, continuing instability leading to non-union, malunion and the frequent need for delayed bone-grafting of the fracture have led to a large proportion of closed tibial fractures being internally fixed. The problem is the difficulty in identifying those fractures that may show a delay in healing. The best option, therefore, is to stabilize all those fractures that are likely to show a delay in union. Severely comminuted and displaced fractures, persistently unstable fractures, high-energy injuries and of course open fractures are those most at risk.

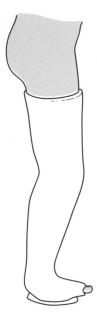

FIG. 10.2   Above-knee walking plaster of Paris cast

Closed fractures – a treatment dilemma?

A significant percentage of closed tibial fractures can be managed conservatively. No one should state that he or she always fixed a certain percentage of fractures. The fact is that different series of fractures may vary widely in the proportions of open, high-energy and unstable fractures contained within the series. Another important consideration is the availability of skill and equipment. Some experts can manage external traction easily if the devices are applied well and the pins maintained by experienced nurses. Plating can do well if soft-tissue damage is minimized at the time of surgery. Conservative management is still an option, but some centres have now begun to lose the skills of traction and serial plastering. There is a consensus today, however, that closed, locked intramedullary nailing is the treatment of choice for the majority of displaced tibia fractures, provided that adequate operative facilities and experience are available.

Conservative management

After an initial closed reduction, a long-leg backslab (or if swelling is minimal a split-to-skin long-leg plaster of Paris) is applied and the leg carefully elevated. The patient should be kept in hospital as large increases in swelling often occur up to 48 hours after the fracture or manipulation and this can lead to muscle death and vessel, nerve and skin problems if the cast is not capable of expansion to accommodate the swelling. Inflexible modern cast materials are particularly bad in this respect. It is important to note that increased pain after treatment of a fracture should not be ignored or treated with increased analgesia.

Immobilization ought to reduce discomfort and therefore increased pain means that the compartment syndrome should always be considered and senior orthopaedic staff consulted immediately.

About 48 hours after manipulation, when pain and swelling have subsided, an above-knee (long-leg) plaster cast can be applied (Fig. 10.2). This extends from just below the groin to the base of the toes. The foot should be held at right angles to the tibia in both planes, and the knee is fixed in a few degrees of flexion to prevent rotatory movements at the fracture site. Minor degrees of residual angulation may be corrected by wedging the plaster at the fracture site (Fig. 10.3). For the first 10–14 days after injury, the leg should be kept elevated, after which, depending on the stability of the fracture in the plaster cast, either a walking heel may be added to the plaster, and the patient can start bearing weight on the leg, or they can be got up and can become ambulant on crutches

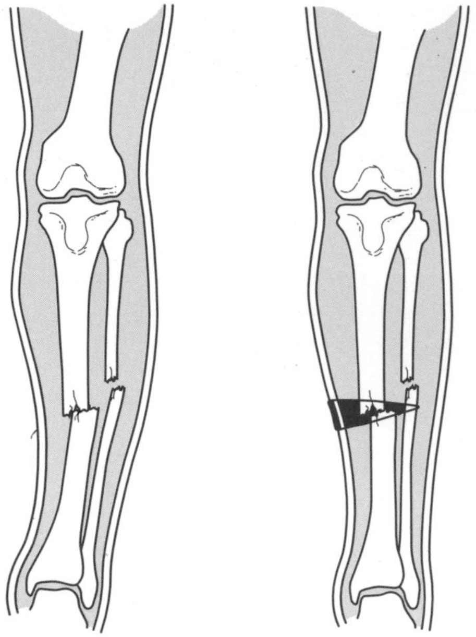

FIG. 10.3 Wedging a plaster cast to correct residual angulation deformity

without bearing weight on the leg. At 8 weeks the above-knee plaster can be reduced to a patellar tendon-bearing (PTB) plaster. In adults, though, immobilization can rarely be discontinued under 12 weeks from the time of injury.

It needs to be noted that, when modern fixation is not available and there is an unstable open fracture or gross comminution, stable reduction or maintenance of length may not be possible using plaster of Paris alone. In these cases about 4 weeks of traction with a pin through the calcaneum or the lower tibia, with the patient's leg on a Braun's frame, may be employed until the risk of redisplacement has passed. Once again, however, as with all conservative management, good results are dependent upon early callus formation. It has been well documented that late instability can cause non-union, and therefore such management should only be used as a last resort.

Fracture fixation

Any attempt to reduce a fracture openly will inevitably lead to further damage to the surrounding soft tissues and the potential for revascularization of the area. This is particularly important in the subcutaneous portion of the tibial diaphysis.

Modern surgical methods of fracture reduction and fixation increasingly try to avoid opening the fracture site. This can be accomplished using either an external fixator or an intramedullary nail; however, it is not possible with plating methods.

Open reduction is indicated when it is not possible to obtain a good position by closed means, if, for example, soft tissues or bony fragments are blocking reduction. It is also absolutely indicated in the presence of an open fracture and in patients with multiple injuries in order to help save life (see Chapter 4) and to make the overall management of the patient easier.

External fixation (Fig. 10.4)

External fixation consists of threaded pins that are attached to a bar and are inserted into the bone away from the fracture site. The external fixation

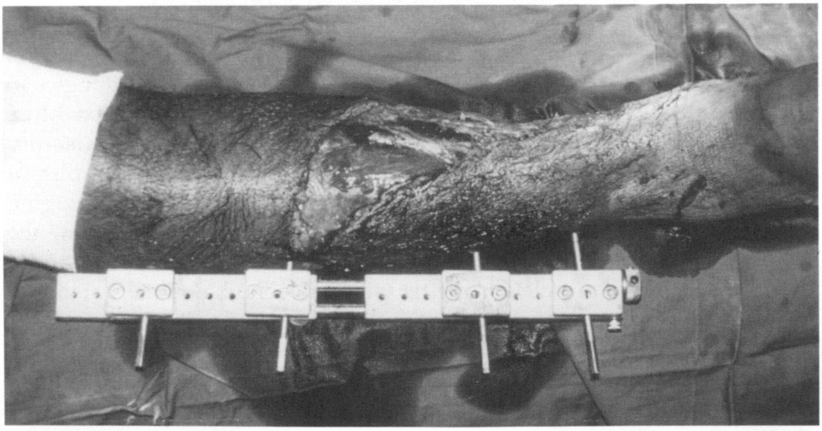

FIG. 10.4 External fixation of an open fracture

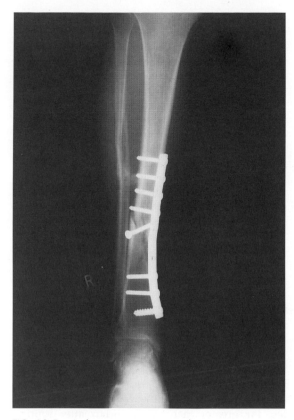

FIG. 10.5 A dynamic compression plate

system is left in place for 6 weeks or more, until there is evidence of callus formation and skin cover has been achieved. The external fixation is then removed and a cast brace applied until the fracture unites. In grade II or grade III open-type fractures it is often necessary to encourage union by means of a cancellous bone graft.

The advantage of this system is that minimal metal is placed near the wound to act as a foreign body. The disadvantages of the system include the need for meticulous pin care and the need for subsequent plaster immobilization.

Plate fixation (Fig. 10.5)

Plate fixation involves exposing the periosteum of the bone and fixing a rigid plate to the bone, compressing the fragments together. With the use of so-called dynamic compression plating, the bone is held so rigidly that external callus does not appear. Hence the fracture unites by primary union rather than by callus formation. This may

take 12 months to occur and therefore the plate should not be removed before that time unless loosening or infection occurs. However, after the fracture has united, bone resorption commences under the plate and therefore the plate needs to be removed 18–24 months after insertion, to allow the bone to regain its structural strength.

The advantages of the system include rigid fixation and early weight-bearing. The disadvantages include the need to open the fracture site, the need for primary bone healing and the need for a second operation to remove the plate.

Intramedullary nail fixation

The treatment of choice today for unstable fractures is intramedullary nailing. The fracture is reduced by applying longitudinal traction under radiographic image intensification control and then a guide wire is passed across the fracture. Reaming of the bone is less frequently used today and a fairly rigid unreamed nail is passed down the bone over the guide wire. The ends of the nail are 'locked' to the bone using 'cross-screws', which give good control of bony length and rotational stability.

The advantages of the system include the avoidance of opening the fracture, good stability, early weight-bearing and improved formation of callus. Despite less 'stress-shielding' of the bone, one disadvantage is that in long bones, the nails should be removed about 18 months after insertion.

A whole new family of different types of nail are now being introduced that can cope with many difficult fracture situations, including 'reconstruction' nails for use in tumour work and in areas such as the supracondylar regions adjacent to knee prostheses.

Open fractures

In the presence of open fractures, the most essential part of the surgical management is the immediate wound toilet. **Very aggressive debridement of dead, damaged and heavily contaminated tissues, including bone, must be carried out within 6 hours**.

Dead muscle is dark and does not contract on pinch testing or electrical stimulation. In severe cases of contamination, multiple debridements and reinspection of tissues must be carried out. Failure to do so in the presence of a metallic implant is risking early infection, including gas gangrene, and late infection, including osteomyelitis. Reduction and immobilization come as a definite secondary consideration. Also, copious lavage and antibiotic cover are essential. **No open wound should be closed completely in any primary closure situation, particularly in the lower limb**.

Soft-tissue cover for the more severe cases of tissue loss is provided in close cooperation with plastic surgical colleagues who have a wide variety of local rotational myocutaneous and free flap techniques at their disposal. Planning for this is carried out during the first inspections and performed as soon as the wound is clean and the bone stabilized. Adequate soft-tissue cover has now been shown to improve the rates of union dramatically and to reduce the risk of infection in these severe fractures.

Whatever method of treatment has been employed, after the fracture has united and external splintage has been discarded, a period of rehabilitation is usually required to overcome residual stiffness and swelling, and also to regain the patient's confidence and restore full function to the limb.

Fractures of the tibia and fibula in childhood

As the inferior tibiofibular joint is rather more mobile in childhood, spiral fractures of the tibia alone are common. Significant displacement is rare and rapid union is the rule. Greenstick fractures of the lower tibial shaft are also common. Treatment in most cases merely consists of an above-knee walking plaster cast, worn for 3 or 4 weeks. However, care must be taken in older children to align the ankle joint properly.

ISOLATED FRACTURES

Fractures of the tibia alone

Fractures of the tibia alone are invariably due to direct violence from a blow, such as a kick in football. Displacement is rarely significant, as the fibula will maintain position. Treatment consists of an above-knee walking plaster cast, later converted to a patella tendon-bearing cast.

Fractures of the fibula alone

If the outer side of a calf is subjected to a severe blow, the fibula may be cracked. The fracture is of no significance, provided it is not a high fibular fracture and the common peroneal nerve is not damaged, because the fibular shaft takes no part in weight-bearing, and supportive treatment by strapping or a walking plaster of Paris from the toes to the knee alone is all that is required. Occasionally the lower fibular shaft may be the site of a 'stress' fracture after repetitive strains, as may occur in occupations such as professional ballet dancing.

If after an injury a fracture of the fibular shaft is discovered, the possibility that this is associated with a diastasis of the inferior tibiofibular joint should be borne in mind and the ankle region should also be carefully examined.

SOFT-TISSUE PROBLEMS IN THE LEG

Compartment syndrome

In all severe soft-tissue fractures of the leg and any fracture involving the tibia, particularly closed fractures, whatever the treatment, the risk of a compartment syndrome is very real. Pain in the leg, far greater than should occur after routine reduction and immobilization of a fracture, is not relieved by opening dressings on an internally fixed fracture or releasing the bandages on a temporary long-leg back-slab.

Poor capillary return and neurological disturbance, such as paraesthesia, are often relieved by releasing a cast or bandaging. However, in compartment syndrome, pain continues to increase because muscle swelling has increased pressure within one or more of four deep fascial spaces within the calf. The critical limit is related to diastolic and local venous pressure and therefore blood can get in but not out of the compartment (Fig. 10.6). The only way to save the muscle from infarction is an emergency multicompartment fasciotomy.

In addition, compartment syndrome can be exercise induced and treatment in severe cases also consists of a fascial release. As with acute post-traumatic cases, pressure monitoring using cannulae inserted into the spaces can provide the diagnosis.

Tendonitis and periostitis

Traction injuries to muscles and tendons, including their origins, insertions and periosteal attachments are common. The differential diagnosis

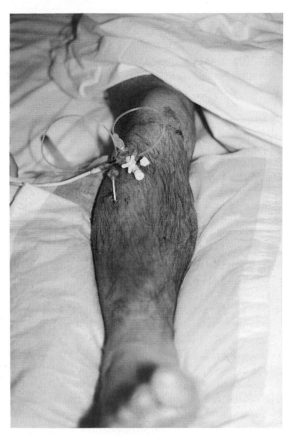

FIG. 10.6 *Monitoring compartment pressure in the tibia*

includes stress fracture and a bone scan is often useful. Treatment is by avoiding weight-bearing on the limb for at least 6 weeks.

There are two bursae related to the insertion of the Achilles tendon to the calcaneum. Patients complain of pain in the heel on dorsiflexion and fluctuation elicited on examination. The overlying skin may be inflamed. Treatment consists of rest, ultrasound and, occasionally, injection of local anaesthetic and steroid into the sheath of the tendon. Similar problems can occur due to a tenosynovitis of the posterior tibial or peroneal tendons. In these patients pain, which may be long standing, is related to walking and there may also be a limp. Tenderness is elicited over the posterior tibial tendon. Ankle movement may be restricted. Rest, ultrasound and, occasionally, local steroid injections bring satisfactory relief.

Surgical decompression of the tendon in its sheath may be required, particularly in patients not responding to treatment, partly to confirm the diagnosis and also to prevent the possibility of tendon rupture.

Rupture of the Achilles tendon

The majority of Achilles tendon ruptures occur in middle-aged 'athletes' in whom the somewhat degenerate tendon separates like two 'shaving brushes' in its midsubstance. Treatment in these cases should be conservative. In the younger athlete and in cases of sharp penetrating objects causing clean cuts of the tendon, operative repair may be indicated. Postoperatively, the management regime should be similar in both cases. A full equinous long-leg non-weight-bearing cast is applied for 4 weeks, followed by 4 weeks' partially weight-bearing in a short-leg semi-equinous cast. A further 2–4 weeks, depending on the age of the patient, in a below-knee weight-bearing cast is then necessary to minimize the risk of re-rupture.

EXAMPLES

Fractures of the tibia

A 20-year-old man comes off his motorcycle sustaining an open fracture to his right tibia. When he is seen in the Accident and Emergency Department he has no other injuries, and X-rays and examination reveal a grade III open tibial fracture.

Questions
- What is the treatment?
- What are the complications?

Answers
- In the Accident Room the fracture is covered and stabilized with a splint. Antibiotics and antitetanus treatment is initiated.
- Within 6 hours from the injuries the patient is taken to the operating theatre and undergoes wound debridement of devitalized tissue, washing out of the wound and stabilization of the fracture, usually with external fixation.
- The wound is left open although the Plastic Surgeon will advise on skin cover usually at the wound inspection 48 hours later.
- The complications are delayed union, non-union and infected non-union.

A 30-year-old woman sustains a closed fracture of the right lower limb after a road traffic accident.
There are no other injuries and she has normal sensation and peripheral pulses in her foot.

Questions
- What is the treatment?
- What are the possible complications?

Answers
- After careful clinical examination of the leg, paying special attention to the state of the skin and the muscle swelling, X-rays are taken.
- These show that there is a fracture of the tibia and fibula, which is by definition a closed fracture.
- The patient is admitted to hospital and the treatment options are to reduce the fracture and immobilize it in a long-leg plaster or to elevate the leg and apply a splint, and on the next available trauma list undertake closed reduction and internal fixation using a locked intramedullary nail inserted into the tibia under X-ray control.
- Complications include compartment syndrome; malunion, non-union and joint stiffness if treated by plaster; and infection and non-union if treated surgically.

11 LOWER LIMB – ANKLE AND FOOT INJURIES

ANKLE INJURIES

The movements of the ankle joint include dorsiflexion and plantar flexion. The movements of the midtarsal and subtalar joints are inversion and eversion. Because the ankle takes all the body's weight, indirect rotational injuries are very common, as the foot is fixed on the ground while the body continues to move forward. Those injuries associated with internal rotation tend to be mainly ligamentous ('sprains'), whereas those due to external rotations tend to be bony.

Injuries resulting from direct abduction or adduction forces are less common, because they are not associated with forward body movement. These are caused by either a fall from a height on to the side of the foot or a sideways blow when the body is stationary.

Lastly, the ankle may occasionally be injured by a direct upward thrust.

Sprained ankle

Because, in the foot and ankle, there is normally a greater range of inversion than eversion movement,

the lateral ligaments of the ankle suffer first in internal rotational injuries. Associated with this, the styloid process of the fifth metatarsal may be avulsed.

The lateral ligament of the ankle is in three parts: the anterior talofibular segment, running forwards from the lateral malleolus; the calcaneofibular portion, running downwards; and the posterior talofibular segment, running backwards.

The first and commonest portion of the ligament to be torn, therefore, will be the anterior talofibular segment. That is what usually occurs in a 'sprained ankle'. Clinically, there will be swelling and bruising over the outer side of the ankle, with tenderness most marked just in front of the tip of the lateral malleolus. The inner side of the joint will appear normal. Radiologically, no bony injury is usually seen, but sometimes a small flake may be avulsed from the malleolus.

If the injury has been more severe, the whole ligament will be torn, in which case tenderness is marked below as well as in front of the malleolus. Also, because the talus itself will have been tilted at the moment of injury, there will have been a fairly extensive tear of the joint capsule, such that some bruising and swelling will probably be present over the inner side in addition. Radiologically, there will be no bony injury beyond an occasional flake avulsed from the tip of the lateral malleolus, though if the ankle is gently inverted at the time the antero-posterior film is taken, a tilt of the talus may be demonstrated.

TREATMENT

If the anterior portion of the ligament alone has been torn, support by adhesive plaster for 10–14 days is indicated. This should extend from the base of the toes to below the knee, the direction of the strapping as it is applied being such that the foot tends to be everted.

If the clinical picture suggests that the entire ligament has been torn through, a below-knee walking plaster of Paris cast that extends from the tibial tubercle to the base of the toes, with the foot at right angles to the leg in both the anteroposte-rior and lateral planes (Fig. 11.1), should be worn for about 6 weeks. Occasionally, direct surgical repair of the torn ligament is undertaken.

It must be remembered, however, that several tendons and their sheaths along with the retinacu-lar fibres can be torn at the same time. For example, the extensor digitorum retinaculum at the front of the ankle can often be strained at the same time as injuries to peroneal tendon, fibular collateral ligament and even tibiofibular ligaments all as part

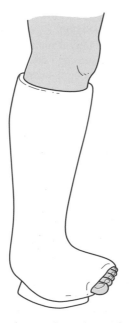

FIG. 11.1   Below-knee walking plaster of Paris cast

of a severe inversion and forced plantar flexion injury. Treatment of such sprains is almost always by immobilization followed by physiotherapy.

Recurrent sprains of the ankle

If there has been a tear of the middle (calcaneofibu-lar) portion of the lateral ligament that has been inadequately treated, some residual laxity will persist. In such cases there will be instability of the joint, such that the patient will complain of the ankle constantly giving way and 'letting them down'. On clinical examination, little that is abnormal may be found though sometimes it may be possible to detect clinically that there is some tilt of the talus on passive inversion of the foot. Radiologically, the abnormal opening of the outer side of the ankle joint may be demonstrated in an anteroposterior film taken with the foot forcibly inverted.

TREATMENT CAN BE CONSERVATIVE

The tendency to repeated inversion may be controlled to some extent if the heel of the shoe is wedged higher or extended on its outer side, coupled with a course of exercises to strengthen the peroneal muscles. Often, however, surgery is required to reconstitute the ligament, using the tendon of peroneus brevis, which is detached proximally from its muscle belly and threaded through a hole drilled in the lateral malleolus.

Classification of ankle injuries

■ External rotation injuries: without diastasis of the inferior tibiofibular joint and with diastasis of the inferior tibiofibular joint;
■ abduction injuries;
■ adduction injuries;
■ vertical compression injuries;
■ fractures due to direct violence.

External rotation injuries

The first time that an injury of this nature was described was in 1769 by Percival Pott, after whom these fractures are named.

Because external rotation of the foot is limited by bones in contact with each other, injuries tend

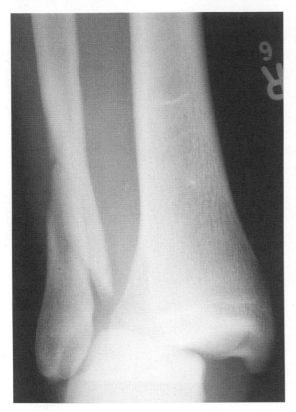

FIG. 11.2 External rotation injury without diastasis

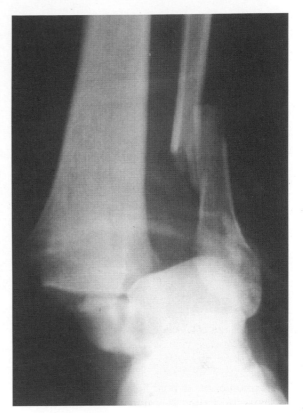

FIG. 11.3 Diastasis of the inferior tibiofibular joint, with fracture of the medial malleolus

to cause fractures of the malleoli. As, however, any displacement also involves the ankle joint, a fracture dislocation is produced. External rotation injuries can occur with or without diastasis of the inferior tibiofibular joint.

WITHOUT DIASTASIS (Fig. 11.2)

An external rotation injury without diastasis is caused by the talus externally rotating in the ankle mortise. There is an oblique fracture of the fibula at the level of the ankle joint. Either the medial malleolus is fractured or the deltoid ligament is ruptured. There may be a posterior malleolar fracture. However, the ankle joint is not totally disrupted because, although the anterior tibiofibular ligament is torn, the strong posterior tibiofibular ligament is intact.

WITH DIASTASIS (Fig. 11.3)

An external rotation injury with diastasis is an uncommon injury in which there is complete

disruption of the ankle joint, with tearing of the medial ligament or a fracture of the medial malleolus along with rupture of the anterior and posterior tibiofibular ligaments. Along with these fractures and ligament tears, there is a fracture of the fibula. This is the fracture dislocation of Dupuytren; the ankle is totally unstable and there is now a true diastasis. Another type of external rotation injury affecting the ankle joint is the Maisonneuve fracture (Fig. 11.4). In this injury there is a medial malleolar fracture and also a fibular fracture at the proximal end of the fibula. These injuries should be treated as though a true diastasis exists and the medial malleolus fixed along with a diastasis screw (Fig. 11.5).

TREATMENT

In a single bone fracture in which only the fibula is damaged, there is no displacement of the talus and treatment consists simply of a protective below-knee walking plaster, worn for about 3 weeks. If there is a fracture of the medial malleolus or a

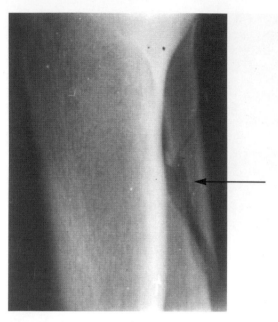
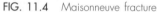
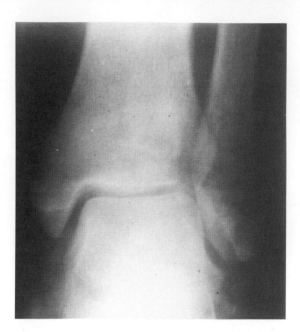

FIG. 11.4   Maisonneuve fracture

disruption of the deltoid ligament, with or without diastasis, reduction is required. This may be either by closed manipulation or by open operation.

In closed reduction the injured limb of the anaesthetized patient is hung over the end of the operating table, thereby relaxing the muscles. The surgeon is seated and the foot is maintained at a right angle to their knee; they use their hands to reverse the displacement by simultaneously pulling the heel forwards, as they internally rotates and adducts the ankle joint. A below-knee plaster cast is then applied. Weight-bearing is deferred until the swelling and reaction to the injury have subsided, usually 4–6 weeks later. Plaster is maintained for 10–12 weeks, after which, as swelling and stiffness may be troublesome, a period of active mobilization using a supporting bandage is usually required. This method is reasonable in the elderly or infirm but requires regular X-rays and repeated application of well moulded plasters to prevent displacement.

Open reduction is indicated in all other patients to ensure a perfect anatomical position. Indeed, manipulative reduction may be impossible because of the interposition of soft tissues between the fragments. On the inner side this consists of a flap of periosteum or the inverted deltoid ligament, whereas on the outer side peroneal tendons may be displaced between the bone fragments. After open

reduction of one or, more commonly, both malleoli, they are fixed by screws and plates (Fig. 11.6).

The posterior fragment usually returns to its normal position when the malleoli are reduced, but this too must be secured at the time of opera-

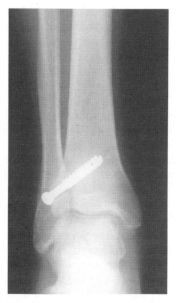

FIG. 11.5   Internal fixation of Maisonneuve fracture using a diastasis screw

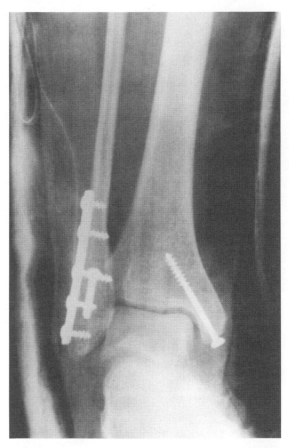

FIG. 11.6   Internal fixation of a medial malleolar fracture

tion, particularly if the fracture involves over one-third of the articular surface of the tibia (Fig. 11.7).

Postoperative management is the same if closed reduction has been employed, except the period of immobilization is much shorter. When a true diastasis occurs not only must the medial and lateral structures be repaired but also the tibiofibular ligament must be given a chance to unite. Hence an oblique screw is passed across the tibia and fibula; it should be removed at 6 weeks.

Injuries due to abduction

In injuries caused by abduction the talus is usually displaced laterally. Both malleoli may be fractured, although an isolated abduction fracture of the medial malleolus may occur without a fracture of the lateral malleolus.

TREATMENT

Undisplaced, isolated fractures of the medial malleoli can be treated conservatively in a well moulded below-knee plaster. However, displaced fractures are better treated by open reduction and internal fixation with a screw, because the fracture displaces in the plaster and the ankle joint needs to be perfectly congruous. After fixing the medial malleolus it is not necessary to fix the lateral malleolus internally, as the ankle joint is now usually stable and can be placed in a plaster cast.

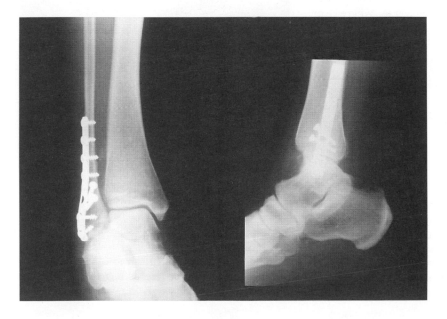

FIG. 11.7   Internal fixation of the tibula in an external rotation injury

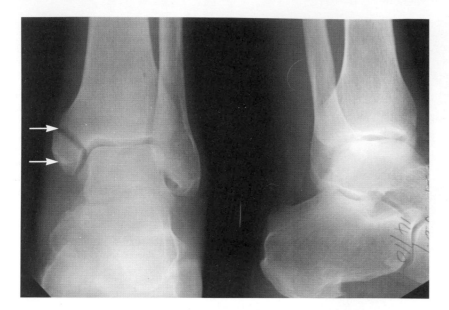

FIG. 11.8   Abduction fracture of the ankle

Injuries due to adduction

The sprained ankle is the commonest variety of an adduction injury and is caused by an inversion twist to the plantar-flexed foot. The management has been discussed at the beginning of this chapter.

Isolated fibular fractures due to adduction injury can usually be treated conservatively although internal fixation of the fibula with an oblique screw may be necessary.

In bimalleolar fractures, which are comparatively uncommon, the talus is displaced medially and both malleoli are fractured. The fracture line in the lateral malleolus is transverse, whereas in the medial malleolus it runs obliquely upwards. Manipulation is unsuccessful because the ankle is unstable and open reduction with internal fixation of both malleoli is necessary.

Injuries due to vertical compression

In a fall from a height when a patient lands on their feet, the calcaneum usually sustains a crush fracture but occasionally, if for some reason the heel is not directly involved, the talus may be driven upwards against the lower end of the tibia, thereby causing a crushing injury to the articular surface. As the patient is likely to twist or to fall sideways upon landing, some lateral or rotational displacement is also usual. Because the articular cartilage is extensively crushed,

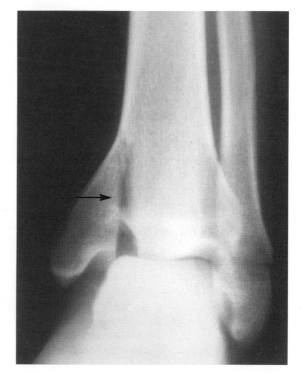

FIG. 11.9   Adduction injury of the ankle joint

damage is greater than the radiological appearance suggests, and severe osteoarthritic changes frequently follow.

TREATMENT

Manipulative reduction by traction and moulding may be attempted and the leg immobilized on a Braun frame. However, internal fixation is advisable in order to restore the anatomy of the ankle joint to as near normal as possible. Weight-bearing must be deferred until the fracture has united. Eventually, however, arthrodesis of the ankle joint may be required.

Ankle injuries in children

Because of the increased mobility in children's feet, ankle injuries are rather less common than in adults. Similarly, because the ligaments are strong and elastic, sprained ankles are not often seen.

EXTERNAL ROTATION INJURIES IN CHILDREN

The usual effect of external rotational strains applied to the foot in childhood will be to cause a fracture separation of the lower tibial epiphysis, together with a greenstick fracture of the lower end of the fibula. As such injuries usually occur when the child is running, some backward displacement is also present.

Treatment

When there is a significant degree of displacement, manipulative reduction similar to that already described for external rotational fractures to the ankle joint in adults is employed (see above). This is followed by application of a below-knee plaster of Paris cast in which weight-bearing can usually be permitted. The cast is worn for a period of between 4 and 6 weeks.

ADDUCTION INJURIES

Because ligamentous tearing is unlikely to occur, the usual result of internal rotational twists or adduction injuries to a child's ankle is also a fracture separation of the lower tibial epiphysis, which is displaced backwards. The fibula often remains undamaged, acting as the axis of rotation of the tibial epiphysis.

These injuries are important because sometimes a crushing force is applied to the inner side of the tibial epiphysis and a fracture extends through the epiphyseal plate – Salter and Harris classification, type IV. This may cause premature fusion of the epiphysis on this side of the bone whereas growth continues on the outer side of the tibial growth plate and in the fibula. As a result a varus deformity of the ankle follows as growth proceeds. This injury is often known as a railings fracture because it is frequently caused by children catching their foot between the bars if they fall when climbing railings.

Treatment

Immediate treatment is the same as that for any other ankle injury and consists of reduction when significant displacement has occurred, followed by a below-knee plaster of Paris cast. Such post-traumatic growth plate premature fusions can be treated early by open epiphysiolysis. However, if growth has ceased, osteotomies of the tibia and fibula may then be carried out to correct the deformity.

TARSAL INJURIES

The bones concerned in this region are the talus and calcaneum. To the latter are attached the powerful calf muscles, via the tendo Achillis.

Fractures of the calcaneum

Fractures of the calcaneum (Fig. 11.10) follow falls from a height onto the feet, and are therefore quite commonly bilateral. They are often accompanied by injuries elsewhere, associated with an upward compression thrust, such as crush fractures of vertebral bodies (notably in the upper lumbar region), or fractures of the base of the skull. For this reason the condition of the lumbar spine should always be checked in patients with calcaneal fractures, and both the heels and spine should be inspected in patients brought in unconscious with basal fractures of the skull.

The clinical appearance is characteristic. There is obvious widening of the heel, with flattening of the longitudinal arch (traumatic flatfoot). In addition, because the plantar fascial attachments to the calcaneum are torn, bruising arising from the fracture haematoma can be seen in the sole of the foot. Radiologically, the bone is crushed, and the disorganization of the subtalar joint can be seen. There is diminution of the angle (Bohler's angle) made by a line that runs along the upper border of the bone, having its apex at the subtalar articular surface. Marked residual stiffness in the subtalar joint is a usual feature.

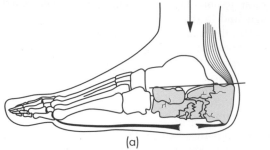
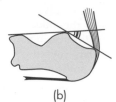

(a)

(b)

FIG. 11.10 (a) Fracture of the calcaneum showing (b) loss of the normal posterior angle

TREATMENT

Most fractures of the calcaneum are minor and usually result in only the posterior part of the bone being injured, with the subtalar joint not being involved. Such cases respond very well to a period of 3–4 weeks in a below-knee walking plaster cast. Alternatively, if there is a large posterior fragment, it should be attached with a screw. The anterior margin of the calcaneum may be avulsed when the tarsus sustains a forced inversion twist. This injury consists of a crush to a bone that is mainly cancellous; reduction of the fracture is difficult to maintain. The main aim of treatment must be to minimize the residual stiffness in the subtalar and midtarsal joints. The patient is therefore kept in a bed with their foot raised on blocks and early mobilization carried out. Weight-bearing is not permitted for 6 weeks. If severe pain persists in the subtalar region, this joint may be arthrodesed. When the bone is not crushed, some surgeons recommend internal fixation and early mobilization to promote subtalar movement. It may therefore be possible to restore congruity of the subtalar articular surface, and bone graft can be used to fill defects.

Fractures of the talus

Major injuries are, fortunately, not very common. The talus, like the carpal scaphoid, receives most of its blood supply from its distal end, the blood entering through the sinus tarsi near its neck. Therefore osteonecrosis of the body of the talus is a notorious complication. (Fig. 11.11.)

The usual fracture site is through the neck of the talus as a result of a forced dorsiflexion injury to the foot. More rarely, as a result of a violent twisting injury, the talus may be dislocated. Most commonly the body retains its relationship to the tibia, but the tarsus is displaced from it at the subtalar and talonavicular joints (plantar disloca-

tion of the tarsus). Sometimes when the neck is fractured the body of the bone is displaced backwards from both the ankle and subtalar joints.

TREATMENT

Fractures of the neck of the talus are reduced by putting the foot into plantar flexion and this position must be maintained until union has occurred. Dislocations should be reduced by closed manipulation if possible as open operation will involve further division of blood vessels to the bone. If osteonecrosis occurs, suggested either by non-union of the fracture or increased body density of the body as seen on X-rays, then bone grafting may be necessary. If painful secondary osteoarthritis occurs then arthrodesis of ankle or subtalar joints may be indicated.

Damage to the articular surface of the talus in the ankle joint must be treated like any other osteochondral fracture. Removal of small loose bodies by arthroscopy or arthrotomy and internal fixation of larger fragments must be carried out in order to preserve congruency. Osteochondritis dissecans of the articular surface may also be treated in a similar way.

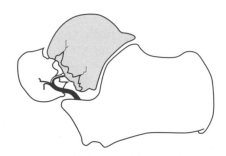

FIG. 11.11 Fracture through the neck of the talus, showing how the blood supply to the body may be cut off

Minor injuries of the talus are common, consisting of flakes of bone avulsed at ligamentous attachments. Treatment consists of protection of the painful area by a cast or strapping for 3–4 weeks.

Fractures of the navicular

Fractures of the navicular (Fig. 11.12) are uncommon fractures, which, if undisplaced, may be treated with a below-knee walking plaster. However, if the fracture is displaced, open reduction and K-wire fixation is necessary. On the other hand, fractures of the tuberosity of the navicular are not uncommon and can lead to quite severe pain and disability. A below-knee plaster is applied for 4 weeks, followed by a period of intensive physiotherapy.

Midtarsal dislocation

Midtarsal dislocation results from a violent rotational twist applied to the forefoot when the heel is fixed. Reduction is rarely difficult but as, in addition to extensive soft-tissue disruption, some damage to the articular surfaces is almost inevitable, later osteoarthritic changes are common. After reduction, a below-knee plaster cast is worn for about 6 weeks, after which a period of intensive active mobilization is usually needed.

Other midtarsal injuries

Injuries to the midtarsal bones may follow direct crushing blows on the tarsus itself, or wrenching forces applied to the foot. They may affect either the inner or the outer side but rarely involve the whole tarsus. Of these, a severe adduction injury that fractures the navicular causing the medial fragment to subluxate is the most serious. In this case primary arthrodesis of the talonaviculocuneiform joints usually gives the best long-term results.

A fracture dislocation of the tarsometatarsal joints also occurs – Lisfranc fracture dislocation – but is fortunately a rare injury (Fig. 11.13). It requires urgent reduction because compression of the dorsalis pedis vessels as they pass between the bases of the first and second metatarsals may cause circulatory insufficiency in the forefoot.

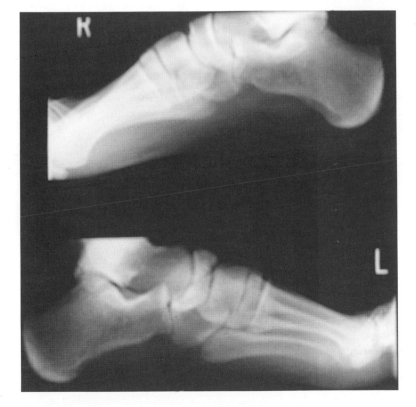

FIG. 11.12   Fracture of the navicular

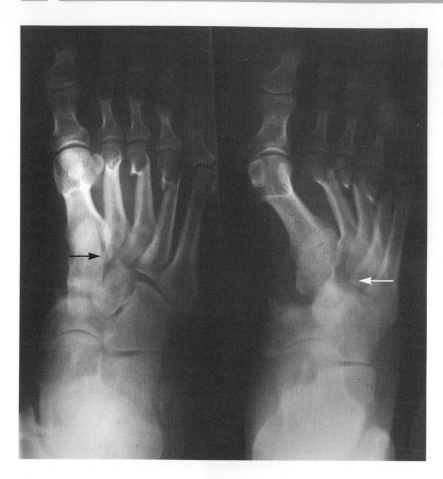

FIG. 11.13   Lisfranc fracture
dislocation

Closed reduction should be attempted, but may not be successful and open reduction may be necessary. Internal fixation is achieved by means of K wires.

INJURIES OF THE FOREFOOT

Injuries of the forefoot consist of injuries to the metatarsals and toes.

Fractures of the metatarsal bases

Fractures of the metatarsal bases, like midtarsal injuries, may follow a wrench or crushing force. They are rarely serious, and often require only a period of supporting strapping applied from the base of the toes to the knee, with a felt pad under the longitudinal arch.

Fracture of the fifth metatarsal base

Fracture of the fifth metatarsal base is a common injury, and is due to an inversion twist of the forefoot, the base of the metatarsal being avulsed by the tendon of peroneus brevis, which is inserted into it. As has been described, it is often associated with a sprained ankle.

TREATMENT

Treatment consists of either supporting strapping or a below-knee plaster cast worn for 2–3 weeks, depending upon the amount of discomfort and soft-tissue damage that is present.

Fractures of the metatarsal shafts

Fractures of the metatarsal shafts are common injuries, often occurring when some heavy object is dropped on the foot. In the central metatarsals displacement is rarely gross, and can usually be accepted. In the first metatarsal good alignment is essential.

TREATMENT

In the case of the second to fifth metatarsals, a below-knee walking plaster cast with a toe platform gives symptomatic relief and should be worn for 3 weeks.

In the case of the first metatarsal, acceptable alignment can usually be obtained by moulding under anaesthesia, after which a below-knee plaster cast with a toe platform is worn for 6 weeks. The first 3 weeks should be non-weight-bearing as any minor softening of the plaster cast may permit redisplacement at the fracture site.

Stress fractures of the middle metatarsals

The second and, slightly less often, the third metatarsal bones are the commonest sites for stress fractures to occur. The incidence is high among army recruits, and these fractures are therefore known as march fractures. They occur in young adults in whom there is flattening of the metatarsal arch such that the heads of the second and third metatarsals take an excessive amount of weight. Usually the patient is an individual who normally leads a semi-sedentary life and who suddenly becomes more active.

Symptoms consist of sudden pain in the forefoot, with slight swelling, aggravated by weight-bearing. X-rays at first are often negative, although usually a hairline crack through the distal metatarsal shaft can be seen if carefully sought. After a few days callus formation can be seen.

TREATMENT

Treatment consists of a plaster cast worn until the main discomfort has subsided (10–14 days), followed by a metatarsal support worn in the shoes and a period of physiotherapy aimed at improving the function of the small intrinsic muscles in the feet.

Injuries of the toes

Dislocations of the metatarsophalangeal and inter-phalangeal joints of the toes occur, but they are much less common than the equivalent injuries in the hand. Manipulative reduction is usually successful and is followed either by 2–3 weeks in a below-knee plaster cast, with a toe platform, or by strapping the injured member to its healthy neighbour.

Fractures due to heavy objects falling on the toes are common. Several toes are often injured simultaneously. Treatment, depending upon the severity of the injury, will consist of either a plaster cast or strapping the injured toe to an uninjured neighbour. In the latter case, the patient will be more comfortable initially wearing shoes with tough leather soles and roomy toecaps.

Crushing of a terminal phalanx accompanied by damage to skin and nail is common, especially in the hallux, and may be treated by a non-adherent dressing and stiff-soled shoe with the toecap cut away.

EXAMPLES

Ankle

A 70-year-old woman falls and sustains an ankle fracture.

When seen in the Accident and Emergency Department with pain and swelling.

X-rays reveal an external rotational injury with a fracture dislocation of the ankle. The fracture involves the medial malleolus.

Question
■ How should this patient be managed?

Answers
■ She should be admitted to hospital for open reduction and internal fixation of the fracture.
■ The fracture needs to be accurately reduced and stabilized to prevent degenerative changes occurring in the ankle joint at a later date.
■ After the operation the patient is mobilized in plaster only partially weight bearing to begin with and she will remain in plaster for about 6 weeks, after which she will have physiotherapy to her ankle to restore function.

Foot

A 25-year-old man presents in the Accident and Emergency Department with a painful right foot, having fallen about 10 feet from the scaffolding on which he was working.

X-rays reveal a fracture of the talus, which is through the neck of the talus.

Questions
■ What is the treatment?
■ What is the prognosis?

Answers
■ The patient needs admitting to hospital, and the limb to be elevated.
■ If the fracture is displaced, reduction and internal fixation will be necessary.
■ If the fracture is undisplaced a below-knee walking plaster would be appropriate and the patient discharged home, non-weight-bearing to begin with.
■ On the whole the prognosis for the undisplaced fracture is good. However, if the blood supply has been damaged, osteonecrosis of the proximal part of the talus, which is involved in the ankle joint, will occur. This leads to pain and disability.

12 CHILDREN'S ORTHOPAEDICS

CONGENITAL MEANS 'PRESENT AT BIRTH'

Congenital conditions may be generalized, affecting all the musculoskeletal system, or localized. Multiple localized congenital abnormalities can coexist because of some intrauterine insult that affected several systems simultaneously.

GENERALIZED CONGENITAL ABNORMALITIES

There are three generalized congenital abnormalities that result from abnormal epiphyseal bone growth: achondroplasia, diaphysial aclasis and dyschondroplasia. Similarly, there are three generalized congenital abnormalities of bone and soft tissue: craniocleidal dysostosis, osteogenesis imperfecta and arthrogryposis multiplex congenital.

Achondroplasia (Fig. 12.1)

Achondroplasia causes severe dwarfing as a result of poor epiphyseal growth. Because the disease mainly involves the long bones, affected individuals have very short limbs, but a trunk and head of normal size. The nose is flattened and the fingers tend to be rather short and of the same length. The vertebral pedicles are short, sometimes causing spinal stenosis.

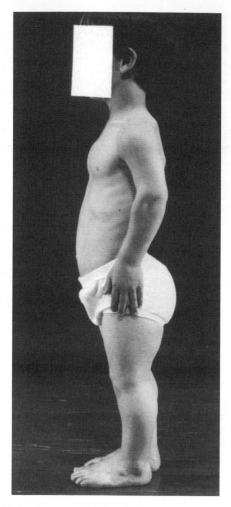

FIG. 12.1 A patient with achondroplasia, showing short limbs

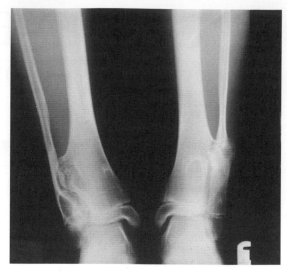

FIG. 12.2 Diaphysial aclasia affecting both tibias

during bone growth. Islands of epiphyseal cartilage rests then remain on the surface of the bone, and as they continue to form bone, outgrowths of bone or exostoses appear. These may be well defined rounded lumps, which gradually elongate and move along the shaft of a long bone as epiphyseal growth proceeds. The projections are covered by bone-forming cartilage cells, and they tend to point away from the end of the bone from which they originated. They stop growing at puberty. At times there is nodular widening of the whole metaphysis. Solitary exostoses are quite common. Multiple diaphyseal aclasia occurs, and is often familiar.

Very occasionally chondrosarcomatous changes occur, and these should be suspected if in adult life one of the exostoses increases in size.

Hypochondroplasia is a less severe variant of the condition.

TREATMENT

Treatment is only necessary if leg lengthening is considered. It takes several operations and 2 years out of the child's life to achieve 10 cm of lengthening. Spinal decompression may be necessary for spinal stenosis in adult life.

TREATMENT

Exostoses should only be excised if they are causing symptoms from pressure, if they are cosmetically unsightly, or if they turn malignant. Most are best left alone.

Diaphysial aclasis (osteochondroma) (Fig. 12.2)

In diaphysial aclasis there is failure of the normal process of remodelling the bone ends that occurs

Dyschondroplasia (Ollier's disease)

Dyschondroplasia is an uncommon condition, when epiphyseal cartilage cells remain behind inside the bone as the epiphysis grows (enchondroma). It causes thickening of the ends and diminution of longitudinal growth. Several bones may be affected in one limb, causing marked shortening. In the metacarpals, metatarsals and phalanges of the hands and feet, the cartilaginous rests produce multiple enchondromata, which look unsightly and can cause pathological fracture.

TREATMENT

Treatment is symptomatic for individual deformities,.particularly of the digits. Solitary enchondromata can be curetted and filled with bone graft. They may weaken the bone and cause fracture, but these fractures unite.

Craniocleidal dysostosis

Craniocleidal dysostosis is a failure of the normal development of membranous bone. Bone arising from cartilage is unaffected.

Clinically, the clavicles are so deficient that these patients can bring their shoulder girdles forward until they almost meet in front. There is also a delay in closure of skull sutures, with a large head. The pubic bones can also be involved, but this is less obvious.

Osteogenesis imperfecta (fragilitas ossium)

Osteogenesis imperfecta is a familiar disorder of collagen. The most striking features are the blue sclera and the fragility of the bones (Fig. 12.3). The teeth may be affected and otosclerosis can cause deafness. There may be dilatation of the aorta and generalized laxity of the ligaments.

There are two main groups: congenital osteogenesis imperfecta and osteogenesis imperfecta tarda. In the former multiple fractures arise *in utero* or during labour; this is often incompatible with life. The latter is a mild type of the disorder that is only recognized later in life. Their fractures must be distinguished from those in 'non-accidental injury' – child abuse with normal bones. They may have a raised urinary hydroxyproline.

TREATMENT

In its milder form, no specific treatment is required. Fractures are treated in the usual way. They heal like any other fracture. In the more

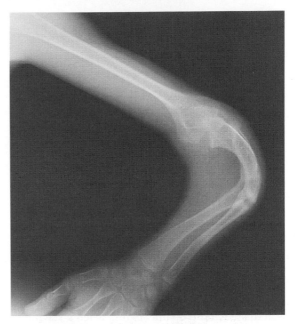

FIG. 12.3 Osteogenesis imperfecta affecting the forearm

severe condition, it is possible to correct or prevent deformity by reinforcing the bone with an intramedullary nail, or an extending nail that allows for growth.

Arthrogryposis multiplex congenital

Children with arthrogryposis multiplex congenital are born with severe multiple joint contractures. All the limbs may be affected or only certain joints. Striated muscle is replaced by fibrous tissue causing marked joint contracture. The hip is often flexed and abducted, and the feet deformed in an equinovarus position. The children are of normal intelligence.

TREATMENT

Treatment is required for the individual joint contractures to restore the joints to the position of optimum function. It is especially important to obtain plantigrade feet by early surgery, but surgery is difficult.

CHILDREN'S HIP DISORDERS

Congenital dislocation of the hip (Fig. 12.4)

The naturally occurring incidence of congenital dislocation of the hip (CDH) is about 1.2 per thousand live births in the UK. It is more common in northern Italy and among Eskimos. It is rare in Africa, perhaps because they carry their infants on their backs with the legs in abduction and externally rotated. Eskimos carry their children with the legs strapped in full extension.

Ortolani and Barlow introduced a birth screening test. The baby is examined with the hips flexed, the index fingers on the outer side of the hip and the thumb over the inner side of the knee. The hip is abducted and palpable 'clunk' is felt if the hip is subluxating in and out of joint. It was thought that with early diagnosis of the subluxating hip and a few weeks in abduction splints to hold the loose hips in place, that the condition would be eradicated. However, many children still present in the early months of life with dislocated hips.

These children are more often girls than boys, often breech presentations at birth, and many have a family history of CDH. Thus, children with a positive family history, breech presentations and those children with a positive Barlow sign at birth are followed up in a high-risk clinic until the surgeon is satisfied that the hips are secure.

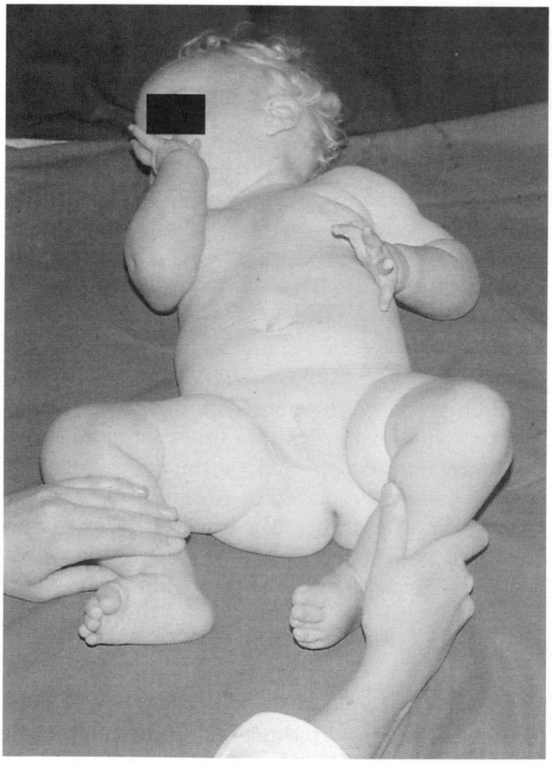

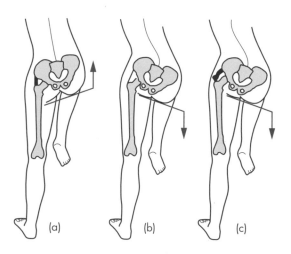

FIG. 12.5 Trendelenburg's sign: (a) negative in a normal hip; (b) positive because of abductor muscle weakness: (c) positive because of joint instability

FIG. 12.4 Dislocation of left hip showing limitation in abduction

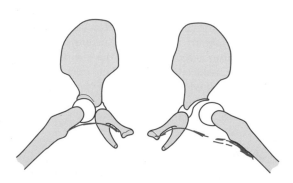

FIG. 12.6 Congenital dislocation of the hip – break in Shenton's line

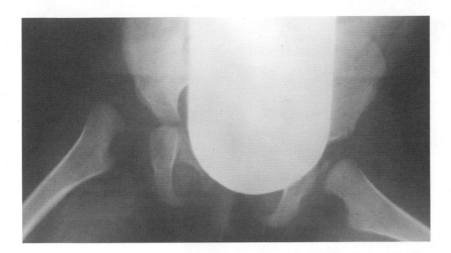

FIG. 12.7 An X-ray of a dislocated right hip showing a break in Shenton's line

PREVENTION

Babies with a positive Barlow sign are treated in abduction splints for a few weeks until the hips are more stable. Other children at risk are observed for any sign of hip dysplasia, to identify CDH as early as possible. The shape of the hip may be examined by ultrasound, and doubtful hips protected in abduction splints.

PATHOLOGY

In CDH it is unusual for the hip to be completely dislocated at birth, but the acetabulum is abnormally shallow so that the femoral head can sublux, and untreated the displacement increases as the baby becomes more active. The acetabulum is shallow, the femoral neck is rotated forward (anteverted) and the labrum acetabulare (limbus) is turned into the joint, obstructing reduction.

CLINICAL

If the condition is not picked up at birth, the child tends not to present until they start to walk. They have a typical 'waddling' gait. The Trendelenburg sign is positive – when they stand on the affected leg, instead of the opposite buttock being raised, it tends to drop (Fig. 12.5). There is no fulcrum to hold the head of the hip in place, and stability is lost. Children with CDH have asymmetrical lower limb skin creases, but so do many normal infants.

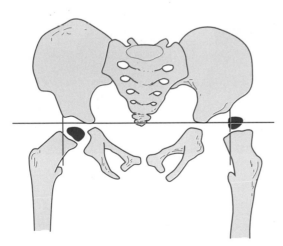

FIG. 12.8 X-ray appearance of a subluxed hip in which the femoral capital epiphysis has appeared

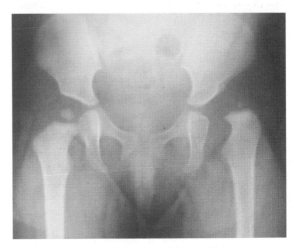

FIG. 12.9 An X-ray showing a dislocated left hip

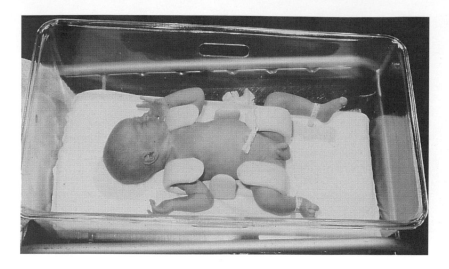

FIG. 12.10 Von Rosen splint for congenital dislocation of the hip

RADIOLOGICAL

Radiological diagnosis is not easy in the early neonatal stage, because the femoral epiphysis may not have appeared. If, however, the legs are held in 45° of abduction, some upward displacement may be seen. This is most easily detected if lines are drawn round the upper border of the obturator foramen of the pelvis and below the femoral neck. Normally the two lines are continuous (Shenton's line), but if there is a step, the head is displaced upwards (Figs 12.6 and 12.17).

Later, when the upper femoral epiphysis is radio-opaque, its displacement is more easily detected. It then lies above a horizontal line drawn through the triradiate cartilage in the acetabulum, and outside a vertical line dropped from its upper border (Fig. 12.8 and 12.9).

TREATMENT

The principles of treatment are first to reduce the hip, and then to maintain it in reduction until the acetabulum is well formed. The hip may be reduced by gentle manipulation in the very young infant, but after a few months surgical reduction is necessary. The adductor muscles are divided, and if the limbus is obstructing reduction, it is excised. Arthrography may be necessary before surgery. The hips are treated very gently to avoid avascular necrosis.

In young infants the hips are maintained in joint with an abduction splint (Fig. 12.10), but an older child will need a plaster of Paris spica applied to hold the limbs in 60° abduction (Fig. 12.11). If the hips are markedly anteverted, they

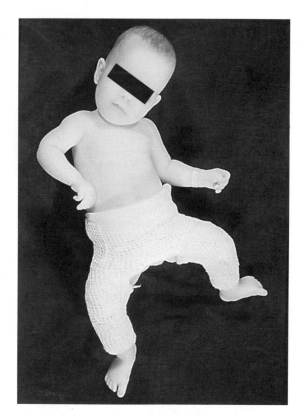

FIG. 12.11 Plaster hip spica for dislocation of the hip

can be maintained in joint by holding the legs abducted and internally rotated in plasters that are joined together by a bar (Bachelor plaster). Immobilization must be longer for the older child.

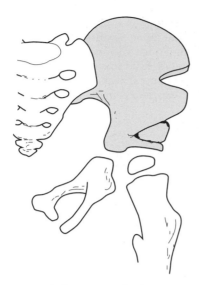

FIG. 12.12   'Shelf' operation for later congenital dislocation of the hip

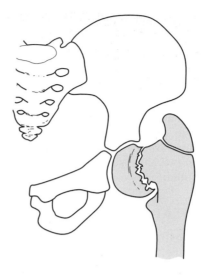

FIG. 12.14   Congenital coxa vera

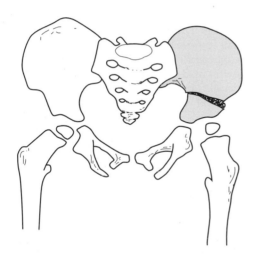

FIG. 12.13   Salter's osteotomy for later congenital dislocation of the hip

Bony surgery may be necessary if after a period
of immobilization the shape of the neck of femur or
of the acetabulum is not satisfactory. The neck of the
femur can be corrected by a femoral osteotomy, and
the shape of the acetabulum improved by a pelvic
osteotomy. A short horizontal cut may be made into
the ilium immediately above the acetabulum, and
the lower portion depressed downwards to cover
the femoral head and held in place by a wedge of
ilium (shelf operation) (Fig. 12.12). Alternatively, the
ilium may be completely divided just above acetab-

ular level, and the whole lower fragment of innominate bone levered downwards, so that the acetabular cavity is rotated into a more horizontal position
– Salter's osteotomy (Fig. 12.13).

An untreated CDH causes an unsightly waddling
gait, but little pain until old age. Thus in a child over
4 years of age with bilateral dislocation, treatment is
often not attempted lest surgical intervention converts
a painless waddle into a painful hip.

Congenital coxa vara (Fig. 12.14)

Coxa vara is a reduction in the angle made by the
femoral neck and the shaft of the femur from the
normal 120° to below 90°. It may be

- congenital;
- infantile, due to an abnormality of the epiphyseal growth plate;
- adolescent, due to a slipped upper femoral
  epiphysis.

In the congenital group, the femoral neck fails
to appear and the head of the femur lies at an
abnormally low position relative to the shaft. This
increases with growth, leading to an extreme varus
angulatory deformity, which represents failure of
a part to develop.

TREATMENT

Treatment is surgical, and consists of a valgus
osteotomy at the upper end of the femur, restoring

the neck to an angle of 120°. The hip will otherwise become arthritic.

Perthes' disease (Fig. 12.15)

Perthes' disease is osteochondritis of the femoral head. It occurs in children between 4 and 10 years of age. Boys are affected more commonly than girls, often in poor socioeconomic conditions. It may be limited to one side, or be bilateral, when the onset on one side will often not coincide with that of the other.

CLINICAL FEATURES

The child usually presents with a limp and pain, which is often referred to the knee. A child complaining of pain in the knee with a limp should always have the hips carefully examined.

There is some limitation of hip movement, notably of abduction and internal rotation. Later, when collapse of the femoral head occurs, there is true shortening.

INVESTIGATIONS

Investigations yield nothing abnormal, except for the X-rays; these show a sequence of changes. First, there is a uniform increase in epiphyseal density, with widening of the joint space. The epiphysis shows signs of fragmentation, followed by osteolytic cavitation in the metaphyseal region. The epiphyseal bone texture finally returns to normal, though often with permanent mushrooming of the femoral head (coxa plana) and widening of a shortened femoral neck. The whole cycle often takes up to 3 years to complete (Fig. 12.16).

TREATMENT

The initial treatment is to rest the irritable hip. At whatever the stage in the process Perthes' disease is detected, there will be pain and loss of movement in the affected hip joint, so bedrest for a few days is sensible to relieve the muscle spasm. When the pain has resolved, the child can be mobilized, initially with the aid of crutches.

If the femoral head is severely affected and there is considered to be a risk of adult osteoarthritis, a femoral osteotomy can be performed.

PROGNOSIS

Childhood Perthes' disease can result in adult osteoarthritis. Unfortunately, it is not clear which hips will proceed to osteoarthritis, although a significant contribution to the understanding of the disease was made by the radiological classification of Catterall. He defined four groups of Perthes' disease based upon X-ray changes, including a group in which the head of the femur is at risk of developing early osteoarthritis.

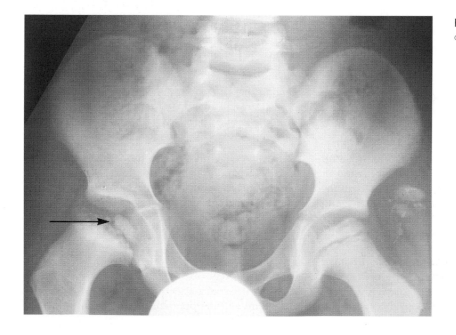

FIG. 12.15   Perthes' disease of the right hip

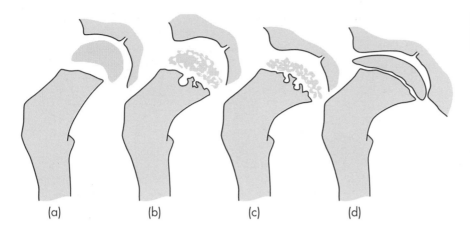

FIG. 12.16 Serial changes in Perthes' disease of the femoral head

(a)   (b)   (c)   (d)

The radiological evidence of healing is worse when the first episode occurs in children over the age of 10, whereas children who present at less than 6 years of age do not usually develop significant arthritis.

Slipped upper femoral epiphysis (adolescent coxa vara)

Slipped upper femoral epiphysis occurs between 12 and 17 years of age, more often in boys than girls, with a ratio 5:1. Twenty per cent are bilateral.

PATHOLOGY

The pathological cause of this condition is unknown. It is believed to be associated with an imbalance between growth hormones and oestrogens. It occurs commonly just before growth ceases, sometimes in the Fröhlich type, overweight, Pickwick boy. Because epiphyses fuse a little earlier in girls than in boys, when girls are affected it is at a slightly earlier age than boys. The displacement is usually gradual, but can be sudden, occurring after an external rotational twist to the limb.

Occasionally, slipping of the upper femoral epiphysis complicates other general conditions of epiphyseal abnormality, such as vitamin D-resistant rickets.

In the presence of generalized growth abnormality, the upper femoral epiphysis alone becomes displaced, probably because it is the only major weight-bearing epiphysis that is constantly exposed to oblique mechanical stresses, and it fails in the same way as a fracture of the neck of femur in the elderly.

CLINICAL FEATURES

The displacement is usually gradual, with the complaint of a limp and pain – the latter is usually referred to the knee. Every adolescent child complaining of pain in the knee should have the hip carefully examined. If the epiphysis is slipping there is an increase in external rotation, with a corresponding decrease in internal rotation. When the child lies on the couch flexing the affected hip is pathognomonic; the knee tends to deviate to the outer side of the chest rather than flexing towards the nipple line. Later, abduction is also limited. The slip may be sudden, after a twisting injury, and the patient is in acute pain, unable to move the leg. It is held in a position of adduction and external rotation.

Slipping of the second hip may occur insidiously while the first is under treatment, so both sides should be regularly examined. Many surgeons will also treat the radiologically normal hip by internal fixation to prevent it too from slipping.

X-RAYS

The initial displacement is backwards, as in the seated position the body weight displaces the epiphysis backwards (Fig. 12.17).

COMPLICATIONS

A displacement epiphysis is a problem, but if avascular necrosis (osteonecrosis) of the epiphysis occurs, it is a disaster. It results from injudicious

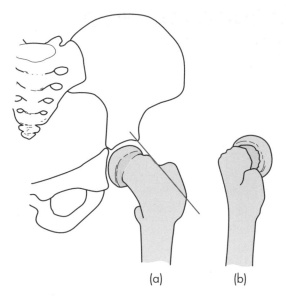

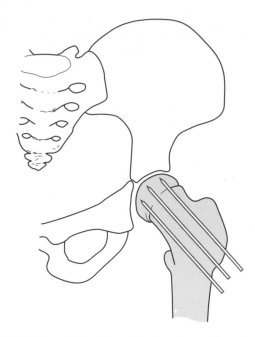

FIG. 12.17   Slipped upper femoral epiphysis: (a) antero-posterior view showing Trethowan's sign, in which a line drawn through the superior border of the femoral neck does not pass through the epiphysis because the latter has slipped; (b) lateral view

FIG. 12.18   Threaded pin fixation for slipped upper femoral epiphysis

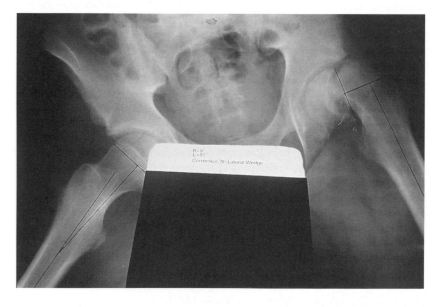

FIG. 12.19   Left slipped upper femoral epiphysis

attempts at reduction either by manipulation or by open operation. This leads to subsequent collapse of the femoral head, very marked stiffness in the joint and osteoarthritis. Marked displacement is to be prevented by early diagnosis, and osteonecrosis avoided by appropriate treatment.

TREATMENT

Treatment is surgical by internal fixation of the epiphysis *in situ* with one or more threaded pins. This prevents further displacement and stimulates epiphyseal fusion. Open reduction is inadvisable for fear of osteonecrosis developing. If slipped epiphysis is diagnosed late then a biplane osteotomy can be performed (Fig. 12.19).

Irritable hip

Hip pain in children of any age is common. It is often associated with a limp and some restriction of hip movement. The pain may be in the knee, with hip pain only at the extreme of hip movement, when the pathology is clearly in the hip and not the knee. For many of these children it is difficult to make a definitive diagnosis. They have pain in the hip, but the pathology is unclear.

The clinician thinks of the following and excludes them by radiography:

■ CDH in the infant and small child;
■ Perthes' disease in children between 4 and 10 years of age;
■ slipped upper femoral epiphysis in those between 12 and 17 years of age.

Some children have a transient synovitis in an otherwise normal hip, which can be demonstrated by ultrasound. Needle aspiration is appropriate, when fluid is removed under pressure. This may occasionally proceed to Perthes' disease. Children with an irritable hip are carefully investigated to exclude other pathology such as bone and joint infection. Frequently, however, investigations are negative, and symptoms resolve with no subsequent problems.

TREATMENT

A few days in bed and a few weeks away from sporting activity is appropriate.

CONGENITAL FOOT DISORDERS

Congenital talipes equinovarus (CTEV)

Talipes (club-foot) means a deformity involving both ankle and foot. In equinovarus deformity, the hindfoot is in equinus and varus, with the forefoot adducted and supinated. (Figs 12.20 and 12.21) The navicular is displaced medially and downwards on the head of the talus. Equinus implies that the heel is tucked upwards. Varus indicates not only that the whole foot is turned inwards, but also that the forefoot is adducted on the hindfoot.

There is probably a genetic predisposition with an environmental trigger. The incidence in the UK is 1 in 1000 live births. Clinically there are two types. First there is a milder form – resolving CTEV – in which full correction to neutral is obtained fairly easily. It is probably caused by the tight position adopted by the feet *in utero*. There is no intrinsic problem, and it gets better without treatment. Second, there is the more severe type – resistant CTEV – in which correction is difficult. Here there is a reduction in calf muscle bulk, with abnormality in the shape of the bones.

The condition is more common in boys than girls (60:40), and is more often unilateral than bilateral (60:40). Ten per cent have a first degree relative with the same condition.

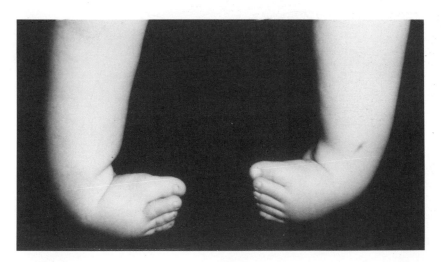

FIG. 12.20 Appearance of congenital talipes equinovarus, anterior view

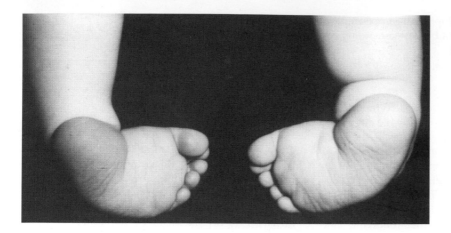

FIG. 12.21 Appearance of congenital talipes equinovarus, posterior view

TREATMENT

The condition is obvious at birth, and treatment should begin straight away. The foot is gently corrected to an improved position and then maintained in plaster of Paris, or strapping (Fig. 12.22). The plaster is changed at weekly intervals, gradually improving the position of the foot. At 6 weeks a decision is made as to whether correction has been obtained. Either the foot is corrected (a resolving CTEV) or the heel is still high (resistant CTEV). The latter requires surgical correction.

The operation releases the tight tissues on the posteromedial aspect of the foot, including the posterior capsule of the ankle joint, and divides the tibialis posterior, flexor hallucis longus and flexor digitorum longus tendons, and lengthens the tendo Achillis. This allows the heel to come down and with the hindfoot correction the forefoot swings into a better position. Some would shorten the peroneus longus, which is slack in the corrected position. Surgery can be carried out in stages, the hindfoot first and a forefoot release later if required, or alternatively in a single one-stage posteriomedial release. In an older child if the foot is not plantigrade, bony surgery may be required. This can be limited either to removal of a wedge from the outer side of the calcaneum – permitting the heel to be everted – or to removal of a wedge from the calcaneocuboid joint, which allows the forefoot to swing outwards.

When deformity persists at maturity, and when the growth rate has slowed down, a triple arthrodesis may be required (Fig. 12.23). Three joints – the subtalar, the talonavicular and the calcaneocuboid – are all fused by removing wedges of bone containing the articular surfaces.

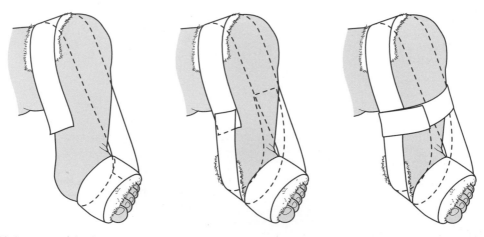

FIG. 12.22 Strapping of the foot in congenital talipes equinovarus

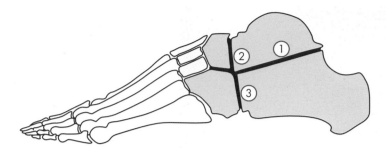

FIG. 12.23   Triple arthrodesis

Congenital talipes calcaneovalgus (CTCV)

Congenital talipes calcaneovalgus is the reverse deformity to talipes equinovarus. The heel points downwards and the forefoot is everted and dorsiflexed. This is a mild postural deformity due to intrauterine pressure on the dorsiflexed foot. Rapid correction is obtained if the baby's feet are left alone.

Metatarsus varus

Metatarsus varus is a deformity situated entirely in the forefoot, which is adducted. There is no hindfoot abnormality. It is not present at birth, but develops in the first few months of life. It is caused by a temporary overgrowth of the outer side of the foot, and it corrects over a couple of years if left alone. It should be untreated except for passive stretching exercises. A few children with persistent deformity will respond to an abductor hallucis release.

Congenital vertical talus

Congenital vertical talus is a rare condition in which the head of the talus is plantar flexed to face downwards into the sole of the foot. It is essentially a dislocation of the head of the talus, which then protrudes into the sole of the foot. There is an equinus heel and dorsiflexed metatarsals. The foot is very stiff.

Treatment involves extensive soft tissue release.

Flat feet (pes planovalgus)

Flat feet may be mobile or stiff.

MOBILE FLAT FEET

Mobile flat feet is normal up to the age of 5 years. After this age, a painless mobile flat foot may be

- due to hypermobility;
- associated with femoral anteversion;
- the result of a neurological condition, such as poliomyelitis or cerebral palsy.

Hence every child who presents with a mobile flat foot should be examined particularly for evidence of hypermobility in other joints. Their hips should be assessed to determine the degree of femoral anteversion, and the central and peripheral nervous system evaluated to identify poliomyelitis or cerebral palsy.

Investigations

Lateral X-rays of the foot may reveal a 'pseudo-vertical' talus in a patient with cerebral palsy.

Treatment

Surgery is reserved for patients with a pes planovalgus deformity from a neurological cause or, occasionally, for excessively hypermobile patients. All the rest are treated conservatively either by reassurance to the parents of children under the age of 5 years and those with femoral anteversion or by the use of a heel support in those patients in whom it is considered necessary.

The surgical treatment consists of stabilizing the subtalar joint by means of a strut graft.

Most patients with mobile painless flat feet do not require any treatment.

STIFF FLAT FEET

Stiff flat feet are a cause for concern, particularly if they are painful as well as stiff. They can be due to

- infection – osteomyelitis or a septic arthritis of the midtarsal joint;
- trauma – a fracture or ligamentous injury;
- congenital – spasmodic flat foot or tarsal coalition; or a vertical talus;

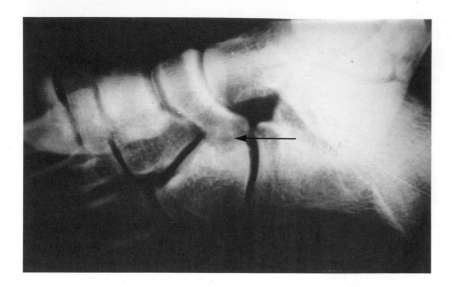

FIG. 12.24   An X-ray showing navicular cuboid coalition

■ arthritis – rheumatoid arthritis or, in adults, osteoarthritis;
■ osteochondritis – Köhler's disease.

Spasmodic flat foot (peroneal spastic flat foot)

These patients present, usually from the age of 10 years upwards, with a painful stiff foot caused by a tarsal coalition.

The initial spasm may be overcome by applying a plaster for a short period. Those patients with a calcaneonavicular bar or navicular cuboid bar (Fig. 12.24), may benefit from excision of the bar, which may only be cartilaginous at an early age.

Talonavicular arthritis tends to develop in early adult life, and in certain patients a triple arthrodesis may be necessary to relieve pain.

Pes cavus

Pes cavus is the reverse of the flat foot and is associated with contractures of the intrinsic muscles of the foot, resulting in claw toes (Fig. 12.25) and painful callosities (Fig. 12.26). The cause is always neurological until proved otherwise and hence pes cavus is a sign of an underlying condition.

AETIOLOGY OF PES CAVUS

■ Poliomyelitis
■ Spina bifida
■ Cerebral palsy
■ Friedreich's ataxia
■ Charcot–Marie–Tooth disease
■ Spinal dysraphism

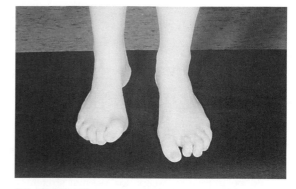

FIG. 12.25   Claw toes in pes cavus

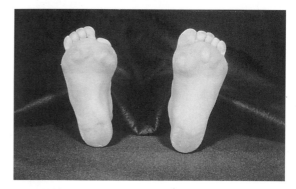

FIG. 12.26   Callosities in pes cavus

■ Polyneuritis
■ Duchenne muscular dystrophy
■ Idiopathic

On examination the whole foot is affected, so there is a relative calcaneus deformity of the heel, which is also often slightly inverted. It is in this type that clawing of the toes is most marked, with hyperextension of the metatarsophalangeal joints such that the phalanges may be dislocated onto the dorsum of the metatarsal necks. This is often due to partial or complete paralysis of the interosseous muscles, and is similar to the claw hand deformity resulting from intrinsic paralysis due to ulnar nerve division.

Pes cavus is rarely seen in early infancy. It usually appears in childhood and progresses until growth ceases. The incidence of spina bifida occulta discovered on routine X-ray is greater than in the population at large, and it has been suggested that tethering of the spinal cord, which normally does not grow in length to the same degree as the vertebral column, may be an aetiological factor.

Symptoms other than clumsiness are unusual in childhood, but later on metatarsalgia, callosities on the toes and disability from the valgus or varus heel may develop.

TREATMENT

Treatment depends upon the degree of deformity, the cause and the rate of deterioration. If there is a neurological cause the deformity may be progressive, because of the muscle imbalance.

While there is active growth of the foot and it is mobile, soft tissue release and tendon transfer may be performed. Later on a calcaneal osteotomy to correct the heel and finally a triple arthrodesis may be necessary.

In the elderly, carefully made supports are useful in relieving pressure. They are designed to distribute weight evenly under the soles of the feet and away from the prominent metatarsal heads.

ABSENCE OF PARTS AND ACCESSORY PARTS

Deficient development may affect any region of the body, but it is most common in the limbs. There are two types. First, there are congenital amputations, which may affect the distal phalanx of a digit or produce complete absence of whole limb. Sometimes these are associated with intrauterine con-

stricting bands, with circumferential deficiency of the subcutaneous tissues. Second, proximal parts of limbs may be absent, such as an absent fibula. This can be associated with a marked inversion deformity of the foot. The outer rays of the foot may also be missing. Absence of the upper part of the femur is associated with gross limb shortening. In the arm, absence of the radius causes the appearance of a 'club hand'. It is often associated with absence of the thumb. Mild congenital shortening of the radius causes dislocation of the inferior radioulnar joint, known as Madelung's deformity.

One side effect of the drug thalidomide was to cause phocomelia, with damage to the developing limb bud during the first months of pregnancy.

Treatment depends upon the nature of the lesion. Limb lengthening can be appropriate.

Accessory digits may vary from small knobs of flesh on the side to complete extra parts. Alternatively, there may also be fully developed metatarsals or metacarpals. The extra digits are usually on the outer side. They are amputated if they cause inconvenience.

ABNORMALITIES OF THE TRUNK

Spina bifida

Spina bifida overta occurs when the neural arch fails to close, and the neural elements are exposed on the surface. There is a serious neurological deficiency below the same segmental level as the bony pathology. Thus the neural arch may be deficient at L1, with complete sensory and motor loss in the lower limbs. In spina bifida occulta, the neural arch is deficient, but the skin is intact, and there is no significant neurological deficit. It is then considered to be an incidental innocuous condition.

Other congenital abnormalities of the spine include wedged vertebrae (congenital hemivertebra), which leads to congenital scoliosis. Vertebrae may be fused together (block vertebrae), which is most frequently seen in the neck, causing a congenital short neck (Klippel–Feil syndrome).

Several ribs may be fused together, which again is a cause of congenital scoliosis. The scapula may fail to descend from the high position in which the limb bud first appears in early fetal life (Sprengel's shoulder).

Torticollis (wry neck)

Torticollis is not the result of a developmental abnormality, but it follows a birth injury to the sternomastoid muscle. There is a muscle haematoma, which produces fibrosis. As a result, during growth, the head is pulled down to one side (torticollis) and if untreated, it will cause facial asymmetry.

Clinically, in the early neonatal stage, a lump is felt in one sternomastoid (sternomastoid 'tumour') from the original birth injury. At a later stage, the muscle contracture pulls the head over to one side. The sternomastoid muscle is tested by inclining the occiput to the opposite shoulder, when the muscle is found to be tight.

TREATMENT

The affected sternomastoid muscle is divided at its origin from the clavicle and sternum, and also at its insertion into the mastoid process.

AFFECTIONS OF THE EPIPHYSIS – OSTEOCHONDRITIS

Epiphyses are the growing ends of long bones. They consist initially of cartilage, but at specific intervals during early growth, depending upon the individual bone concerned, osseous centres appear within the cartilage. These grow until the only remaining cartilage is the epiphyseal plate, which ossifies at the cessation of growth, and the articular cartilage of a synovial joint.

At certain sites several separate osseous centres appear at the growing ends of bones. Those that do not directly articulate with the neighbouring bones, for example the greater trochanter, are known as apophyses.

Certain epiphyses fail to develop normally, which may be the result of ischaemic necrosis. The bone becomes ischaemic, deforms and then slowly it is reconstituted.

Pathology

The epiphysis first becomes more dense than surrounding bone as a result of an impaired blood supply. Then the avascular bone alters shape as it begins to collapse. Later, as new blood vessels grow into the area, its texture recovers, but the shape remains distorted.

In theory, any epiphysis may be affected, but in practice the condition is largely restricted to certain sites:

- *the femoral head – Perthes' disease* (see above);
- *the head of the second or third metatarsal – Freiberg's disease;*
- *the ring epiphysis of vertebral bodies – Scheuermann's disease;*
- *the tarsal navicular – Köhler's disease;*
- *the carpal lunate – Kienböck's disease;*
- *osteochondritis of the femoral head (Perthes' disease).*

Osteochondritis of a metatarsal head (Freiberg's disease)

The second or third metatarsal head is affected with changes occurring in adolescence. There is pain at the base of the affected toe and in the sole of the foot under the metatarsal head. Symptoms are often mild, and the condition is missed until osteoarthritic changes develop in adult life.

Radiological changes consist of flattening and fragmentation of the metatarsal head (Fig. 12.27).

TREATMENT

Treatment is symptomatic, relieving pain by protecting the metatarsal head with a below-knee walking plaster or a metatarsal support worn in a firm shoe. Athletic activities are curtailed until the pain settles.

If symptoms recur later in life from osteoarthritis, similar conservative treatment is usually effective; if not, a metatarsal osteotomy to elevate the metatarsal head can relieve the pain.

Osteochondritis of vertebral body epiphyses (Scheuermann's disease; adolescent kyphosis)

In osteochondritis of vertebral body epiphyses, several vertebrae are affected, usually in the thoracic region. Onset is at the time of puberty, when the ring epiphyses that surround the margins of the vertebral bodies appear.

There are complaints of minor backache, and parents or teachers notice a 'round shouldered' posture. The pain settles, leaving a kyphosis that is a cosmetic rather than functional problem.

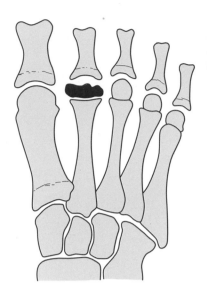

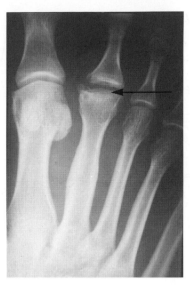

FIG. 12.27   Freiberg's osteochondritis of a metatarsal epiphysis

Radiologically, the epiphyses appear fragmented with apparent narrowing of the disc spaces anteriorly. Later in life there is some wedging of the affected vertebrae with a generalized kyphosis.

TREATMENT

A course of exercises will encourage the best posture. A spinal brace is not very effective. Surgical intervention is rarely required, but occasionally with a severe kyphotic deformity, osteotomy and spinal fusion with instrumentation is recommended.

The intermittent thoracic pain in childhood settles. Individuals are left with a kyphotic posture which is a cosmetic rather than functional problem.

Osteochondritis of the tarsal navicular (Köhler's disease)

Köhler's disease (Fig. 12.28) is an example of osteochondritis affecting the main bony nucleus rather than an epiphysis. It usually occurs in children around 5 years of age. Clinically, they complain of pain in the foot and they develop a limp. There is some tenderness over the navicular bone.

Radiographs show a dense navicular bone, which is flattened to a disc. Later, the bone returns completely to its normal shape.

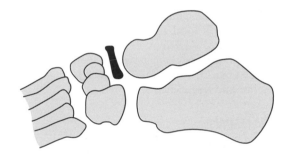

FIG. 12.28   Köhler's osteochondritis of the tarsal navicular

TREATMENT

A below-knee walking plaster of Paris cast is worn until the pain disappears.

Avascular necrosis of the lunate (Kienböck's disease)

Kienböck's disease also occurs in the main bone nucleus, but it differs from other forms of osteochondritis, inasmuch as this condition occurs in an adult bone. Its pathology follows the same cycle as other forms of osteochondritis. The probable cause is minor trauma to the lunate, interrupting the blood supply and precipitating osteonecrosis.

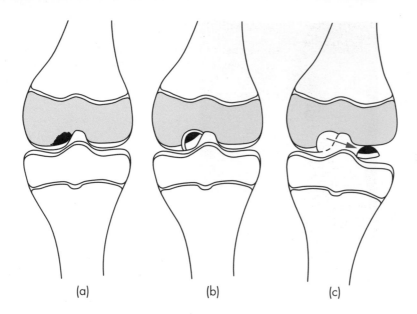

FIG. 12.29 The formation of a loose body in osteochondritis dissecans, involving the knee joint

(a)   (b)   (c)

CLINICAL FEATURES

Osteonecrosis of the lunate occurs in young adults. They complain of increasing pain and stiffness in the wrist, with localized tenderness in the region of the lunate.

Radiographs are characteristic. Initially they show increased density in the lunate, which later becomes irregular and fragmented.

TREATMENT

At an early stage, the hand is immobilized in a scaphoid type of plaster cast for 3–6 months. Later, if symptoms persist because of degenerative change, the lunate may be excised. Sometimes a prosthesis replaces the excised bone. If there are severe osteoarthritic changes in the wrist, arthrodesis gives a better result.

Osteochondritis dissecans

In osteochondritis dissecans a piece of the articular surface of a bone with its overlying cartilage becomes separated and eventually exists as a loose fragment within the joint (Fig. 12.29). The bone usually dies but because the cartilage is nourished by synovial fluid, this survives. The cartilage may extend to surround the bone. It usually occurs towards the end of the growing period, and the lower ends of the femur and humerus are most frequently affected. It occurs less commonly in the body of the talus and the head of the femur.

CLINICAL FEATURES

The patient is often a boy between 12 and 18 years of age who complains of discomfort on certain positions of the knee. These symptoms persist until the loose body separates. There is then sudden locking, and spontaneous unlocking of the joint. The locking will recur, but in different positions, depending where the loose body is opposed between the articular surfaces.

Locking from a loose body in the knee differs from the locking due to a meniscus injury, which always occurs in the same position with pain at the same site. Sometimes, the loose body is palpated in the suprapatellar pouch, or on the lateral or medial side of the knee. It slips away from the palpating fingers to be lost in the joint – 'joint mouse'.

In the elbow, locking is less painful and transient because the weight of the forearm distracts the bone ends. Loose bodies in osteochondritis dissecans are a common cause of osteoarthritis of the elbow and consequent restriction of movement of the elbow. In the hip and ankle, loose bodies are less likely to cause locking because they only occasionally become jammed between the articular surfaces; pain is then the predominant feature.

Radiographs are characteristic. At an early stage the separating portion will be seen as a dense fragment of bone surrounded by a clear line. In the knee this is usually on the medial femoral condyle near the intercondylar notch, slightly behind the midline (Fig. 12.30). In the

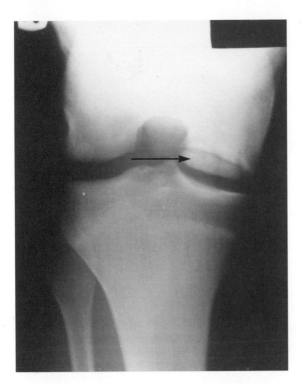

FIG. 12.30 Osteochondritis dissecans of the medial femoral condyle

elbow it usually arises from the capitulum of the humerus. If the separating fragment is large, it may break into two or more smaller pieces.

TREATMENT

If detected before separation, some surgeons will recommend avoiding sporting activity until the symptoms resolve, whereas others will carry out arthroscopy, and drill the area to promote revascularization.

Later, when the fragment has separated as a loose body, it is removed arthroscopically. Usually the sharp edges of the cavity are pared down.

Summary
Congenital disorders of the musculoskeletal system may be generalized, or affect only a localized part; treatment is required for deformity, generally to improve function but occasionally for cosmoses such as leg lengthening in children of short stature. Painful lumps should be excised in diaphysial aclasia and dyschondroplasia. Fractures through weakened bones in osteogenesis imperfecta heal in the usual manner, but need care to prevent deformity.

Disorders at the hip in children can cause painful arthritis in later life and require early and accurate diagnosis. Hip pathology should be suspected in every child with knee pain. Treatment of congenital talipes is usually rewarded with excellent function.

EXAMPLES

Generalized congenital abnormalities

Questions

History A 16-year-old boy complains to his general practitioner that he has noticed a lump on the inner side of his right thigh. It was tender when he was kicked during a football match.

X-ray He is referred to hospital for an X-ray, which shows an osteochondroma (diaphysial aclasis) projecting from the medial lower femoral epiphysis into the inner thigh.

Examination The hospital doctor notices that the lump is much bigger when palpated than it appears to be on the X-ray.
   A full musculoskeletal examination does not reveal any other bony swelling.

Treatment He is told that he has an innocent bony swelling, but because it is tender and is interfering with sport the bony swelling is removed.
   The specimen is sent for pathological examination. Histology confirms it is a benign osteochondroma.

Answers

The general practitioner would suspect an osteochondroma; possible malignance must always be considered. A short history of swelling requires prompt referral for X-ray.

The lower femur and the upper tibia are common sites for osteochondroma.

The radiolucent cartilaginous cap covering the bony spur is responsible for the lump being larger clinically than it appears on the X-ray.
   Multiple osteochondroma are not uncommon.

Chondrosarcomatist changes affecting the cartilaginous cap are very rare. He has a short history because he was only aware of the lump when it was kicked. It has probably been present for many years.
   Osteochondroma are generally only excised because of their inconvenience.

Children's hip disorders

Questions

History A 14-year-old boy is sent to hospital by his general practitioner complaining of pain in the right knee. He has been limping for 10 days.

Examination When examined by the casualty officer the right knee is normal. The right leg is 1 cm short. When flexing the right hip, the femur falls into external rotation. Internal rotation is limited and painful. He is rather obese and is pubertal.

X-ray Anteroposterior X-ray of the hip shows a small display of slip of the upper femoral epiphyseal. This is more marked, however, on the lateral view.

Treatment He is referred to the orthopaedic surgeon who operates the following day inserting three pins across the femoral epiphysis of both hips (the slipped right epiphysis and the normal left epiphysis).

Answers

Sudden onset of pain in the knee and the limp should alert the doctor to the possibility of hip pathology. Both joints are supplied by branches of the obturator nerve.

The short leg and an external rotation deformity in a 10–18 year old is compatible with a slipped upper epiphysis. Endocrine factors are often important in slipped upper femoral epiphysis.

The backward slip of the epiphysis is greater than the downward slip.

The slipped epiphysis is not reduced but left slightly displaced for fear of precipitating osteonecrosis, and the epiphysis is fixed *in situ* to prevent increasing deformity. The opposite hip has a 30 per cent chance of slipping and is therefore treated prophylactically.
   The patient walks out of hospital after 7 days. The pins will be removed in 2 years time.

13 ARTHRITIS

'Arthritis' is a term used to describe any joint lesion. It may be caused by a local pathology, or by a generalized condition affecting many joints and other systems. There are three types of arthritis:

- *osteoarthritis* (arthritis): this results from age-related changes and the effects of repeated mechanical stresses and strains. Therefore it is weight-bearing joints that are usually affected.
- *inflammatory arthritis*: many joints and the periarticular tissues are simultaneously affected by inflammatory changes. Rheumatoid arthritis is the most common inflammatory joint problem.
- *infective arthritis*: there is a causative infective organism; this is discussed in Chapter 16.

OSTEOARTHRITIS

Osteoarthritis is a degenerative condition, in which there is mechanical damage to the articular cartilage. There is an imbalance between the natural wear and the repair process of the cartilage. It is a non-inflammatory disorder of joints. Degenerative changes occur in the joints as a result of ageing and might be considered physiological. In the spine, degenerative change is beneficial in supporting a system that might become unstable. In elderly persons some degree of osteoarthritis is present in all joints, and this may not cause any problem. It is unwise, therefore, to tell a patient that they have 'arthritis', solely because X-rays show some degenerative change. Symptoms occur particularly in weight-bearing joints if the process is exaggerated.

AETIOLOGY

Osteoarthritis in excess of the normal age-related degenerative change can occur:

In some patients the cause of osteoarthritis in an isolated joint remains unknown.

Some patients have an unexplained tendency to develop osteoarthritis that affects several joints. The terminal interphalangeal joints in the fingers are often also involved, with nodular thickenings – 'Heberden's nodes'.

Osteoarthritis may be secondary to other conditions:

- previous fractures involving the joint surface, or causing malalignment and therefore excessive joint wear;
- joint instability from ligament injury;
- loose bodies in the joint;
- congenital abnormalities (CDH, epiphyseal dysplasia);
- childhood pathology (Perthes' disease, slipped epiphysis);
- osteonecrosis;

- obesity;
- Paget's disease of the bone;
- neuropathies, causing unprotected joint stress;
- metabolic and endocrine disorders (alcaptonuria, acromegaly, and the mucopolysaccharidoses).

PATHOLOGY

The pathological process begins with a breakdown of the articular cartilage. It becomes roughened and eroded, exposing bare bone. The process may not be entirely mechanical, as the synovium releases intracellular enzymes, lysozymes producing hyperaemia, and degradation enzymes and mediators, such as interleukin-1, which may affect the chondrocytes.

The underlying subchondral bone becomes sclerotic with grooves on its surface – eburnation (Fig. 13.1). Cystic spaces may simultaneously appear beneath the sclerotic bone surface. Remodelling of the joint architecture can occur, which in the hip increases the size of the head of the femur – coxa magna – or causes the acetabulum to protrude into the pelvis – protrusio.

As the process continues, new cartilage and bone develop at the joint margins, producing osteophytes. These may break away and, if they have no soft-tissue attachment, become loose bodies in the joint. Fibrosis develops in the joint capsule, restricting joint movement and causing pain when it is stretched.

In some patients it is believed that the bone is primarily at fault. As in Paget's disease, the bone is abnormally stiff, and it fails to absorb stress. These forces are transmitted to the articular cartilage, which in turn fails under load.

CLINICAL FEATURES

The two main complaints are of pain and stiffness. The onset is insidious, with joint pain developing for no apparent reason in a middle-aged or elderly individual. Symptoms may develop in a younger person, if there is a previous history of joint pathology. At first the pain may only occur when the joint is stretched at the extremes of movement, then it becomes troublesome on weight-bearing. For some patients weight-bearing pain is only experienced when the last thin covering of articular cartilage is worn away, that is, when they begin to walk bone rubbing on bone. Patients are then surprised at the sudden onset of pain in a hip that, radiologically, is quite degenerate. Finally the joint is painful even at rest, disturbing sleep. As

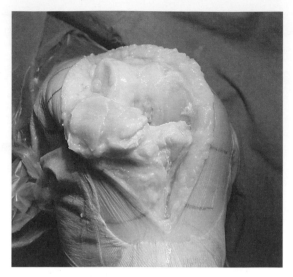

FIG. 13.1   *Osteoarthritis of the knee*

the disease progresses, the joint can become ankylosed and totally stiff, and the pain may then dramatically improve. The joint movement becomes increasingly restricted, because of fibrosis of the capsule. A fixed deformity occurs when a full joint range cannot be achieved. It can be more limited in one direction than another. Pain causes muscle spasm, and the more powerful muscle groups restrict movement to a greater degree than their less powerful antagonists. Thus in the hip the flexors, adductors and external rotators are stronger than their opponents, and the hip develops a fixed flexion/adduction external rotation deformity. In the knee, the hamstrings are stronger than the quadriceps and the knee develops a fixed flexion deformity; it loses the important final degrees of extension.

For some patients their main complaint is not the pain and stiffness, which may be tolerable, but rather the loss of independence. This is a major problem for the elderly.

On examination, the abnormal gait is obvious. The patient with osteoarthritis of the hip has an antalgic (pain relieving) gait, leaning towards the affected hip as they walk. This transference of the centre of gravity towards the affected side, although increasing the energy requirements of walking, reduces the lever arm on the hip joint, and therefore reduces the load bearing of the joint. Neither do they fully extend the hip as they walk. The diagnosis can often be made from the pattern of the patient's gait. In osteoarthritis of the knee the pattern is different, with the patient adopting a short stepping gait to avoid too much knee movement.

Stiffness will be noted from the gait pattern or from direct examination of the joint. There is often joint crepitus due to the irregularities in the opposing articular surfaces. This can be felt or heard on movement of the joint. In the more superficial joints, osteophytes and bony thickening is palpable and a small effusion may be present due to synovial irritation. Soft-tissue synovial thickening or local heat would suggest an inflammatory arthritis rather than osteoarthritis. Muscle wasting rapidly follows and is an index of joint function. The girth of the thigh measured 10–12.5 cm above the knee joint, will be reduced in unilateral osteoarthritis of the hip or knee.

INVESTIGATIONS

Blood investigations will be normal because osteoarthritis is not a constitutional disease. Radiographs are characteristic. First the joint space is narrowed, from a reduction in the thickness of the articular cartilage (Fig. 13.2). Cystic changes appear in the subchondral bone with increased density and sclerosis. There is marginal osteophyte formation, and steady remodelling of the joint, altering its normal morphology.

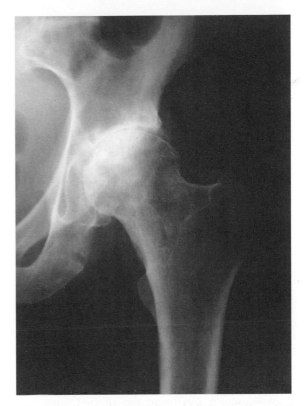

FIG. 13.2   An X-ray of a hip in a patient with rheumatoid arthritis

TREATMENT

Treatment depends upon the individual joint affected, the symptoms and, most important, the disability, which varies with each individual patient. The symptoms do not match the degree of X-ray changes, some patients having severe pain with minimal degenerative changes, and others having gross changes radiologically, but fewer symptoms. It is not possible to reverse the pathology that has already occurred in the joint. The natural history, however, is for the symptoms to fluctuate, with periods of pain and periods of less disability, but with a steady deterioration. Every patient needs counselling about the natural history, and the therapeutic options.

Conservative treatment is recommended first. It aims to control the symptoms caused by the changes already present and to limit as far as possible the progress of the pathology. It can be subdivided into local and general measures.

Local treatment consists of the use of exercises such as swimming and cycling to improve the tone of muscles acting upon the affected joint. This tries to retain the range of movement and protect the joint from some of the minor strains to which it is subject in the course of everyday life. Heat also is employed in some form, either as warm clothes or a hot water bottle at night in an effort to relax muscle spasm and relieve some of the local pain. In the physiotherapy department, heat is a preliminary to exercise activity. A walking stick may help to control pain and help the patient to compensate for the disability.

General treatment uses analgesics, usually the soluble aspirin type, when pain is troublesome. They are particularly appropriate at night if pain affects sleep. Limited courses of anti-inflammatory drugs can help, but may have unpleasant gastrointestinal side effects. An obese patient should lose weight to reduce the strains on affected joints. For young patients, resettlement in more suitable employment may extend the useful life of the degenerate joint.

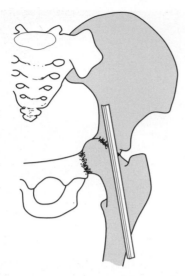

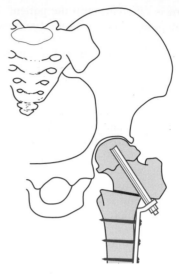

FIG. 13.3   Arthrodesis of the hip, recommended for trauma in the young patient or for infection

FIG. 13.4   Intertrochanteric displacement osteotomy of the hip, recommended for the young arthritic hip only

Operative treatment depends very much upon the individual joint. There are three surgical operations for arthritic joints: arthrodesis, arthroplasty and osteotomy.

Arthrodesis, by fusing the affected joint, will completely relieve the pain (Fig. 13.3). However, there is the cost of reduced function. Neighbouring joints and contralateral joints must be in good condition to compensate for the stiffened joint.

Arthroplasty (making a false joint) aims to restore a useful range of painless movement.

An osteotomy seeks to correct a deformity, or to redistribute the stress across a joint (Fig. 13.4). Osteotomy may also alter the haemodynamics of the subchondral bone and relieve troublesome rest pain, thought to be due to intraosseous venous hypertension.

The hip

Osteoarthritis of the hip is a very common condition, and perhaps the major cause for elective orthopaedic admission. Its cause is usually unknown. It is more common in rural communities. Sometimes it is secondary to a known disorder of the hip such as congenital dislocation, Perthes' disease, slipped epiphysis, the late results of rheumatoid arthritis or trauma. It can occasionally be preceded by osteonecrosis from excess steroids, alcohol abuse, deep sea diving or immune suppression. However, more often there is no known cause.

Clinically, the patient complains of pain and stiffness. The pain occurs on movement, and when it is severe it wakes them at night. Walking distance is limited. Patients with osteoarthritis of the hip joint have difficulty reaching down to cut their toenails or put on their shoes and socks.

Examination reveals a classic antalgic gait. The thigh muscles are reduced in bulk. The range of movement is carefully recorded with the patient lying supine on a couch – flexion, fixed flexion,

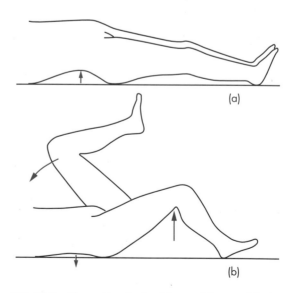

FIG. 13.5   Thomas' test for fixed flexion deformity of the hip

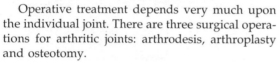

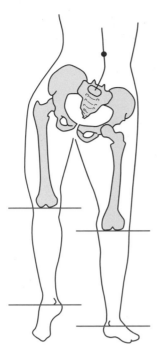

FIG. 13.6   Apparent shortening due to adduction deformity of the hip

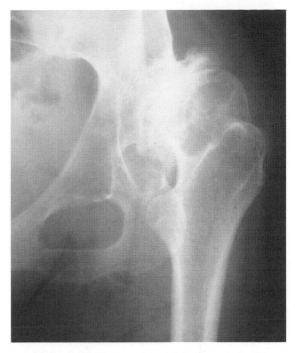

FIG. 13.7   X-ray of osteoarthritis of the hip, producing true shortening of the leg

external and internal rotation, abduction and adduction. Fixed flexion (or loss of full extension) is measured by Thomas' test. The patient fully flexes the opposite hip, which flattens the lumbar spine abolishing the normal lumbar lordosis. The other hip should normally still be extended with the thigh resting on the couch, but if there is loss of full extension (fixed flexion), the thigh will have lifted from the couch (Fig. 13.5).

The leg may be short. This can be apparent shortening as a result of fixed adduction of the hip. The pelvis is then tilted to accommodate the fixed adduction, and the leg appears to be short compared with the opposite side (Fig. 13.6). There may in addition be some true shortening of bone from remodelling. The superior aspect of the head of the femur can be resorbed and the hip displaced upwards (Fig. 13.7). Shortening is measured as the difference in length from the umbilicus to the respective medial malleolus. True shortening is measured as the difference in length from the anterior superior iliac spine to the respective medial malleolus, when the two hips lie in the same degree of adduction.

Once the deformity and the movement of the joint are known, the vascular system should be examined and the neurological state assessed.

Before surgery is contemplated, the general condition of the patient is evaluated, particularly the cardiovascular state and the presence of prostatic symptoms.

CONSERVATIVE TREATMENT
General

General conservative treatment has been described above, and includes analgesics, anti-inflammatory drugs and reduction in the amount of activity of the patient both at work and in the home.

Local

Physiotherapy can help in the form of exercise and short-wave diathermy. A walking stick in the hand opposite the arthritic hip significantly reduces the load on the hip. If the main hip symptom is pain during the extension phase when walking, a 1 cm raise to the heel of the shoe can be of benefit, particularly if there is fixed flexion of the hip.

SURGICAL TREATMENT

Total hip replacement (THR) is the operation of

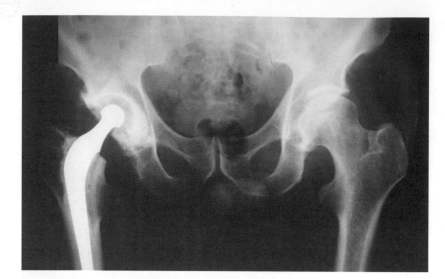

FIG. 13.8 Charnley total hip replacement

choice. Occasionally arthrodesis or osteotomy are appropriate procedures, but the excellent results to be expected by arthroplasty from a THR have largely made the other operative options superfluous.

Historically, THR has developed via using an interpositional metal cup to cover the femoral head in the 1930s, to replacing the femoral head alone in the 1940s. Charnley and McKee independently developed the concept of a THR in the 1960s. They replaced the femoral head and the acetabulum, an advance made possible by the advent of bone cement (Fig. 13.8). With only relatively minor modifications, this concept has remained unchanged for 35 years.

The hip is exposed from the front, the side or the back. The hip is then dislocated, the head of femur excised and the acetabulum reamed. An acetabular cup is inserted into the deepened acetabulum and a metal femoral component into the prepared proximal femur. These are fixed to the bone with bone cement, and the hip is then reduced. The patient can usually be taking a few steps the next day.

The benefits are enormous, usually with relief of pain and a mobile hip. However, there are always surgical risks and these must be discussed with every patient before operation.

COMPLICATIONS OF THR

Eighty-five per cent of patients are well satisfied with their hip replacement. However, there are complications, particularly infection, pulmonary emboli and late mechanical failure of the prosthesis.

Infection after a primary hip replacement is uncommon and is less than 2 per cent, but when it does occur it is disastrous. The prosthesis has to be removed in order to eradicate the infection. There will be long periods in hospital and no guarantee that repeat surgery will be successful. Thus considerable care is taken to avoid infection.

Because infection can be blood-borne, a bacterial analysis of the urine is necessary before surgery. Patients are routinely covered with perioperative prophylactic antibiotics. The operation is carried out in a clean air operating suite. A careful surgical technique is essential, with gentle tissue handling. Postoperative haematoma with its potential for abscess formation is avoided by good haemostasis. Later infection can occur from bacteraemia although it is more likely to be due to pathogens introduced at the time of surgery being 'activated' and multiplying at a later stage. Antibiotic cover is required for infected tooth extraction.

Intraoperative death can occur when the bone cement is introduced into the shaft of the femur. A combination of factors may result in hypotension and cardiac arrest. These may include a chemical reaction of the cement and showers of small bone marrow emboli entering the venous circulation at the time.

Technical error during surgery may damage vessels or major nerves, and incorrect placement of the prosthesis runs the risk of postoperative dislocation.

There is a 30 per cent risk of deep venous thrombosis, which may be somewhat reduced by giving prophylactic anticoagulants preoperatively.

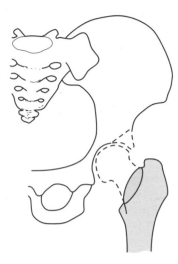

FIG. 13.9   Pseudoarthrosis of the hip (Girdlestone)

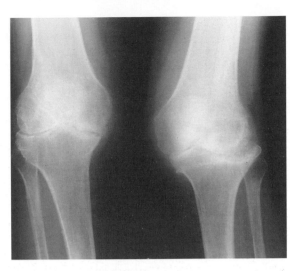

FIG. 13.10   Osteoarthritis of the knee joint in a patient with rheumatoid arthritis

About 1 per cent of patients will develop a pulmonary emboli.

Aseptic loosening will occur in every hip replacement if the patient lives long enough. The average life expectancy of a THR is about 10 years, but youth, an energetic lifestyle, obesity and the male gender are particular risk factors for premature loosening of the hip. For this reason, these patients need careful counselling, and it may be appropriate for them to continue longer than others with conservative treatment. When aseptic loosening does occur, it can be treated by a revision operation, although the overall success rate of revision is only 70 per cent.

Excision arthroplasty (Girdlestone arthroplasty) is an operation that consists of excision of the head and neck of the femur and the upper rim of the acetabulum, leaving a false joint – a pseudoarthrosis (Fig. 13.9). This produces a mobile though unstable joint, which is painless. It is appropriate as an intermediate procedure after removing an infected prosthesis. If the infection can be eradicated after an excision arthroplasty, a new revised THR is possible.

The knee

The knee is the largest joint in the human body nd is subject to great strains. For this reason ordinary wear and tear is considerable and internal derangements that upset the mechanics of the joint are common. Both 'primary' and 'secondary'

osteoarthritis frequently occur. Common predisposing factors are deformities such as genu varum and valgum, osteochondritis dissecans and recurrent dislocation of the patella. In addition, later osteoarthritis can follow trauma – residual ligamentous laxity in either the anteroposterior or the lateral plane and mechanical upsets due to long-standing meniscus injury. Osteoarthritic changes are often first restricted to one part of the joint.

CLINICALLY

The patient complains of pain when walking and sometimes at rest. The fear of losing independence is often a major concern. They have an antalgic gait, limping with a flexed knee. They may stand with a valgus or varus deformity as a result of remodelling of the bone. Joint laxity may be apparent as they stand, with the knee giving way into valgus. The thigh is wasted, and there may be an effusion. The range of movement is limited, usually with fixed flexion and loss of full flexion. There is bony thickening and crepitus as the knee is flexed. Often the patella is relatively immobile (Fig. 13.10).

CONSERVATIVE TREATMENT

Surgery is unnecessary for those patients with minimal disability or for those who respond to conservative treatment. Physiotherapy can teach them to maintain good quadriceps tone. Reduction in body weight, and the use of a walking stick

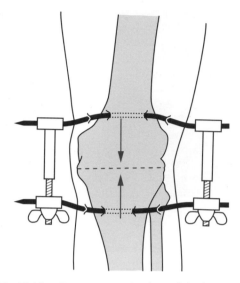

FIG. 13.11   Compression arthrodesis of the knee

reduce the load on the knee. Analgesics and anti-inflammatory drugs may also be helpful. Occasional injections of intra-articular steroids will give periodic relief of pain. An arthroscopic wash-out will also give quite dramatic pain relief to some patients, probably by temporarily changing the metabolic activity of the surface synovial cells.

SURGICAL TREATMENT

Arthrodesis, osteotomy and arthroplasty can all be appropriate surgical procedures for osteoarthritis of the knee. However, arthroplasty is the most commonly performed of these operations.

Osteotomy

In patients under the age of 70 years in whom the joint remains mobile but there is pain and defor-mity, a tibial wedge osteotomy is helpful. The osteotomy may be medial or lateral, to correct a valgus or varus deformity.

Arthrodesis

Arthrodesis relieves pain but is a disability in itself, and can be achieved by using compression (Fig. 13.11). However, it now tends to be a salvage procedure after failed total joint replacement.

Arthroplasty or total knee replacement (TKR)
(Fig. 13.12)

Unconstrained prostheses
In unconstrained prostheses, femoral and tibial surfaces of the knee are replaced, the femoral component being metal and the tibial plastic. These surface replacements are used when the ligaments are intact. Unicompartmental replace-ments are indicated if one compartment is healthy. The positioning of the prosthesis with correct alignment and tension is critical. A few degrees of malalignment can lead to failure.

Semi-constrained prostheses
When the degenerative joint is unstable the larger semi-constrained prosthesis helps stabilize the joint by its shape. It is applicable when the disease is more

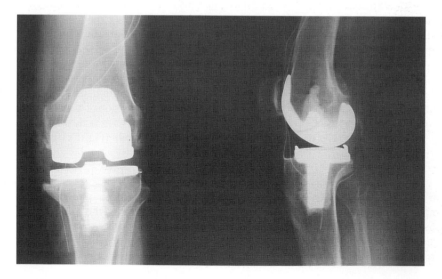

FIG. 13.12   Total knee replace-ment

advanced. There are many different designs. The articular surface of the patella can also be replaced.

Hinge prostheses

Historically, hinge prostheses were the first knee joints to be designed. They tended to fail because the knee is not only a hinge; when flexed, it is able to rotate. This introduces large rotational shear forces on a constrained hinge, with a high risk of aseptic loosening and the loss of bone stock, such as is found in patients undergoing revision arthroplasty. They are also appropriate in tumour excision surgery, in which custom-made prosthesis replace large parts of a limb.

Complications

The complications of knee arthroplasty are similar to those for hip replacement: infection, technical difficulties, deep venous thrombosis and late loosening. There is a greater risk of infection, probably because the prosthesis is more superficial.

The operation usually achieves pain relief, a knee that will fully extend and flex to just above 90°, and a leg that is stable. The failure rate is similar to that of hip replacement.

There are times when knee revision surgery fails and the only procedure available for good function is an amputation. In spite of encouraging results from TKR, these risks have to be explained to every patient.

Other joints

THE UPPER LIMB

In the upper limb, the symptoms of osteoarthritic changes are not so severe. Degenerative changes follow trauma, but tend not to cause the disability found in the weight-bearing joints. Minor changes rarely require very active treatment.

Primary osteoarthritis of the shoulder joint is treated conservatively. Total shoulder replacement can be used, especially if symptoms are severe and keeping the patient awake at night.

In the elbow osteoarthritis may follow trauma. Loose bodies from separated osteophytes can cause intermittent locking and require excision, and total elbow replacement can be performed in the more severe situations (Fig. 13.13). Osteoarthritis of the wrist or carpus after fracture of the scaphoid, with subsequent osteonecrosis, may require surgery. The joint between the base of the first metacarpal and trapezium is another common site for painful osteoarthritis, but this usually responds to conservative treatment – rest and occasional steroid injections. Keinböck's disease, in which the lunate becomes avascular, can cause wrist pain. The terminal interphalangeal joints are affected with generalized osteoarthritis and Heberden's nodes. Symptoms are rarely severe, the changes often being noticed by chance in patients who complain of osteoarthritic changes elsewhere.

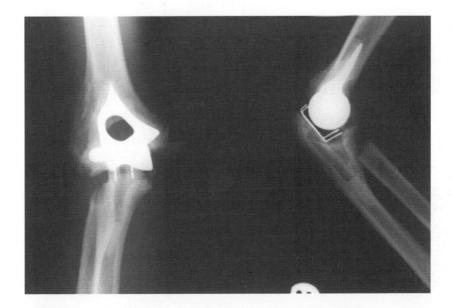

FIG. 13.13 An X-ray of a Souter total elbow replacement

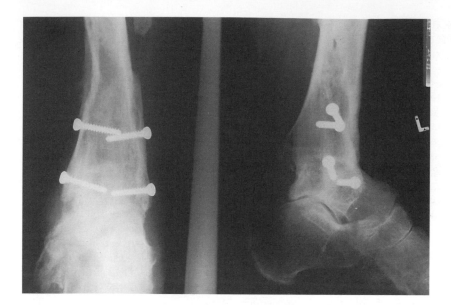

FIG. 13.14   Arthrodesis of the ankle joint

THE LOWER LIMB

In the lower limb, osteoarthritis of the ankle usually follows severe fractures involving articular surfaces. If symptoms prove severe enough, arthrodesis gives good results (Fig. 13.14). Osteoarthritis of the tarsus may be due to deformities such as incompletely corrected congenital talipes equinovarus or trauma. Carefully made arch supports to distribute the weight evenly are often sufficient to control symptoms. If this fails, 'triple arthrodesis' will be effective. Osteoarthritis of the metatarsophalangeal joint of the big toe can also occur.

THE BIG TOE

Of the toes, the big toe is the most important, because the weight is largely taken on the first metatarsal head when standing, and when walking the thrust of the big toe is the most powerful in driving the body forwards.

Most abnormalities of the big toe result from malalignment of the first metatarsal, which may take two forms. First, it may tend to resemble the first metacarpal in the hand, and to point medially (metatarsus primus varus). As a result the toe deviates laterally, leading to the condition known as hallux valgus (Fig. 13.15). This deformity is increased by the bowstring effect of the tendons. Associated with this, the metatarsal head does not take full weight, so the transverse arch is reversed.

Alternatively, the big toe may assume a more horizontal line than the other metatarsals (metatar-

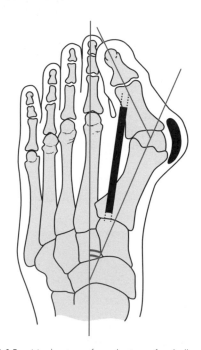

FIG. 13.15   Mechanism of production of a hallux valgus

sus primus elevatus). As a result of this, the big toe is held slightly flexed, so that it can take weight; this, in turn, increases the stresses upon the first metatarsophalangeal joint such that osteoarthritic changes occur, and the joint becomes stiffer; this condition is known as hallux rigidus.

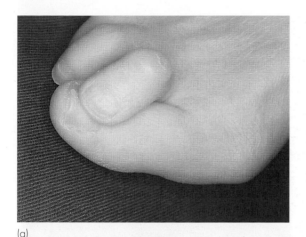

(a)

FIG. 13.16 (a) Patient with hallux valgus with a hammer toe; (b) X-ray of the hallux valgus

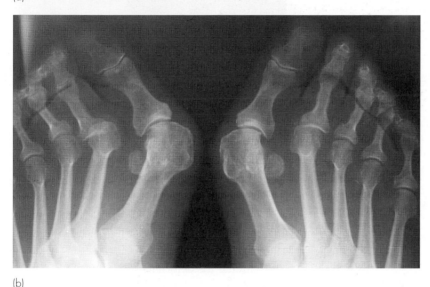

(b)

Hallux valgus

The presenting symptom in hallux valgus is usually pain over the prominent metatarsal head. This is due to rubbing from shoes, and leads to an adventitious bursa (bunion), which may become inflamed or even frankly septic. In addition, metatarsalgia may be troublesome and, if the big toe is markedly deviated, it may cause symptoms from deformity of the second toe, which tends to override the first (Fig. 13.16). There is usually a family history of hallux valgus.

Treatment

Treatment depends upon the age and general condition of the patient. In the very elderly and those with poor circulation, treatment is symptomatic. Surgical shoes, made to accommodate the deformed toes and incorporating metatarsal supports, usually help. In all others, surgery is indicated to deal with the bunion and correct the valgus deformity of the toe, though it is not possible to restore normality. A common operative procedure (Keller's operation) consists of excision of the base of the proximal phalanx and of the prominent metatarsal head on the medial side. This relieves the pressure symptoms but leaves the toe as an inefficient lever (Fig. 13.17).

In younger adults and adolescents (Fig. 13.18) it may be possible to correct the basic deformity by osteotomy of the distal metatarsal shaft, the head being moved laterally and rotated to correct the

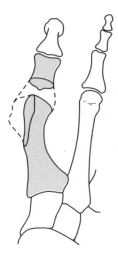

FIG. 13.17   Keller's excision arthroplasty for hallux valgus

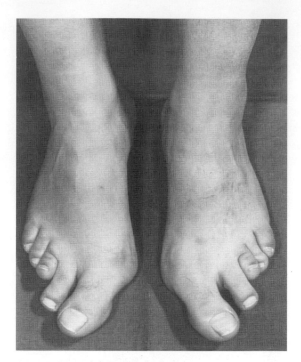

FIG. 13.18   Adolescent hallux valgus

valgus deformity in the toe itself. Another method is to deal with the soft tissues; the bunion is excised, the adductor hallucis tendon is detached from the phalanges and inserted into the metatarsus and the lateral sesamoid is removed. In addition, the resulting 'hammer toe' deformity in the second toe has often to be treated surgically (see below).

Hallux rigidus

Hallux rigidus is osteoarthritis of the first metatarsophalangeal joint. Symptoms are due to pain on movement of the joint, particularly dorsiflexion, and exostosis formation on the dorsum of the metatarsal heads, which in turn leads to adventitious bursa formation similar to, but at a different site from, that occurring in hallux valgus.

Treatment

As with hallux valgus, Keller's operation gives good results in relief of pain in the joint itself, but by impeding the toe's function as a lever, increases the liability to metatarsal pain. It is therefore a useful operation in middle-aged individuals, but in younger patients an attempt to preserve toe function is also desirable. This can be achieved by arthrodesis of the metatarsophalangeal joint, thereby in effect increasing the relative length of the metatarsal bones and leaving the patient with a short single-jointed toe.

THE LESSER TOES

The toes are liable to develop deformities very similar to those occurring in the fingers. In the latter, however, these result from definite injuries to the extensor apparatus whereas in toes they appear to develop spontaneously, possibly being aggravated by footwear.

Hammer toes

The hammer toe deformity, which most frequently involves the second toe because it is often the longest, consists of fixed flexion at the proximal interphalangeal joint, with hyperextension at the distal interphalangeal and metatarsophalangeal joints. It is often seen in conjunction with a hallux valgus.

Clinically, presenting symptoms are due to a painful corn over the prominent head of the proximal phalanx. In addition, owing to dorsal subluxation at the metatarsophalangeal joint, there may be painful callosities under the metatarsal head.

Treatment

A felt pad applied behind the corn may relieve some of the pressure from shoes, and help from a chiropodist is also often useful, but surgery provides the only satisfactory answer. Best results are obtained by fusion of the joint in an extended position, which can be done by converting the head of the proximal phalanx into a peg and fitting this into a hole bored into the base of the middle phalanx (spike arthrodesis). Alternatively, when the passive flexion of the metacarpophalangeal joint is full, excision of the proximal interphalangeal joint may be performed.

Mallet toe

Mallet toe is a flexion deformity of the terminal joint, similar in appearance to a mallet finger (Chapter 7). The cause is not clear and sometimes several toes are affected. Pressure from shoes causes painful corns to develop over the prominent head of the middle phalanx. Sometimes corns also appear on the tip of the toe.

Treatment

Chiropodist's padding may help to control a painful corn, but if it is really troublesome, excision of the head of the offending middle phalanx or amputation of the tip of the toe gives good results.

Adducted fifth toe

Adducted fifth toe is a deformity often present since infancy. The fifth toe is adducted over the fourth toe, and as a result pressure symptoms may follow.

Treatment

In children and young adults the deformity may be corrected by division of the tight dorsal capsule of the metatarsophalangeal joint and extensor tendon, coupled with a V/Y-plasty which enables the skin to be elongated. In older patients the toe should be amputated if it is troublesome.

Subungual exostosis

Subungual exostosis is an outgrowth of bone from the tip of the terminal phalanx, which pushes the nail upwards and causes reactive thickening in the surrounding skin. The big toe nail is that most commonly affected.

Treatment

Treatment consists of gouging the bony lump, sometimes trimming back the nail in order to provide adequate exposure.

The spine (see Chapter 15)

Degenerative change commonly occurs at the lower cervical (C5/6/7) and lower lumbar (L3/4/5) regions of the spine, where there is considerable segmental stress. These changes are almost universal in elderly people. There is good correlation between degenerative changes in the neck and the lower back. These changes may be considered protective in stabilizing the spine.

Osteophytes can, however, compromise the nerve roots and be responsible for pain in a root distribution – root entrapment syndrome. There may be associated nerve root signs: diminished reflex, motor weakness, muscle wasting and sensory loss.

Degenerative spondylolisthesis tends to occur in middle life at L4/5 level, more often in women than in men. There is a forward displacement of one vertebra on another. It can cause back pain, and if the vertebral canal is developmentally small, the neural content of the canal be compromised giving root pain or sometimes neurogenic claudication.

Degenerative lumbar scoliosis also occurs in middle life, with a gradual increase in the scoliosis. It too gives back pain and sometimes root pain or claudication if the vertebral canal is already small.

Treatment

Treatment focuses on the sum and the degree of disability. If back pain is the main problem, this is managed conservatively, or occasionally by surgery to stabilize the spine. If there is a neurological problem, decompressive surgery is necessary when conservative management fails.

INFLAMMATORY ARTHROPATHIES

In inflammatory joint conditions although the joint pathology is usually the dominant feature, this is only part of a generalized disorder. There is systemic disturbance with a raised erythrocyte sedimentation rate, and other tissues are usually involved.

The inflammatory joint diseases can be classified into two groups.

- Seropositive arthritis: rheumatoid arthritis, Felty's syndrome and Sjögren's syndrome;
- Seronegative arthritis: ankylosing spondylitis, Reiter's syndrome, reactive arthritis, psoriatic arthropathy and arthropathy of inflammatory bowel disease.

Rheumatoid arthritis

Rheumatoid arthritis is a generalized disease, more common in women than men, and, although it can present at any age, it usually appears in early middle life.

PATHOLOGY

The disease primarily affects the synovial membrane, which becomes oedematous with inflammatory changes. There is usually a moderate joint effusion. Proliferating synovial tissue affects the edges of the articular cartilage, which become eroded. The subchondral bone becomes affected. The pathology extends to the extra-articular soft tissues with gradual disorganization of the joint and deformity.

The synovial sheaths of the tendons can be affected, with the tendons also becoming involved and sometimes rupturing from attrition.

CLINICAL FEATURES

Usually many joints are involved, but occasionally only one joint is significantly affected. The symptoms may be episodic or steadily progressive. The onset is usually insidious, with vague joint pains often associated with general malaise. There may be morning stiffness. The disease initially involves the small peripheral joints of the hands and feet. In some patients it may progress no further, but in others it will spread to the wrist, knees, shoulders, hips, elbows, ankles, cervical spine and the temporomandibular joint.

SIGNS

The affected joints are swollen as a result of synovial thickening and sometimes a small effusion. There is a boggy sensation when palpating the joint and the skin is usually warm. The first joint to be infected is frequently the index metacarpophalangeal joint followed by the remainder of the metacarpophalangeal joints. As a result of joint instability the fingers drift into ulnar deviation. Tendon imbalance and rupture can produce swanneck and boutonnière deformities of the fingers and a Z-deformity of the thumb. Synovial thickening of the extensor tendon sheaths will produce swelling at the back of the wrist. Involvement of the wrist joint can cause sequential rupture of the extensor tendons of the fingers, beginning first with a dropped little finger.

The skin is paper thin and easily damaged. Rheumatoid nodules can occur, particularly on the extensor surface of the proximal forearm. Thickening of the flexor tendon sheaths in the fingers will cause trigger finger.

Involvement of the subtalar joint will cause a painful valgus foot. Rheumatoid arthritis of the knee and hip causes painful arthritis and flexion contractures.

As the disease progresses the inflammatory component tends to burn out leaving a degenerate joint radiologically indistinguishable from osteoarthritis.

EXTRA-ARTICULAR FEATURES

- Weight loss and fever
- Keratoconjunctivitis sicca (Sjögren's syndrome)
- Rheumatoid lung
- Neurological features:
  a) cervical cord compression, from atlantoaxial subluxation, producing long tract cord signs
  b) entrapment syndromes (e.g. median nerve compression)
  c) peripheral neuropathies
- Anaemia
- Rheumatoid nodules
- Vasculitis.

In children juvenile rheumatoid arthritis is described as Still's disease and has a poor prognosis. It may appear as a mono- or polyarthritis, sometimes with iridocyclitis and pericarditis and frequently hepatosplenomegaly. It can lead eventually to amyloid disease. The combination of rheumatoid arthritis with splenomegaly and neutropenia in adults is known as Felty's syndrome.

INVESTIGATIONS

In patients with rheumatoid arthritis the erythrocyte sedimentation rate is usually raised; this can be used to monitor the activity of the disease. Patients are seropositive if the IgM rheumatoid factor is demonstrated. They are often anaemic. X-rays will demonstrate some reduction in the joint space as a result of erosion of the articular cartilage. There will be subchondral osteoporosis and, subsequently, bone destruction and deformity.

Treatment

Treatment is conservative or surgical.

Conservative treatment

This focuses on the patient's general health, nutrition and elimination of septic foci. The rheumatologist will recommend drugs such as aspirin, paracetamol, indomethacin, gold, penicillinamine, antimalarials (e.g. chloroquine) and sometimes steroids. Physiotherapy is appropriate, with heat to relieve joint pain and stiffness. Wax baths are particularly helpful; the patient places their hands in warm wax and exercises the fingers by removing the hardened wax. Splints particularly at night can relieve pain and discourage the development of deformities. Intra-articular steroid injection can produce remarkable pain relief but this is usually temporary and too frequent injections can cause severe cartilage destruction.

Surgical treatment

This can involve synovectomy, arthroplasty, arthrodesis, tendon surgery and nerve decompression.

A synovectomy means excision of the proliferating synovial tissue from the joints or tendon sheaths. It is sometimes appropriate in the hands, feet and knees. The rationale depends on the assumption that the inflamed synovial tissue causes articular cartilage damage, therefore it is an appropriate procedure early in the course of the disease when synovial swelling is gross. It improves the cosmetic appearance and relieves some of the pain.

An arthroplasty is an excision of the joint. The pathological joint can be replaced with an artificial joint or alternatively a space may be left for fibrous tissue to recreate a false joint. In the hands, silastic joint replacement is effective in the metacarpophalangeal joints of the fingers. There is usually a remarkable improvement in the cosmetic appearance, correcting the ulnar drift, and often some relief of pain, but functionally the patient cannot perform much better after surgery than they did before. In the hip and the knee, joint replacement is similar as for patients with osteoarthritis. In the shoulder and elbow, joint replacement is effective in relieving pain and improving movement but the indications are less frequent in these larger upper limb joints. Excision arthroplasty by removing the head of the radius or the lower end of the ulna can improve function.

Arthrodesis is helpful in selected joints with rheumatoid arthritis. It is more important that the thumb is a stable prop rather than an unstable mobile structure and therefore arthrodesis at the base of the thumb can be appropriate. It is sometimes helpful to arthrodese the neck if an unstable

cervical spine is causing damage to the spinal cord. Cervical fusion can be life saving.

Tendon repair is necessary when the extensor tendons sequentially rupture at the back of the wrist. There may be a sharp prominence of bone at the head of the ulna, which damages the extensor tendons, and therefore the head of the ulna is usually excised. Trigger finger is treated by division of the flexor tendon sheath.

Carpal tunnel decompression is necessary when the median nerve is compressed at the wrist.

Ankylosing spondylitis

Ankylosing spondylitis is an arthropathy that tends to be progressive, leading to bony ankylosis. It begins in the sacroiliac joints and spreads to the spine, particularly in young men. Women can also be affected.

CLINICAL FEATURES

The onset is insidious, with low back pain and stiffness that is worst after rest. It initially affects one side of the lower back first and then the other, sometimes radiating into the back of the thigh. It is worse in the morning and after sitting in a chair, and the symptoms tend to improve with activity. The disease can affect only the sacroiliac joints or, alternatively, it can spread over a number of years to affect the lumbar and thoracic spine, the costovertebral joints with restriction of chest expansion, the shoulders, hips, knees and, occasionally, the temporomandibular joints. The spine becomes ankylosed and stiff and frequently deformed in a marked kyphosis. If the hips are also affected with a fixed flexion deformity, this tends to exaggerate the stooped posture. At a late stage, breathing is entirely abdominal and, because of the restricted chest expansion, this compounds the risk of respiratory infection.

INVESTIGATIONS

The erythrocyte sedimentation rate is raised providing a useful guide to the disease activity. The HLA-B27 antigen is usually present in patients with ankylosing spondylitis, though of course patients can possess this antigen without having the disease. Radiographically, the joints first affected are the sacroiliac joints with loss of clarity of the joint outline. These joints subsequently become fused. As the vertebral bodies are affected they become square in shape. Ossification of the anterior and posterior longitudinal ligaments create the appearance of a bamboo spine. It is not uncommon for an ankylosed spine to spontaneously fracture causing back pain. A bone scan is probably the most useful investigation to identify early pathology in the sacroiliac joint before radiological changes are apparent. The patient is advised to sleep on a hard bed without a pillow in order to minimize the progression of the thoracic kyphosis. Hydrotherapy is useful in maintaining joint mobility. Long-term anti-inflammatory drugs can reduce the progression of the disease. If the hip joints are affected, total hip replacement is effective. Osteotomy of the spine is occasionally indicated in the presence of severe spinal deformity.

Reiter's syndrome

Reiter's syndrome is a triad of arthritis, conjunctivitis and urethritis, and it usually follows a venereal infection with non-specific urethritis. It is more common in men.

There is asymmetrical involvement of the joints, particularly the knees, ankles and metatarsophalangeal joints. X-rays show erosion of the articular cartilage and a periosteal reaction. Its progression is similar to that of rheumatoid arthritis.

Reactive arthritis

Reactive arthritis is an aseptic synovitis in the presence of some other infection in a predisposed individual. For example, aseptic synovitis can occur in rheumatic fever, caused by haemolytic streptococci. Other organisms associated with a reactive arthritis are *Salmonella* and *Shigella*. *Campylobacter* and *Yersinia* are also associated with arthritis, and it also occurs in meningococcal infection. It is the lower limb joints that are usually inflamed. Antibiotics are not required for the aseptic synovitis except for the treatment of the primary condition. Anti-inflammatory drugs are useful in combination with resting the joint in the acute phase, and physiotherapy during rehabilitation.

Psoriatic arthropathy

Psoriasis is a common skin condition of unknown aetiology. It manifests by scaly, hyperkeratotic, pruritic skin lesions found particularly around the elbow and knees. The nails and nail beds can also be infected.

A polyarthritis can be associated. Its prognosis is usually better than that of rheumatoid arthritis.

OTHER JOINT CONDITIONS

Joints may be secondarily affected in other types of disease.

Neuropathic (Charcot's) joints

Neuropathic or Charcot's joints occur in neurological diseases in which there is loss of normal proprioceptive and pain sensation. The normal appreciation of pain and the protective response is absent, resulting in bone destruction, new bone formation and deformity. The joint is swollen and unstable with radiological features of exaggerated degenerative arthritis. The joints most commonly affected are the knee, hip, ankle, shoulder and elbow.

The responsible neurological lesions are either neurosyphilis (tabes dorsalis) or syringomyelia, the latter generally affecting the upper limb joints. This is usually treated by an orthoses to support the joint. Surgery is usually accompanied by poor results because the patient cannot voluntarily protect the surgically treated joint.

Gout

Patients suffering from gout have an abnormality of purine metabolism with a raise blood uric acid. Sodium biurate crystals are deposited in the soft tissues, particularly around the smaller joints.

CLINICAL FEATURES

The patient is usually middle-aged with sudden severe pain in a joint. The metatarsophalangeal joint of the big toe is the usual joint to be first involved, although no joint is immune. The joint is hot, red, and swollen with shiny skin, and it is acutely tender. It is painful both with exercises and at rest, causing sleepless nights. The swelling subsides after a few days, only to recur again sometimes in a different joint. The condition can be activated by trauma or surgery.

The affected joint will steadily become degenerate in association with the deposition of urate crystals. Such deposits can also occur in other soft tissues, particularly in the ears or on the back of the forearm where they are known as tophi.

The kidney can be affected, sometimes with renal failure.

Treatment

Treatment is medical with anti-inflammatory drugs or uricouric agents. The joint is rested in the acute phase. Surgery is not indicated because it will often provoke a new attack.

Pseudogout (chondrocalcinosis)

Pseudogout is an acute inflammatory arthritis in older patients caused by calcium pyrophosphate crystals within the joint. The articular cartilage calcifies, particularly in the knee.

Haemophilia

Haemophilia is a blood dyscrasia in which, as a result of a deficiency in the clotting mechanism, there is a tendency to bleed from minor trauma. Haemarthrosis occurs in the major joints. With recurrent interarticular bleeding, fibrosis is followed by severe damage to the articular cartilage, with resultant stiffness and deformity. The disease occurs only in males, being transmitted by female carriers.

TREATMENT

Patients are informed of the risk and necessity for treatment in specialized units. Anti-haemophiliac globulin is required. The haemarthrosis is treated by rest and protective splintage. Fresh blood or cryoprecipitate may be required to replace the deficient clotting factor.

Synovial chondromatosis

Synovial chondromatosis is an uncommon condition that can affect any joint. The synovium proliferates forming multiple cartilaginous nodules, which are shed as loose bodies into the joint. These may calcify.

TREATMENT

Treatment involves not only removal of the loose bodies, but synovectomy to prevent their recurrence.

Summary
Osteoarthritis of the hip is one of the most common musculoskeletal disabilities. Total hip replacement will usually produce excellent results. Risks, however, must be discussed with each patient. Late loosening is quite common after 12 years. The operation is therefore delayed if possible in the younger patient and in the obese, in whom conservative treatment is recommended. In osteoarthritis of the knee, joint replacement is equally effective when conservative treatment fails. Rheumatoid arthritis is the most common of the inflammatory joint disorders. It is a systemic disease affecting multiple joints requiring a lifetime of treatment. Appropriate surgery can maintain useful function and independence.

EXAMPLE

Osteoarthritis of the hip

Question

History   A 63-year-old woman was referred by her general practitioner for an orthopaedic opinion about her painful osteoarthritic right hip. She could only walk half a mile because of pain. She could not reach down to cut her own toe nails and the pain was keeping her awake at night.

Examination   She weighed 14 stone and was limping heavily with a short right leg. There was a 20° adduction deformity, a 20° external rotation deformity and 30° of fixed flexion on the right side.

Investigations   X-rays showed loss of joint space osteophytes, cystic formation and bone sclerosis.

Surgery   The dieticians helped her lose weight. Hip replacement was successful. She could sleep at night, reach down to her feet and manage her own shopping.

Answer

Night pain was the main reason for referral.

Gross degeneration of the hip with thickening of the capsule and pain had caused fixed deformity and an apparently short leg. The true length of the femur was not significantly reduced.

She is advised to avoid further obesity to increase the life expectancy of the hip replacement and delay the need for surgery to the opposite asymptomatic hip, which has already shown signs of degenerative change.

SOFT-TISSUE PROBLEMS

TENDONS AND THEIR SHEATHS

Tenovaginitis

Tendon sheaths are liable to mild chronic inflammatory thickening known as tenovaginitis. The entrance to the tendon sheath is usually the site at which thickening is most marked. The cause is usually unknown; occasionally, repeated mild traumatic irritation may be a factor, as sometimes the patient can recall doing some repetitive movement involving some strain a short time before the onset of symptoms. Rarely, particularly if more than one site is affected simultaneously, tenovaginitis may be the first sign of rheumatoid arthritis. Indeed, synovial inflammation frequently plays a part in the inflammatory process.

The tendon sheaths in the hand are one of the most common sites, either where the finger or thumb flexors enter their synovial sheaths at the level of the metacarpal head (trigger finger or trigger thumb) or where the abductor pollicis longus (APL) and extensor pollicis brevis (EPB) cross the lower end of the radius at the wrist deep to the corresponding part of the extensor retinaculum (de Quervain's disease).

In trigger finger or trigger thumb the patient becomes gradually aware of a clicking sensation at the base of the affected digit, with some local tenderness. It is usually worse in the morning. Gradually this increases, until eventually on flexion the finger snaps suddenly shut, and then only with difficulty can it be extended, which it also does with a snap. When this occurs very definite thickening can be felt opposite the entrance to the sheath. A similar condition is encountered in infants, when the mother notices an inability to extend the interphalangeal joint.

Treatment consists of an injection of long-acting steroid suspension into the tendon sheath, which may abort the process and afford lasting relief. When, however, it has reached the stage of frequently becoming stuck, surgical division of the constricting sheath along with excision of the proximal 1 cm of the front of the tendon sheath is a simple operation that gives very satisfactory results. In infants, an open operation is required and it is particularly important to identify the digital nerve to the thumb, before the constricting sheath is divided and a portion excised, because the structures are so small.

Tenovaginitis of the EPB and APL at the level of the radial styloid is known as de Quervain's disease. The patient complains of pain at the base of the thumb, localized to the radial styloid, which is aggravated when the thumb is extended. The range of movement is not sufficient to result in clicking, but a definite localized lump can be felt corresponding to the retinaculum.

Treatment in the early stages can once again be a steroid injection, but failure of such measures ought to be followed by division of the tendon sheaths, which again usually gives good results. The terminal cutaneous branch of the radial nerve lies nearby, and therefore should be looked for and avoided.

Carpal tunnel syndrome

In which the median nerve is compressed by a thickened flexor retinaculum (transverse carpal ligament), is usually idiopathic. However, there are some obvious causes, such as osteoarthritis of the wrist, a malunited fracture of the lower radius, ganglia, myxoedema, pregnancy or rheumatoid arthritis. Clinical features include pain, numbness and paraesthesia in the palmar aspect of the thumb, index, middle and radial side of the ring fingers corresponding to the area supplied by the median nerve. Symptoms at night characteristically wake the patient and are relieved by movements. In severe cases, the thenar muscles are somewhat wasted. The condition must be differentiated from the nerve root irritation secondary to cervical spondylosis.

Treatment can be wrist splintage initially but cure can be obtained by open division of the transverse carpal ligament; arthroscopic division of the transverse carpal ligament has proved useful.

Traumatic tenosynovitis

Traumatic tenosynovitis consists of an inflammatory reaction around a tendon as a result of repetitive movements that impose a strain upon it, particularly if performed by an individual who does not normally use that muscle group very much. This usually affects the deep extensors of the wrist on the radial side, although it may occur over the front of the ankle. The patient is usually a fit young adult who has been using the affected limb excessively, often repetitively. Pain on active

movement or passive stressing is the complaint; on examination, in addition to slight local tenderness, swelling and some crepitus can be found.

Treatment consists of rest in a cast or splint for about 3 weeks, after which cautious mobilization and restriction of activity is continued for up to 6 weeks. Steroid injections and local physiotherapy regimes such as ultrasound, heat and interferential treatment may also be used. Anti-inflammatory agents may be given systemically or topically. The same principles of treatment apply whether the sheath of the tendo Achilles, the peroneal tendons or the posterior tibial tendons are involved.

Infective tenosynovitis

Infective tenosynovitis is a serious condition with tendon sheaths in the hand and wrist being those most commonly affected. Acute suppurative tenosynovitis results when organisms enter the tendon sheath either as a result of a direct wound or, more commonly, due to deeper extension of a subcutaneous digital infection. Once infection is in the tendon sheath, it rapidly spreads through its length. In the index, middle and ring fingers this extends from the distal interphalangeal joint to the metacarpal head, but in the little finger the sheath is continuous with the common flexor sheath at the wrist. In the thumb, the tendon sheath also extends to wrist level. There is severe pain in the affected finger, which will be hot and swollen on the palmar aspect throughout its length. It will be held semiflexed, and any attempted movement, active or passive, is acutely painful. Some general constitutional upset is also present.

Treatment by urgent drainage is required. An incision is made into the distended tendon sheath proximally and distally and the pus evacuated. It is then frequently irrigated with the appropriate antibiotic solution. Systematic antibiotics are given in addition. As soon as the acute phase has subsided, cautious gentle mobilization is commenced to minimize adhesion formation between the tendon and its sheath. In the case of the little finger and the thumb, an incision proximally near the wrist is often also required. Chronic infective tenosynovitis can be due to the tubercle bacillus. In this case infection is bloodborne, as with other tuberculous lesions. The flexor tendon sheaths at the wrist are those usually affected. Surgical excision of the entire affected tendon sheaths, followed by cautious gentle mobilization, gives best results.

MUSCULOTENDINOUS LESIONS

At certain sites, where a large muscle group is attached to a bony prominence and where there may have been a history of acute or repetitive trauma, rupture of muscle and tendon fibres can occur. A bony prominence such as the epicondyle of the elbow, the lower pole of the patella or the origin of the longitudinal plantar ligament in the heel are examples of such sites. Stress is concentrated at these points and acute or gradual rupture of the tissues results in chronic inflammation and scar tissue formation.

Flat sheets of tissue, such as the rotator cuff muscles in the shoulder, can also be chronically subject to excessive forces, resulting in their failure. Acute injuries such as to the trapezius muscle in the neck in a 'whiplash' injury may also lead to painful scar tissue formation.

The relatively inflexible scar tissue that remains may then itself be subjected to repeated insults and healing is retarded. In advanced cases slow failure of these tissues results in total degeneration. Healing is then extremely slow as the inflammatory response cannot remove such tissue, thereby preventing the formation of stable scar tissue. A chronic condition is then created, which can be poorly responsive to conservative measures such as steroid injections or rest. However, even stable scar tissue can cause aching sensations and may be subject to increased sensitivity in cold weather.

'Tennis elbow' and 'golfer's elbow'

These terms are used to describe a point of tenderness at the lateral (tennis) or medial (golfer's) epicondyle of the humerus at the elbow. However, these may be induced by industrial exertions as often as by sporting pursuits. Indeed, activities such as typing are more likely to cause lateral epicondylitis, and use of a hammer or screwdriver, a medial epicondylitis, than any membership of a sport's club.

Clinical features include marked local tenderness, usually just in front of the epicondyle. Passive stretching or active contraction of either the extensor muscles for a lateral condition or the flexor muscles for the medial condition will induce pain. Pronation and supination will also be painful

(Mill's manoeuvre). The differential diagnosis ought to include pain referred down the arm in patients with cervical spondylosis. X-rays of the affected area are usually normal.

Initial treatment consists of rest, including advice for the modification of work practices. If this fails, an injection of 1–2 ml 1% local anaesthetic and an anti-inflammatory steroid suspension into the tissues adjacent to the damaged area can afford rapid relief. Such an immediate response to the local anaesthetic is a good diagnostic sign, but the patient must be warned that the steroid may take up to 3 weeks to work. It must be remembered that direct injections of several millilitres of fluid into an already inflamed tendon or muscle is an extremely painful manoeuvre and may do more harm than good to already compromised tissue.

If injection therapy and voluntary use of a sling fail, a period of rest with the elbow flexed to a right angle in a cast for 4–6 weeks should be tried. Should all else fail, open stripping of the common extensor attachment to the lateral epicondyle and elbow capsule is required. This may remove degenerate scar tissue and reactivate the healing process. Alternatively, a local neurotomy may be performed.

'Frozen shoulder' and 'painful arc'

The shoulder is a shallow ball-and-socket joint with superior stability being derived from bony structures, including the acromion, clavicle and coracoid, and also strong ligaments between the bones. Stability in other directions is largely dependent upon the muscles and tendons. The muscles that are inserted into the tuberosities of the humerus ensheath the humeral head and thereby form the 'rotator cuff'. The supraspinatus segment of the cuff is subject to the greatest mechanical strains. The shoulder is also surrounded by a flexible capsule like any other joint. Thickened bands within the capsule form a complex of ligaments that supports the humeral head like a sling. The subacromial bursa lies beneath the acromion and deltoid, and thereby allows the supraspinatus tendon to glide freely.

Pain and stiffness due to inflammation and contracture of any of these tissues will result in a so-called 'frozen shoulder'. However, because of combinations of wear, subluxation and swelling of soft tissues, the greater tuberosity makes contact with the acromion, and pain during abduction will

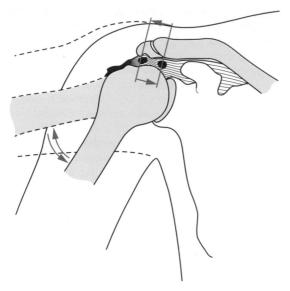

FIG. 14.1   Representation of the cause of 'painful arc' in supraspinatus tendinitis

occur. When the arm is elevated beyond this point so that the bones are no longer touching, pain will be relieved. This is known as a 'painful arc' syndrome (Fig. 14.1).

Supraspinatus tendinitis

Because of inflammation within the rotator cuff, there will be pain in the shoulder on active resisted abduction and some limitation of movement in all directions. 'Painful arc' (90°–140° abduction) is a feature. On palpation, a tender spot will be felt just below the tip of the acromion, but no other abnormality may be found. The results of X-ray and blood investigations will be within normal limits but investigations such as MRI scans can be useful to inspect for tears of the muscle.

Treatment can be by use of a steroid injection into the subacromial space. In addition, local heat, ultrasound and gentle exercises should be prescribed. In patients with persistent pain, partial acromionectomy or division of the coracoacromial ligament may be of help. More generalized conditions such as 'frozen shoulder' (periarthritis), in which all shoulder movements are restricted and painful, should be referred for intensive physiotherapy preceded by a short period of rest in a sling until the acute inflammation settles down. As soon as the pain starts to diminish, exercises should commence, preceded by heat to reduce the muscle spasm. At first these should consist of gentle swinging (pendulum exercises) of the arm within the limits of pain. These passive range of movement

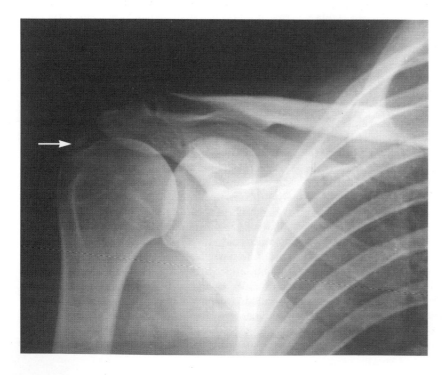

FIG. 14.2 Calcification in the supraspinatus tendon

exercises can then be followed by a progression to active assisted shoulder movements.

The differential diagnosis in such cases must include careful consideration as to whether the shoulder pain might be referred from the cervical spine. Indeed, pain from the fifth and sixth cervical roots often causes spasm of the rotator cuff musculature, which in turn leads to a degree of periarthritis, so that both conditions may be present together.

Occasionally, calcific deposits form within the supraspinatus tendon in degenerate fibres, near its insertion into the greater tuberosity (Fig. 14.2). In the acutely painful stage, steroid injections and even aspiration of the calcified material give dramatic relief from pain. Surgery may occasionally be indicated, involving a general debridement, possible rotator cuff repair and a subacromial decompression, including division of the coracoacromial ligament.

Bicipital tendinitis

The tendon of the long head of the biceps exits through the anterior part of the shoulder joint, to pass via the bicipital groove into the upper arm. Inflammation of the tendon sheath adjacent to the shoulder and in the bicipital groove of the humerus is a largely under-diagnosed condition. It responds well to steroid injection and a short period of immobilization in a sling.

As age increases, degenerative changes take place in the tendon, which becomes frayed and may rupture. There will be tenderness over the humeral head, which will be aggravated if supination of the forearm is attempted against resistance with the elbow flexed. Rupture of the tendon of the long head of the biceps may occur after an interval, or, in an elderly man, may take place quite spontaneously, often with very little pain, so that sometimes it is discovered by chance. The appearance is characteristic as, when the elbow is flexed or the forearm pronated, a marked bridge will appear over the lower part of the biceps muscle. When in the painful phase, the arm should be rested. If rupture of the long head has occurred, this should be accepted, as surgical repair is very difficult and there is no real disability.

Plantar fasciitis

Plantar fasciitis is a condition that usually occurs in middle-aged men, consisting of pain under the heel. Onset is insidious, and the cause is usually obscure. It can occur in rheumatoid arthritis, gout and ankylosing spondylitis. Sometimes it may be bilateral. The tender spot is most commonly just anterior to where the weight is taken, and corresponds to the site of attachment of the plantar fascia to the calcaneum. The pain is aggravated by weight-bearing and, provided no pressure reaches the tender spot, is often almost absent at rest. It is characteristically worse on first taking weight on getting out of bed.

X-rays are usually normal. Occasionally a spur is seen pointing forwards at the site of attachment of the plantar fascia, but these also occur in symptomless heels, so their significance is doubtful.

Spontaneous remission usually occurs after 1–2 years. Soft heel cups and soft padded longitudinal arch supports relieve pressure and reduce traction on the tender area and marked pain reduction is often obtained. A local injection of steroid gives rapid relief.

BURSITIS

Bursae occur wherever the skin crosses a prominent bone and is subject to pressure. In some areas, such as the patella, the tibial tubercle, the olecranon, the ischial tuberosity and the greater trochanter, bursae are found in all individuals. However, a bursa is liable to form, enlarge and become inflamed over any bone that is abnormally prominent, for example those occurring as part of the bunion in hallux valgus.

Prepatellar bursitis ('Housemaid's knee')

Prepatellar bursitis results from pressure on the knee when kneeling on a hard surface. Clinically, there will be a tender fluctuant swelling over the kneecap, with crepitation on palpation, creating the erroneous impression of underlying fractures of the patella. Treatment consists of aspiration after which a pressure bandage is applied. If recurrence rapidly follows, excision of the bursa may be necessary.

Tibial tubercle bursitis ('Clergyman's knee')

'Clergyman's knee' is an infrapatellar bursa, and follows pressure form kneeling upright on a hard surface. Treatment is the same as for housemaid's knee.

Olecranon bursitis ('Student's elbow')

'Student's elbow' occurs after prolonged pressure of the point of the elbow on a hard surface, such as a desk or table. Treatment is as for housemaid's knee.

Ischial bursitis ('Weaver's bottom')

Pain over the ischial tuberosity may follow prolonged sitting on a hard surface. Cushions, steroid injections and local heat and ultrasound therapy will relieve symptoms.

Greater trochanteric bursitis

Fascia lata and the iliotibial band rubbing over a prominent greater trochanter will cause a bursitis in this area. Rest, avoidance of pressure on the area, heat, ultrasound and steroid injections will help.

GANGLIA

Ganglia are common, but their aetiology is still not completely understood. They are cystic swellings containing jelly-like material, which cause pain on movement and other mechanical symptoms.

Ganglia can form in many sites, particularly in the hand and foot. Dorsal ganglia on the wrist always arise from the capsule on the back of the scapholunate joint and communicate with that joint through a tortuous duct that acts as a valve.

Treatment consists of either aspiration of the ganglion or surgery. The operation is justified if the ganglia are painful or disfiguring, but removal must involve excision of the ganglion down to its source in the joint. Removal of part of the capsule of the joint is usually required.

Ganglia on the front of the wrist often lie close to the radial artery. Like ganglia on the back of the wrist, they can arise from the scapholunate joint, but usually come from either the scaphotrapezial or radioscaphoid joint. Injections are not advised because of the proximity of the radial artery. When surgery is indicated, the ganglion should be excised along with its duct down to the joint, including part of the joint capsule.

Ganglia on the front of the fingers are small firm swellings like peas. They arise from the synovial cavity of the flexor tendon and should be excised in continuity with the part of the fibrous flexion sheath from which they arise. Ganglia at the back of the distal interphalangeal joints are called mucoid cysts and are found in older patients with degenerative changes in the underlying distal interphalangeal joint. These cysts frequently recur after excision; surgery to the cyst alone is inadvisable.

Ganglia in other sites can cause pressure on nerves, for example the ulnar nerve of the wrist, and can also be found within bone.

DUPUYTREN'S CONTRACTURE

Dupuytren's contracture is a condition affecting the palmar aponeurosis, in which thickening, fibrosis and contracture occur; the cause is not known. It affects men more than women, and heredity appears to play a part, in that it is more common in Celtic races. It is also found in epileptics and in alcoholics with cirrhosis of the liver. It has also been found to be associated with diabetes.

CLINICAL FEATURES (Fig. 14.3)

Dupuytren's contracture usually starts in middle age, on the ulnar side of the palm. The first sign is a small hard subcutaneous nodule near the base of the ring finger, in the distal palmar skin crease. As it extends, the skin gets increasingly puckered and adherent, and thick subcutaneous strands can be felt, corresponding roughly to the bands of the palmar aponeurosis as it splits on either side of the base of the finger. Eventually the metacarpophalangeal and proximal interphalangeal joints become pulled down, the distal joint remaining unaffected. Both the ring and little fingers may be affected equally, but usually one is more involved than the other. In time, in severe cases, the condition spreads to affect the middle finger, and later the index. Occasionally, nodules occur early at the base of the thumb and index fingers.

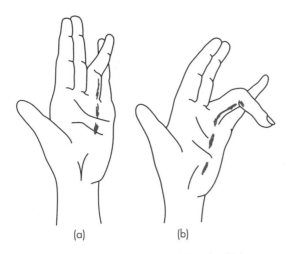

FIG. 14.3 Dupuytren's contracture: (a) early; (b) late

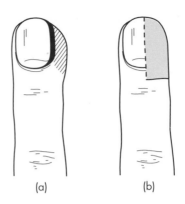

FIG. 14.4 A paronychia: (a) before surgery; (b) after excision and drainage

Often in people prone to Dupuytren's contracture, there is subcutaneous thickening over the dorsum of the proximal interphalangeal joints, known as 'knuckle-pads'. Rarely, the plantar fascia of the foot is also affected.

TREATMENT

Surgery affords the only cure. This must involve excision of all the affected palmar fascia. Skin flaps are raised by careful dissection, and the digital nerves must be carefully dissected free where they pass through the tight band.

When there is a gross flexion deformity of one digit, permanent contracture of the joint capsules may also have occurred, in which case a stiff finger will remain, and amputation gives the best result.

Postoperatively, when sound skin healing has been achieved, a prolonged course of mobilizing exercises, careful stretching and splintage is required to restore full movement.

HAND INFECTIONS

The hand, being the part that is most subjected to injury, is peculiarly liable to infection as a result of some minor trauma such as a prick. In addition, because of its specialized nature, hand infections differ from the boils and abscesses met elsewhere in the body. Tendon sheath infections have already been discussed earlier in this chapter. Other sites

requiring consideration include infection of the nail beds, the finger pulp and the potential deep spaces in the palm, situated between the metacarpals and interossei on one side and the flexor tendons on the other. The causative organism is usually *Staphylococcus aureus* or *Streptococcus pyogenes*, although after an animal bite other pathogenic organisms can be found, including *Pasteurella* species.

Nail bed infection (paronychia) (Fig. 14.4)

Paronychia usually begins as an infection of one side of the base of the nail fold, from whence it spreads across beneath the nail fold, and sometimes also under the base of the nail itself.

TREATMENT

In early cases, local incision, rest and the administration of broad-spectrum antibiotics may abort the attack. If the infection has spread, however, the nail fold must be raised by incisions on either side, and often the base of the nail itself must also be removed.

Pulp space infection

Pulp space infections follow direct inoculation of organisms, as by a prick. Because the finger pulp has many strands connecting the skin to the bone, spread of pus does not at first occur and considerable tension is built up. This, coupled with the normal large number of sensory nerve endings in

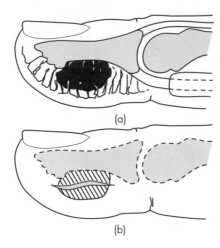

FIG. 14.5   Pulp space infection of the finger: (a) site of pus formation; (b) incision for drainage

a fingertip, makes a pulp space infection extremely painful. In addition, unless the tension is rapidly relieved, osteomyelitis of the terminal phalanx may follow.

TREATMENT (Fig. 14.5)

In early stages it may be possible to abort the attack with antibiotics. If the abscess is obviously pointing beneath the surface a direct incision is required, but otherwise, to avoid scarring on the sensitive fingertip, a lateral incision should be made.

Deep fascial space infections

Because the potential space deep to the flexor tendons is divided into two parts by a vertical septum running along the length of the third metacarpal, there are two 'spaces' – that on the radial side being known as the thenar space, and that on the ulnar side being known as the mid-palmar space. The spaces extend superficially to the webs between the fingers. Injections may reach these spaces by direct inoculation as a result of wounds at the bases of the digits, or as a result of spread proximally from more superficial lesions (Fig. 14.6).

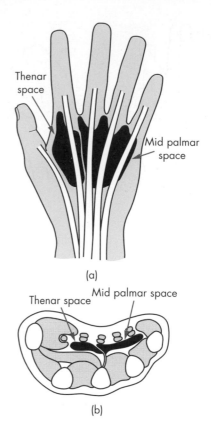

FIG. 14.6   Anatomy of the palmar fascial spaces: (a) anteroposterior view; (b) in section

CLINICAL FEATURES

Because the infection is deep, pointing of the pus is unlikely to occur until late. There will be marked pain and swelling in the palm of the hand, with stiffness of the fingers and oedema of the dorsum of the hand. In thenar space infections there will be swelling in the web of the thumb.

TREATMENT

Drainage is by incisions into the web spaces either between the thumb and index finger in the case of thenar space infections or between the middle and ring or ring and little fingers (depending upon where the swelling is most marked) in the case of the mid-palmar space.

EXAMPLE

Musculotendinous lesions

A 60-year-old man presents with pain in his right shoulder, which has developed suddenly. He is unable to lift his arm above about 60°, because of the pain.

Questions
■ What is the possible diagnosis?
■ What is the treatment?

Answers
■ A painful arc syndrome is due to
  (a) supraspinatus tendon inflammation
  (b) fracture of the greater tuberosity
  (c) acromioclavicular joint degeneration
■ Treatment after arranging for X-rays is to inject the subacromial space with steroids and local anaesthetic, followed by physiotherapy to the arm and shoulder.
■ Restrictions of all movements suggest frozen shoulder. (Don't forget that scapular movement allows for 60° of shoulder abduction.)

15 SPINE

THE SPINE IN HEALTH AND DISEASE

Human beings are unique among primates in adopting the upright posture. This places considerable stress on the lumbar spine, but its form is a remarkable match to its function. The spine has three distinct functions. The first is its strength to support the upright posture, the second is its mobility, enabling function in a variety of postures and the third is the protective function for the spinal cord and the cauda equina below L2.

Strength

Each vertebral body with a cortical shell and inner cancellous structure is ideally designed to provide strength and lightness of weight. The lower vertebrae are larger than those more proximal with the greater cross-sectional area in the lower spine to match the greater load. The intervertebral discs that permit largely sagittal movement in the lumbar spine, rotation in the thoracic spine and combined movements in the neck, are also remarkably strong. The annulus is arranged in multiple layers of parallel collagen fibres alternately orientated at 60° to the vertical. This radial ply effect causes the disc merely to bulge when subjected to axial load. If a patient falls from a height landing on the feet, the vertebral bodies will fracture before a healthy disc is injured.

Mobility

The intervertebral disc is the largest avascular structure in the body (Fig. 15.1). It is composed of a lattice of collagen interspersed with very large molecules of proteoglycan. The high osmotic pressure attracts water into the disc with the nucleus having 90 per cent water concentration. The water content of the disc reduces to 70 per cent in later life. There is an equilibrium between the osmotic pressure attraction water into the disc and the hydrostatic pressure extruding water from the disc. In recumbence, fluid is imbibed into the disc with a gain of about 17 mm in height after 1 hour of recumbency. This diurnal change has some nutritional benefit, particularly for the transport of small molecules.

Many discs develop fissures, which are frequently symptomatic. A disc protrusion occurs when a fragment develops within a fissure and then only a small axial load can extrude the fragment usually in a posterior direction. This will cause the posterior annulus to bulge – protrusion – and sometimes the annulus will tear completely – herniation. If the fragment of disc ruptures completely through the annulus to lie within the vertebral

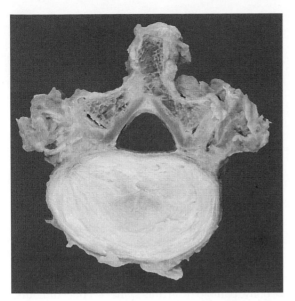

FIG. 15.1 A lumbar vertebra showing a normal lumbar disc

canal, this is called a sequestration. The patient may experience the first symptoms of disc protrusion when the annulus suddenly bulges with stretching of the pain sensitive peripheral fibres, or when the fragment completely herniates into the vertebral canal. They usually believe this is a significant injury when in fact the pathological process has been developing asymptomatically for years.

Protection

The vertebral canal is the important segmental tunnel of bone that protects the spinal cord and, below L2, the cauda equina. There is usually 30 per cent more room within the vertebral canal than is occupied by the dural contents, which provides a margin of safety for any compromising lesion. Thus a disc protrusion can bulge backwards into the vertebral canal giving some back pain but not affecting the cauda equina, provided the vertebral canal is of adequate size.

Thirty per cent of individuals will have a symptomless disc protrusion by the time they reach 60 years of age. Only a minority who develop a protrusion will have nerve root problems because of a small vertebral canal. Similarly, degenerative osteophytes can develop at the edge of the vertebral canal without affecting nerve function, and segmental movement can occur with vertebral displacement (spondylolisthesis) without any neurological

problem. However, some individuals have a constitutionally small vertebral canal and these are the ones at risk of neurological complications when other pathologies encroach into the canal.

The vertebral canal reaches maturity at a very early age. The area of the canal and the midsagittal diameter is of adult size by 1 year of age, which suggests that if there are environmental factors affecting the canal size, these must operate very early in life. Maternal and child health-care programmes may thus have significance for back pain in later life. In general, however, the spine's design is ideal for its function. It is strong, mobile and protective and only when environmental insults damage the bone, affect disc nutrition or stunt the canal's growth do problems arise.

- Failure of bone (fracture) – see Chapter 5
- Failure of the motion segments (backache)
- Failure of protection (neurological compromise)

THE MOTION SEGMENT AND BACK PAIN

PATHOLOGY

The motion segment is a three joint system: the intervertebral disc and the two facet joints. Segmental movement permits smooth restrained motion but if there is excessive or erratic motion, this can be a cause of chronic back pain. This is difficult to discriminate from other causes of back pain (painful facet joints, painful end-plates, strained ligaments and muscles). They are sometimes grouped together as mechanical back pain when the cause is believed to be a mechanical problem and when symptoms are aggravated by mechanical strain. The exact cause of the pain is generally unknown.

CLINICAL FEATURES OF CHRONIC BACK ACHE OF MECHANICAL ORIGIN

The pain is in the lumbar region, sometimes referred to one or other side, sometimes round the pelvis or into the thighs. It can be constant or intermittent and is aggravated by bending, lifting, carrying, standing and walking far and it is often improved by lying down. Lumbar movements may be limited; the painful segment is usually tender to spinal palpation. There are usually no abnormal neurological signs.

SPONDYLOLISTHESIS

When a vertebra is displaced in the sagittal plane, this is described as spondylolisthesis. There are 5 types of spondylolisthesis:

- dysplastic (Fig. 15.2)
- isthmic (Fig. 15.3)
- degenerative
- traumatic
- pathological.

The degree of slip is graded from I–IV.

I   <25% slip
II   25–50% slip
III 50–75% slip
IV   >75% slip.

It can be a cause of mechanical back pain. Isthmic spondylolisthesis occurs when there is a bilateral defect in the neural arch (pars intra-articularis). If there is a defect without displacement, it is described as spondylolysis and when there is anterior displacement of the vertebra it is a spondylolisthesis. The condition occurs in 5 per cent of the population, probably as a result of a stress fracture in childhood. There is a familial predisposition. It is generally asymptomatic. When a pre-existing defect is strained it can produce temporary back pain or sometimes long-standing back pain requiring spinal fusion. Degenerative spondylolisthesis occurs usually at L4/5 level, particularly in middle-aged women when the degenerate facet joints do not satisfactorily restrain shear. The fourth lumbar vertebra displaces slightly forwards, and with an intact neural arch this can cause a spinal stenosis, sometimes with back pain and sometimes with root pain. If pain is severe the spine is both decompressed and fused.

DIFFERENTIAL DIAGNOSIS

Back pain is a symptom of many different pathologies that need to be excluded:

- non-spinal causes – gynaecological, renal, pancreatic and aortic aneurysm;
- bony pathology in the spine – bone tumours, primary and metastases, multiple myelomatosis, leukaemia, osteomyelitis and tuberculosis;
- intradural and extradural tumours.

MANAGEMENT OF PATIENTS WITH CHRONIC BACK PAIN

Back pain of mechanical origin has a lifetime prevalence of about 70 per cent. It is generally temporary and self-limiting, sometimes requiring a day or two

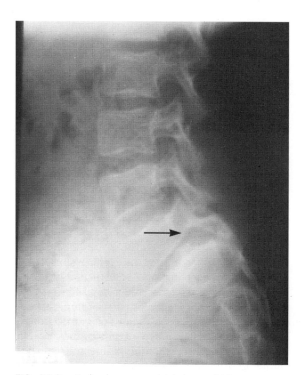

FIG. 15.2   A dysplastic spondylolisthesis of L5

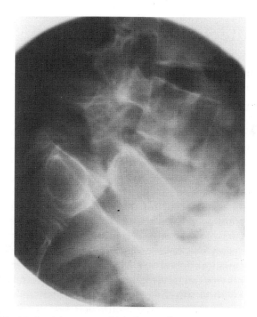

FIG. 15.3   Isthmic spondylolisthesis of L5

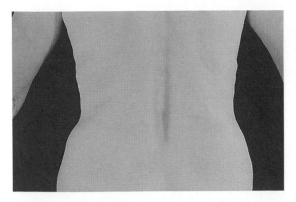

FIG. 15.4 Low back pain patient with muscle spasm

in bed. However, in a few patients it can be a chronic problem (Fig. 15.4) and management is then difficult. Therapeutic options are physiotherapy, rehabilitation to strengthen the spine, back school for education and a temporary corset. Failure of conservative management may require spinal fusion (Fig. 15.5) or ligament reinforcement.

NEUROLOGICAL COMPROMISE

There are three common neurological problems associated with lumbar spine pathology: disc protrusion, root entrapment from lateral canal stenosis and neurogenic claudication. They have well defined criteria and are easily diagnosed.

Disc protrusion

PATHOLOGY

The disc is either bulging or there is a sequestrated fragment of disc that has herniated through the annulus, compressing the nerve against the neural arch (Fig. 15.6).

SYMPTOMS

The pain is first experienced in the back as the annulus stretches and tears. If the nerve root is compressed, the root pain is then felt in the buttocks and down the back of the thigh to the calf, often with pins and needles in the foot. The root pain is often made worse by coughing.

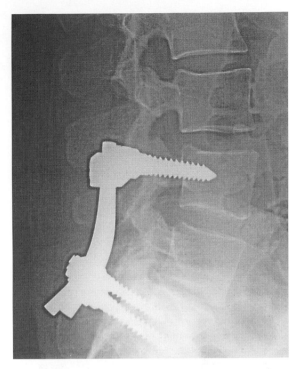

FIG. 15.5 Spinal fusion using bone grafts and pedicular fixation of the spine

SIGNS

There are two important signs. The first is limited straight-leg raising. With the patient lying supine and the head resting on one pillow, the examiner puts a hand under the heel and lifts the straight leg off the couch. In health the straight leg should be easily raised to 90° of flexion. In the presence of a symptomatic disc protrusion, the leg may only raise up to 30 or 40°. This root tension sign is pathognomonic of a disc protrusion. The second important sign is a trunk list. When standing the patient is tilted over to one side, usually to the left. This is not due to a short leg or to a structural scoliosis because the list disappears if the patient lies down or if gravity is abolished. This sign is present in about 50 per cent of patients with disc protrusion and is specific for a protruding disc. Nerve function may be severely affected with reduction of the knee or ankle reflex, some reduction in sensation in the appropriate dermatome (big toe – L5, outer foot – S1). There may be motor weakness of dorsiflexion of the big toe. These abnormal nerve function signs are signs of dysfunction. They confirm nerve root pathology but not its cause.

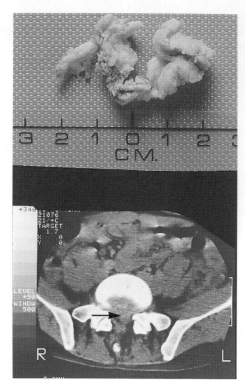

FIG. 15.6   A sequestrated disc and the preoperative CT scan

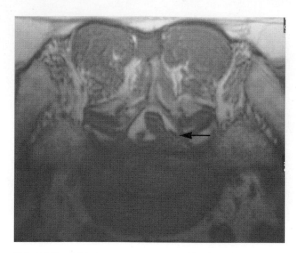

FIG. 15.7   MRI showing sequestrated lumbar disc

MANAGEMENT

Most patients with a symptomatic disc protrusion causing root symptoms will improve with a few days bedrest. It becomes an emergency if there is such a massive disc protrusion that the nerves to the bladder are affected. The patient either cannot pass urine or is incontinent because of damaged sacral roots, which is associated with perianal anaesthesia. However, in the absence of these signs, the patient can be safely nursed in bed at home and most will make a steady recovery over a week or two. When there is no improvement in the straight-leg raising after 3 or 4 weeks, surgery is indicated. After appropriate imaging (MRI or CT) (Fig. 15.7) the disc protrusion/sequestration is surgically removed.

Root entrapment from lateral stenosis

PATHOLOGY

The pathology is in the root canal – the lateral part of the vertebral canal that extends to the intervertebral foramen and contains the nerve root and the posterior root ganglion. Space can be at a premium and when the root canal is constitutionally small and is then compromised by degenerative change from the facet joint or a degenerate rim of disc, the nerve root can become symptomatic.

SYMPTOMS

The pain is felt in a root distribution, in the back of the thigh into the calf and foot. This is generally quite severe and because of the degenerative change the patient is usually in mid to late adult life. Unlike the pain in disc protrusion, it is not aggravated by coughing.

SIGNS

Signs are usually few. Lumbar extension is often limited because this further narrows the root canal, but straight-leg raising is good and the patient does not have a trunk list. If the root is badly damaged there may be a weak reflex, some sensory loss or motor weakness.

MANAGEMENT

Although the small root canal and the degenerative change remains, many of these patients will make a steady recovery with the pain settling down over a few months. If the pain is severe, an epidural injection of steroid can help. Surgical decompression of the root canal may be necessary in certain patients.

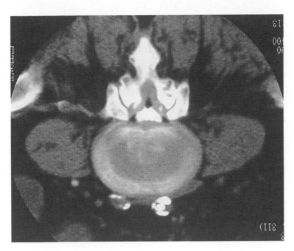

FIG. 15.8   CT showing spinal stenosis

Neurogenic claudication

PATHOLOGY

Patients with neurogenic claudication have spinal stenosis usually at two levels. If the central canal is stenosed at around venous pressure at two levels, the intervening segment of the cauda equina becomes congested with a build-up of metabolites in the nerve roots. At rest this is no problem but with exercise there is a failure of arterial vasodilatation. The arterial vasodilatation of the cauda equina, which is normally associated with motor activity, fails and there is impairment of bilateral motor conduction when walking. Sometimes there is a single level central canal stenosis and a more distal unilateral root canal stenosis, which causes congestion of one nerve root and produces unilateral claudication when walking. Neurogenic claudication rarely occurs under 50 years of age.

SYMPTOMS

These patients have had quite a long history of back pain and a shorter history of discomfort in their leg(s) when walking. They have no symptoms in the legs at rest but after walking 30–100 m, the leg(s) become(s) uncomfortable, heavy and tired and after walking a little further they have to stop. After a period of rest the symptoms settle and they can walk again. Leaning forward seems to help because it increases the available space in the vertebral canal. They are better walking up a hill, stooping forwards, than down a hill leaning backwards and they can often cycle in comfort. The effect of posture on the symptoms is in contradistinction to intermittent claudication from peripheral vascular disease. Sometimes the two types of claudication coexist.

SIGNS

There are few abnormal signs apart from an inability to extend the spine. Many patients will have a 'Simeon stance', standing with the hips and knees flexed, slightly stooping forwards. There are generally no abnormal neurological signs. Imaging with MRI, CT or myelography will confirm the spinal stenosis (Fig. 15.8).

MANAGEMENT

Most patients with neurogenic claudication require no more than reassurance that the symptoms having reached a plateau will probably not increase. These patients do not develop a serious neurological problem, they do not go off their legs and they often learn to accept their limitations. In a few patients calcitonin 100 units 4 times a week for 4 weeks may improve the blood supply to the nerves and can have a long-standing effect. Surgical decompression will improve the walking distance in the disabled patient.

THE CERVICAL SPINE (Fig. 15.9)

Many of the conditions found in the lumbar spine are also found in the cervical spine and include:

- infection: osteomyelitis and disc space infection
- neoplasms: benign and malignant
- trauma.

Local causes of disorders of the cervical spine include intervertebral disc protrusion, and chronic cervical disc degeneration with or without nerve root entrapment – cervical spondylosis.

Intervertebral disc protrusion

In the neck, disc lesions are most common at the lower two spaces, between C5/6 and C6/7 vertebrae, which is where the mobile part of the cervical spine joins the more rigid thoracic spine. An

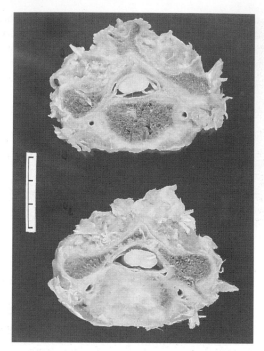

FIG. 15.9 Cross section of the anatomy of the cervical spine

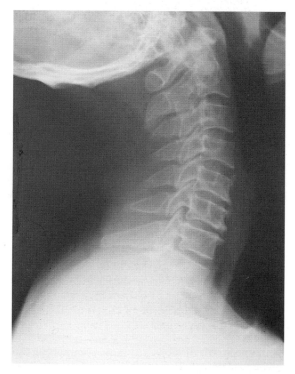

FIG. 15.10 Lateral x-ray of the neck showing cervical spondylosis

acute cervical disc prolapse is relatively uncommon, the patient presenting with an acute pain in the neck. They are unable to move their neck, and if the disc sequestrates there may be pain radiating into the upper limb, from nerve root compression.

Clinical examination reveals a stiff neck with clear neurological signs if the nerve roots are compressed. Unless the cord is compressed there will not be any long tract signs.

INVESTIGATIONS

These include plain X-rays of the cervical spine and MRI if the pain does not resolve and surgery is indicated.

TREATMENT

As in a lumbar disc prolapse, the majority of patients will respond to conservative treatment:

- rest
- sedation and analgesics
- cervical traction, if necessary.

If the pain persists, or if the spinal cord is compromised, or the root pain is not resolving, surgical decompression of the disc is required. The affected disc is removed by the anterior approach.

Cervical spondylosis (neck pain)

Degenerative changes of the lower intervertebral disc occur frequently; indeed, they may be visible on X-ray and yet be symptomless. However, as in the lumbar spine, disc degeneration can result in instability which can lead to neck pain and nerve root pain.

The patients are usually within the age range of 40–60 years and may present with neck pain, headaches and arm pain. About 60 per cent of these patients also have associated low back pain. On examination they have limitation of rotation, with pain on extension. There may be a localized tender spot in the spine or shoulder, and they have paraesthesia along the affected dermatome. Clear signs of muscle wasting and of sensory and reflex loss are not common.

INVESTIGATIONS

The most information can be achieved from lateral X-rays of the cervical spine in flexion and

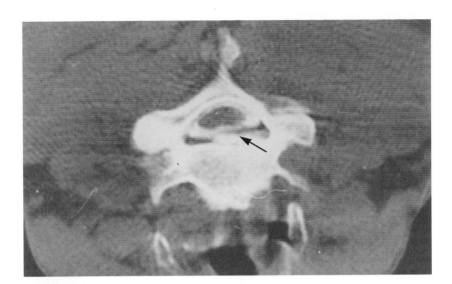

FIG. 15.11   A CT scan with contrast of the cervical spine, showing osteophyte encroachment of the nerve

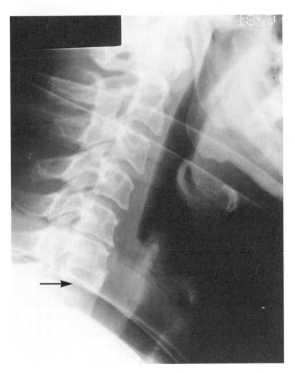

FIG. 15.12   Anterior cervical fusion between C6 and C7

TREATMENT

The vast majority of patients with this common condition are best treated conservatively:

- rest the neck in a collar
- physiotherapy
- analgesics
- non-steroidal anti-inflammatory drugs (NSAIDs).

In selected patients anterior decompression and interbody fusion will bring relief of their symptoms (Fig. 15.12).

SCOLIOSIS

Scoliosis is a deviation of the spine from the sagittal plane, and may be due to an abnormality in the spine itself (structural) or because the spine is held tilted (postural). Curves are of two types: primary, resulting from the causal pathology; and secondary, of which there may be two – one above and one below the primary – to compensate for the main curve.

Postural scoliosis

Postural scoliosis may be caused in a number of ways. The tilt in the lumbar spine resulting from the muscle spasm associated with an acute disc prolapse, already described in this chapter, is an example of this. The more common cause of a permanent postural scoliosis is that which results

in extension (Fig. 15.10). Other investigations, if surgical treatment is considered, include nerve conduction studies, MRI or CT scanning with contrast (Fig. 15.11).

from the natural attempt to compensate for an inequality in leg lengths. In the latter case, in all but minor differences in leg lengths, structural alteration in the shape of the vertebrae follows, so what was at first postural becomes structural. When a postural curve is present, if the cause is removed the spine will completely straighten itself.

Structural scoliosis

Scoliosis can lead to impairment of respiratory function and to backache in middle age; idiopathic scoliosis presents a particular cosmetic problem as well. Structural scoliosis may be subdivided into several groups.

CONGENITAL

The cause of congenital scoliosis is some gross structural abnormality, such as the congenital absence of half a vertebra (hemivertebra) or fusion of several ribs on one side. The deformity is usually obvious at birth, hence the term congenital. Congenital spinal deformities are rigid, and if there is a growth asymmetry they progress steadily, with an accelerated rate of progression at the adult growth spurt. Unsegmented bars are the most notorious, and can lead to spinal cord compression because of unequal growth.

Treatment

Treatment is surgical in curves over 50°, and particularly in those congenital fusions in which there is an unsegmented bar. Surgery may be either by a posterior fusion *in situ* or by vertebral excision and posterior fusion combined with internal fixation.

NEUROMUSCULAR

Neurogenic

When the muscles on one side of the spine are paralysed, a curve will develop. Naturally, if the paralysis occurs before growth has ceased, the deformity will be more marked than if it occurs in adult life. Common causes of paralytic scoliosis are anterior poliomyelitis, severe spina bifida with a meningomyelocele (Chapter 19) and, less commonly, neurofibromatosis and syringomyelia. Neurogenic scoliosis may arise in children with cerebral palsy and spinal muscular atrophy (Fig. 15.3). Paralytic curves are characterized by the fact that a large number of vertebrae are involved in

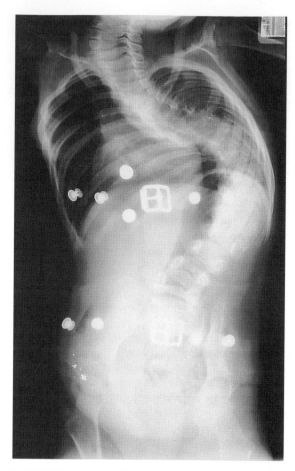

FIG. 15.13   An X-ray of neurogenic scoliosis in a child with spinal muscular atrophy, who is standing in a brace

the primary curve. If the paralysis is severe the deformity may be gross.

Scoliosis associated with neurofibromatosis is probably due to a combination of local paralysis of the small muscles of the spine and the tumour of the nerves forcing open the intervertebral foraminae. These curves often appear to be very sharply angulated.

Myopathic

Muscular weakness such as occurs in Duchenne muscular dystrophy (Chapter 19) can lead to scoliosis and kyphoscoliosis.

Treatment

The treatment is by surgery, which is extensive because the whole curve needs to be corrected. This can be done by anterior spinal fusion combined

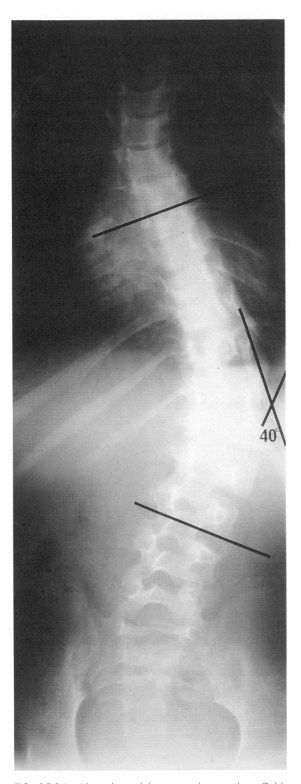

FIG. 15.14 Idiopathic adolescent scoliosis with a Cobb angle of 40°

with instrumentation, by a posterior spinal fusion combined with instrumentation or by both anterior and posterior spinal fusion with instrumentation.

IDIOPATHIC

The most common example of scoliosis developing in childhood is labelled 'idiopathic', as the causal pathology remains obscure. In the primary curve not only is there a lateral bend but also the vertebrae themselves are rotated, the bodies being displaced further to the side than the neural arches. This, in the thoracic region, results in the ribs in the convex side being very prominent posteriorly, the resulting rib hump thereby exaggerating the deformity. On the other hand, if the primary curve is in the lumbar region it is much less noticeable, and may pass unobserved until secondary degenerative osteoarthritis causes backache in middle life.

Idiopathic scoliosis can be divided according to the age of presentation:

- infantile – up to 3 years;
- juvenile – between 4 and 10 years;
- adolescent – 10 years onwards.

There is an important genetic factor in the aetiology of idiopathic scoliosis and the incidence is around 2:1000 children. However, infantile idiopathic scoliosis occurs mainly in boys, whereas in adolescent idiopathic scoliosis, girls predominate.

In general, the earlier in life the curve appears the more potential there is for deformity to become severe. In adolescent idiopathic scoliosis, after the growth spurt the curves tend to deteriorate and deformity can become quite marked. It is obviously relevant to determine when the spinal deformity first appeared and also vital to know whether there is pain. Essentially, idiopathic curves should not be painful.

CONNECTIVE TISSUE DISEASES

Examples of connective tissue diseases that cause structural scoliosis are Marfan's syndrome and Osteogenesis Imperfecta.

TRAUMA

Scoliosis can develop after a fracture or after an extensive laminectomy.

Investigations

X-rays are important to measure the angle of the curve and to detect any bony deformity (Fig. 15.14).

These X-rays should include the whole spine and iliac crests, and should be anteroposterior and lateral.

Cobb's angle is the maximum angle between the vertebral bodies on each end of the structural curve and is the record of the angulation of the curve.

The maturity of the skeleton is assessed by the appearance of the iliac crest apophyseal line.

Treatment

Treatment may be conservative or operative.

Conservative treatment consists of exercises and spinal supports. The supports can be used to hold the curve until surgery is indicated.

However, if there is an increasing curvature in the growing child or there is asymmetry of the trunk producing a severe deformity, operative intervention is advocated. The precarious blood supply of the spinal cord, particularly at the level of the scoliosis, must be considered. Methods of treatment available include fusion of facet joints on both sides of the curve and instrumentation with metal rods along the vertebral column to correct the curve.

Anterior fusion may also be used, particularly in thoracolumbar or lumbar scoliosis, in which correction of the curve can be achieved.

Summary

Back pain is the most common single cause of absenteeism from work. Most episodes settle down naturally over a few days. In chronic low back pain it is difficult to identify the exact pain source. Treatment is therefore difficult. It might involve analgesics, physiotherapy, manipulative treatment, educational advice, energetic exercise programmes, the pain clinic or surgery. Pain affecting the leg is easier to diagnose – disc protrusion or root entrapment from degenerative change – and the natural history of these root pathologies is good. Surgery is required in a minority. Bladder dysfunction is the only absolute indication for urgent disc surgery. Neurogenic claudication usually affects the elderly, and is due to a two-level spinal stenosis.

EXAMPLE

Neurological compromise

Question	Answer
History A 33-year-old factory worker helped a colleague to lift a heavy component and experienced sudden pain in the lower back. He left work early. His doctor visited him at home and the next day advised him to stay in bed.	Sudden onset back pain resulting in going to bed is often caused by disc protrusion, stretching the posterior annulus.
Progress 3 days later he was no better. The pain radiated down the left leg to the foot. It was aggravated by coughing.	After a few days the protrusion may compress one of the nerve roots, causing root pain.
Signs he could not stand up straight but was listing to the left. Straight-leg raising was 60° on the right and 30° on the left. The left ankle was reduced.	The root tension sign of limited straight-leg raising is the most important sign in disc protrusion.
Management The patient was given analgesics and advised to rest at home (not strictly in bed).	There is no urgency about referral to hospital provided there are no urinary symptoms such as loss of bladder control suggesting a central disc protrusion and cauda equina compression.
At 2 weeks The leg pain had settled down. Straight leg raising was 90° on the right and 70° on the left.	With continued improvement a good prognosis can be expected. This episode may well settle down. Further recurrences can be expected. Physiotherapy advice in a 'back school' is appropriate.

The cause of bone infection is either direct contamination of an open fracture or at surgery, or alternatively infection may be indirect and blood-borne from a distant primary source. It may be acute or chronic.

ACUTE HAEMATOGENOUS OSTEOMYELITIS

Acute haematogenous osteomyelitis is an acute infection of bone from blood-borne pathogenic organisms.

PATHOLOGY

Organisms will enter the bloodstream causing bacteraemia from any focus of infection, but usually these bacteria do not survive. If, however, they reach devitalized tissue the body's defence is impaired and they can cause a secondary infective lesion. A haematoma may result from trivial trauma and provide such a devitalized site for acute haematogenous osteomyelitis. Acute osteomyelitis occurs most frequently in the metaphysis of long bones in children and,

perhaps because the knee is prone to minor trauma, the lower end of the femur and the upper end of the tibia are most commonly affected. The responsible organisms are *Staphylococcus aureus*, *Streptococcus pyogenes* and *Pneumococcus*. However, *Haemophilus influenza*, *Escherichia coli*, *Proteus vulgaris*, *Pseudomonas aeruginosa* and *Salmonella* are sometimes isolated.

The medullary cavity cannot expand, and considerable tension builds up in the metaphysis, forcing pus through the Haversian canals to form a subperiosteal abscess. The underlying bone surrounded by pus is then deprived of its blood supply. Unless pus is evacuated early, a segment of bone will die and eventually separate as a sequestrum (Fig. 16.1).

The raised periosteum continues to form new bone, which surrounds the sequestrum. This new layer of bone is known as an involucrum. The abscess eventually bursts through the periosteum tracking to the surface as a sinus. By the time a sequestrum has formed the disease has reached the chronic stage and is difficult to eradicate. This should be prevented by early diagnosis and adequate treatment.

CLINICAL FEATURES

Acute haematogenous osteomyelitis usually affects the long bones in children or adolescents but

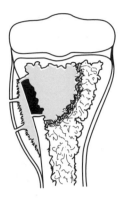

FIG. 16.1 Chronic osteomyelitis showing the formation of a sequestrum and involucrum

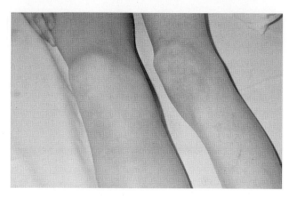

FIG. 16.2 Acute haematogenous osteomyelitis of the right tibia, the leg is swollen and acutely tender

osteomyelitis of the spine tends to occur in adults. The child complains of a sudden onset of very severe pain in the limb with toxaemia and a high temperature. A small infant is unable to localize the pain and presents simply as a fretful child with a high pyrexia. They refuse to walk, are anorexic and obviously toxic. The affected bone is acutely tender but because the child is fretful it is often difficult to localize the site of tenderness. The clinician must gain the child's confidence and gradually palpate from areas peripheral to the suspected lesion until the maximum site of tenderness is identified. In the early stages when the infection is within the metaphysis there is no significant local heat or swelling (Fig. 16.2). However, these signs rapidly follow as a subperiosteal abscess develops. It is often possible to obtain a history of some minor injury a few days earlier or of an apparently insignificant infective lesion such as a sore throat or a skin pustule.

The epiphyseal growth plate is a barrier to the spreading infection, which tends to track to the surface of the bone (Fig. 16.3). However, at some anatomical sites the metaphysis is intra-articular. Thus osteomyelitis of the hip or of the elbow can track into the adjacent joint causing suppurative arthritis. Joint movement is then markedly restricted and the joint is swollen. Acute suppurative arthritis of the hip can occur in the newborn from a primary focus at the umbilicus. This diagnosis must be considered in every newborn child with a pyrexia of unknown origin. Delay in the diagnosis will result in avascular necrosis (osteonecrosis) of the head of the femur and an arthritic hip for life.

X-rays are unhelpful when trying to make an early diagnosis. It takes 3 weeks before subperiosteal new bone is identified on an X-ray and by this time

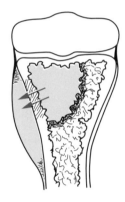

FIG. 16.3 Acute osteomyelitis showing the subperiosteal abscess

chronic osteomyelitis has developed. When on X-ray there is bony rarefaction, the changes are irreversible. The diagnosis of acute haematogenous osteomyelitis is made clinically from the history and examination. It is supplemented by investigations.

INVESTIGATIONS

The white blood cell count will show a marked leucocytosis, and it is usually possible to obtain a positive blood culture of the causative organisms. The erythrocyte sedimentation rate (ESR) or C-reactive protein is high. A ^{99m}TcMDP (methylene diphosphonate) bone scan or diagnostic ultrasound scan will detect early bone changes.

TREATMENT

The two mainstays of treatment are rest and antibiotics. The limb is placed in a splint and the child is given appropriate systemic antibiotics. The antibiotics of choice (before identifying the organism from the blood culture) depend on the local policy of each hospital for the systemic treatment of *Staphylococcus aureus*. It usually involves two intravenous antibiotics. When the organism has been identified it may be necessary to change the antibiotic regime, but by that time the infection will usually have been brought under control. Antibiotics are continued for a period of 6 weeks.

Provided appropriate antibiotics have been administered at an early stage, surgery is unnecessary. Usually, 18 hours of antibiotics produces a dramatic improvement with the child developing an appetite and the pyrexia subsiding. However, if after giving antibiotic therapy for 18 hours there is no systemic improvement, it is necessary to operate and drain the pus. The periosteum is incised at the appropriate site and pus extrudes. The wound is then closed without a drain. Decompressing the metaphysis rapidly relieves the severe pain and there is a marked clinical improvement.

CHRONIC OSTEOMYELITIS

Chronic osteomyelitis occurs when there has been a delay in the diagnosis of acute haematogenous osteomyelitis or inappropriate treatment, or both. Irreversible changes develop in the bone with the formation of a sequestrum surrounded by a involucrum. The organisms lie dormant in avascular necrotic areas, occasionally becoming reactivated, resulting in a flare-up. The bone is thickened and sclerotic, often containing a sequestrum within an abscess cavity (Fig. 16.4).

CLINICAL FEATURES

After inadequate treatment of acute osteomyelitis the bone may develop a quiescent phase that can last for months or years. There may be no symptoms, though scars of previous sinuses and abscesses are usually present. At intervals a flare-up occurs. It may follow minor trauma to the affected region or occur spontaneously. The bone rapidly becomes painful with constitutional upset and pyrexia. There is local redness, swelling and heat. The scar of an old sinus frequently breaks down to discharge purulent material.

There may be a prolonged discharge of pus with no other symptoms and then the sinus may close. However, pus remains in the bone and it builds up in pockets to flare up again from time to time throughout life.

Chronic osteomyelitis is occasionally complicated by amyloid disease, and a squamous cell carcinoma can develop in chronic ulcerated skin.

TREATMENT

It is very difficult to provide a permanent cure for chronic osteomyelitis. Organisms can be identified

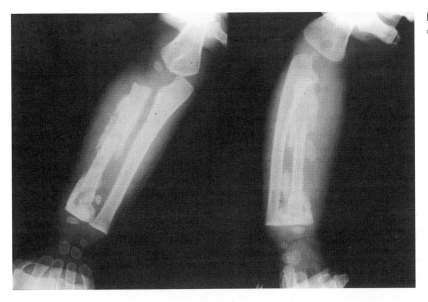

FIG. 16.4 Chronic osteomyelitis of the radius

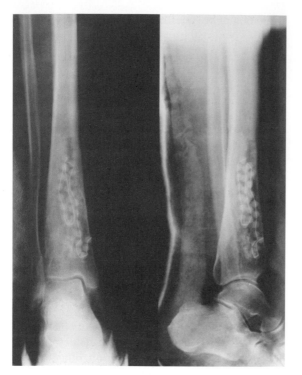

FIG. 16.5   Chronic osteomyelitis with cement beads

from a discharging sinus or from a blood culture and appropriate antibiotics are given. However, although these are often successful in treating the acute flare-up, they are unable to penetrate the dead sequestrum and organisms tend to lie dormant until they are reactivated at a later stage.

Sinus tracks can be visualized by taking X-rays of radio-opaque material injected into the sinus (sinogram). It is then possible to trace the sinus surgically and drain a deeper abscess. If there is an obvious sequestrum, it is removed with excision of surrounding necrotic bone and scar tissue. The operation is as radical as possible, leaving a wide depression that can be filled by a muscle flap or a bone graft. It is important not to leave a dead space. Antibiotic cement beads (Fig. 16.5) are a useful method of providing slow release antibiotic in high concentration at the infected site, and they are placed in the freshly cleaned cavity beneath the muscle graft.

BRODIE'S ABSCESS

Brodie's abscess is a form of chronic osteomyelitis that occurs without any preceding symptoms.

There is a persistent boring pain in the metaphysis of a long bone with little or no constitutional upset. X-rays show a circumscribed cavity in the metaphysis with opaque margins. A Brodie's abscess is treated by opening the cavity, clearing out the sterile pus and curetting the margins. If the cavity is small, it is identified before surgery by inserting a guide wire under X-ray control.

OTHER BONE INFECTIONS

Bone infection is a late complication of typhoid fever. The vertebral column and major long bones are particularly at risk. Typhoid osteomyelitis occurs usually when the generalized disease is resolving. The radiological appearances are similar to those seen in tuberculosis (see below).

TREATMENT

Treatment consists of prolonged administration of the appropriate antibiotic, and surgery to drain the abscess.

PYOGENIC INFECTION OF THE SPINE

Haematogenous discitis

Primary discitis can occur in children and adolescents. The first symptom is back pain and the spine is very stiff as a result of muscle spasm. In the early stages an X-ray is normal but an MRI scan will show vascular changes of the adjacent vertebrae. A ^{99m}TcMDP scan will also confirm changes in blood flow. A needle biopsy may identify the organism.

TREATMENT

Treatment is rest in bed, and antibiotics; rarely is surgical drainage necessary.

Iatrogenic discitis

Iatrogenic discitis can follow any surgical treatment of an intervertebral disc such as surgical discectomy or a percutaneous technique to treat or investigate a disc. During the postoperative period the patient experiences severe back pain with muscle spasm. There must be a high level of suspicion in order to make this diagnosis. It is confirmed by an MRI scan.

Pyogenic vertebral osteomyelitis

In contrast to haematogenous osteomyelitis of the long bones, which affects children, spinal osteomyelitis tends to occur in adults. These patients usually have a low resistance from chronic liver or renal disease or from AIDS. They complain of back pain and stiffness. The spine is tender. There may be a pyrexia. Plain X-rays are not helpful in the early stage but the diagnosis is confirmed by MRI or ^{99m}TcMDP scan, or both. It is important to make an early diagnosis and institute treatment before an epidural abscess develops, compressing the spinal cord.

TREATMENT

Appropriate antibiotic therapy is selected after a blood culture or spinal aspiration. Vertebral collapse with or without neurological compromise, requires anterior decompression and spinal fusion.

JOINTS – INFECTIVE ARTHRITIS

A joint is infected from one of three routes: first by the bloodstream from a distant focus, second, by direct spread from osteomyelitis of a metaphysis that is within the joint capsule and third, as a result of direct inoculation by a penetrating wound through the skin.

Acute septic arthritis in children

Like acute osteomyelitis, this is usually caused by *Staphylococcus aureus*. It is seen most often in children as a complication of acute osteomyelitis. It occurs in those sites at which the metaphysis is within the joint capsule. It has serious consequences because the pus destroys the articular cartilage, causing bony or fibrous ankylosis.

CLINICAL FEATURES

There is severe pain in the affected joint with general malaise and a raised temperature. The joint is hot, tender and swollen with marked restriction of movement as a result of muscle spasm, and it is usually held completely rigid. As the synovial cavity becomes distended with purulent fluid, fluctuation is elicited. An abscess may eventually form and rupture through the skin, leaving a chronic discharging sinus.

INVESTIGATIONS

X-rays at an early stage are normal. Later there is some rarefaction of the adjacent bone followed by subarticular irregularity. There is a polymorphonuclear leucocytosis in the blood, and the erythrocyte sedimentation rate is markedly elevated. A joint aspirate provides fluid filled with polymorphs from which the causative organism may be cultured.

TREATMENT

The patient is put to bed, the joint rested in a splint and a systemic course of broad-spectrum antibiotics commenced. When the sensitivities of the organism are known, the antibiotics may be changed to more appropriate drugs. The joint is repeatedly aspirated until the effusion subsides, washing out the joint with sterile saline. Antibiotic is left in the joint. Open drainage may be necessary if the pus cannot easily be aspirated but this should be avoided if possible for fear of increasing residual stiffness. Mobilization is encouraged once the infection is under control.

Acute septic arthritis of the newborn

The hip is the joint most commonly affected, the causative organism being either a staphylococcus or a streptococcus. The primary focus is often in the umbilicus. The head of the femur may sequestrate and the epiphysis be discharged through a sinus in the groin, leaving an unstable hip. The gait is subsequently identical to that of unreduced congenital dislocation of the hip.

CLINICAL FEATURES

The baby is obviously unwell but, because the hip joint is not near the surface, the site of infection may be unrecognized until an abscess forms in the buttock or thigh. When pathological dislocation occurs the limb becomes markedly short, and the growth is impaired.

TREATMENT

The limb is splinted in abduction, the joint is aspirated and the infection treated with systemic antibiotics. Surgical reconstruction is complex and difficult when irreversible bony changes have occurred.

Gonococcal arthritis

Gonococcal arthritis is a complication of gonococcal urethritis. There is an acute inflammatory reaction, often in several joints simultaneously. It usually appears a few weeks after the onset of the disease. The affected joints are acutely painful, hot and swollen, but the constitutional upset is much less marked than with other forms of acute infective arthritis.

TREATMENT

Treatment is similar to that for acute septic arthritis – aspiration, rest and appropriate antibiotics.

Brucellosis (undulant fever)

Brucellosis is an uncommon disease of bone and joints. It is produced by Gram-positive bacilli that are both non-mobile and non-sporulating. The bacteria infect humans through the skin, conjunctiva and the gastrointestinal tract.

It may occur as an acute febrile illness which then becomes chronic. In the acute form, a child may present with a short history of knee pain and significant synovial swelling. There is a recurrent fever and, although the white blood cell count is not significantly raised, there is a relative lymphocytosis with a high ESR or C-reactive protein. The brucellosis titre is elevated.

Treatment is with antibiotics, e.g. co-trimoxazole, tetracycline or streptomycin, alone or in combination.

TUBERCULOSIS OF BONE AND JOINT

PATHOLOGY

As a result of improvements in hygiene and standards of living throughout the world tuberculosis is less frequent than it was a generation ago. It can occur in the elderly and those who have reduced resistance, and it still remains an important cause of chronic bone and joint infection in developing countries.

The organism may be either the human or the bovine tubercle bacillus, but more commonly the former, and it reaches the bony site from a primary focus in the lungs or the alimentary tract. The primary focus may be small and unrecognized and sometimes totally quiescent. Tuberculous bacilli may infect bone (tuberculosis osteitis) or synovial membrane (tuberculous synovitis), but frequently both bone and the neighbouring joint are affected together.

The tubercle bacillus first causes an inflammatory reaction with typical tuberculous giant cells. This is soon followed by tissue necrosis, and the formation of a tuberculous (cold) abscess – caseation. These cold abscesses track along the tissue planes, eventually reaching the surface as a chronic sinus, sometimes at a distance from the bony focus. Secondary infection with pyogenic organisms will then develop. There is eventually a fibrous ankylosis of the affected joint and when secondary pyogenic infection occurs it is converted to a bony ankylosis.

CLINICAL FEATURES

Tuberculosis causes a constitutional disturbance with loss of weight and general lassitude. Often there is an evening rise of temperature causing the characteristic 'night sweats'. There are local features of pain, particularly on movement of the affected part, with muscle spasm. This leads to deformity. There is also muscle wasting and swelling at the site of the lesion.

INVESTIGATIONS

The ESR and the C-reactive protein are raised. Estimations at regular intervals provide a useful guide to the progress of the disease. The white count usually shows a lymphocytosis. Bacteriological examination of the sputum and early morning urine samples will often reveal the presence of tubercle bacilli even when there is no clinical evidence of active disease in the respiratory or genitourinary tracts. Pus should be cultured and tested for acid-fast bacilli. A Mantoux test, which consists of the intradermal injection of dead tubercle bacilli, provides useful negative information. If the patient has never been in contact with tuberculosis, there will have been no antigen–antibody reaction and a local lesion is then unlikely to be tuberculous. A positive reaction, however, merely confirms that the patient has at some time formed antituberculous antibodies.

X-rays of the affected area show, in the early stages, bony rarefaction and loss of trabecula pattern. Later there is bone destruction with erosion of articular surfaces. Soft-tissue swellings may also be visible, particularly in cold abscesses of the spine.

TREATMENT

Treatment is subdivided into general treatment of the patient and local treatment of the affected part.

General treatment of the patient

General treatment involves building up the patient's strength and resistance to the tubercle bacillus by rest, fresh air and good food. In addition, a course of antituberculous chemotherapy is commenced and continues for 9 months. This therapy consists of at least three antibiotics: rifampicin, isoniazid (isonicotinic acid hydrazide, INAH) and para-aminosalicylic acid (PAS). Ethambutol can be substituted for PAS.

Treatment of the spine (Pott's disease)

The spine is the most common part of the skeletal system to be affected by tuberculosis, the disease usually occurring in the thoracic or lumbar

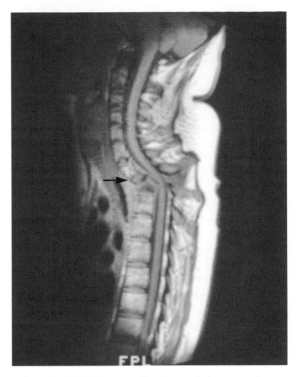

FIG. 16.7   MRI showing tuberculosis of the cervical spine with destruction of T_1 vertebra

regions. The initial focus is in a vertebral body, adjacent to the disc, and it soon spreads across the disc destroying it and involving the adjacent vertebral body (Figs 16.6 and 16.7). A paravertebral abscess of caseous material develops around the vertebral bodies, producing a fusiform shadow on the X-ray. In the lower dorsal and lumbar regions this pus commonly spreads into the neighbouring psoas sheath and then tracks down the psoas muscle to form a psoas abscess. It produces a swelling in the iliac fossa and can then spread deep to the inguinal ligament, forming a sinus in the thigh. This is one of the differential diagnoses of a swelling in the groin. It may be the first sign of tuberculosis, the thoracic lesion having been unrecognized. If the thoracic vertebral disease spreads posteriorly, it can affect the spinal cord with either pus or granulation tissue or with tuberculous bony debris. It can then cause paraplegia.

Clinical features

Tuberculous disease of the spine can occur at any age and at any level, but is most common in adolescents and young adults. There is gradual

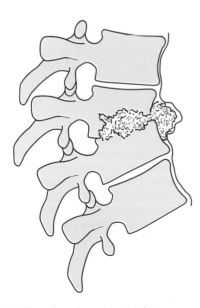

FIG. 16.6   The tuberculous spine (early)

development of back pain. The spine is stiff with muscle spasm, and later, a kyphotic deformity can occur due to a collapse of vertebral bodies. There may be wasting of the erector spinae muscles and soft-tissue swelling. A psoas abscess will produce an abdominal swelling sometimes extending to the femoral triangle in which reciprocal fluctuation may be felt.

Complications

There are two important groups of complications; the first are from pressure on the spinal cord (Pott's paraplegia) and the second are those that follow the immobilization treatment.

Pott's paraplegia

The spinal cord may be involved at any stage in the course of the tuberculous disease of the thoracic spine. The onset is usually insidious with motor weakness or sensory impairment in the lower limbs and sometimes with loss of bladder or bowel control. Patients with thoracic spine tuberculosis are assessed by regular neurological examination because, once it has developed, neurological damage is often irreversible.

Those liable to develop neurological complications often show a well marked globular paravertebral abscess shadow, indicating that the pus is under pressure.

Complications due to immobilization

These take three forms: first, hypostatic pneumonia due to accumulation of secretions at the lung bases; second, urinary infections and the formation of calculi, and third, pressure sores.

Antituberculous chemotherapy has significantly improved the management of skeletal tuberculosis. Surgery is often now unnecessary if the diagnosis is made early. The patient is treated with antibiotics and a spinal support in the form of the surgical brace or plaster jacket. Advanced disease may require spinal fusion to prevent further vertebral collapse.

Neurological complications are treated by anterior spinal decompression and bony fusion supported by metal instrumentation. Posterior decompression by laminectomy is unwise because this destroys the last remaining area of spinal stability.

Treatment of tuberculosis of joints

Tuberculosis can affect any of the joints of the body, particularly the hip, the knee and the shoulder. The principles of management for these joints are the same as for the spine – antibiotics and rest

at least in the initial periods. The affected part is rested by splinting. It is placed in the best position of function lest the joint stiffness becomes permanent. If the disease does not settle with rest and antibiotics, surgery is necessary with antituberculous cover. A sequestrum may be identified on CT and healing is unlikely to occur until this is excised. Once there are signs of improvement, early mobilization is encouraged to regain good function. Surgery is necessary if the disease is advanced, in which case arthrodesis provides both good function, and total joint replacement can also be performed to restore function.

INFECTION AFTER TOTAL JOINT REPLACEMENT

Total joint replacement is now one of the most common causes of bone infection. On the whole it is uncommon after primary joint replacement, occurring in about 2 per cent of patients. If local or blood-borne infection colonizes one of these areas, the body's defence is inadequate and a chronic osteomyelitis develops. The hip becomes painful, red and swollen with a discharging sinus.

The risk of infection after joint replacement is reduced by using ultraclean air operating systems, perioperative prophylactic antibiotics, careful tissue handling to minimize operative trauma and eradicating any urinary infection that might cause bacteraemia.

ULTRACLEAN AIR SYSTEMS

The late Sir John Charnley introduced ultraclean air systems to reduce infection after total hip replacement. Most conventional operating theatres are ventilated with air filtered at the rate of 20 changes per hour and maintained at a positive pressure in relation to their surroundings. Charnley's purpose-built system has 300 or more changes per hour, which are combined with unidirectional laminar flow. With this system postoperative infection can be reduced to less than 1 per cent.

ANTIBIOTICS

Antibiotics are administered intravenously in high doses at the time of surgery. Cefuroxime 1.5 g intravenously with two further doses of 750 mg intra-

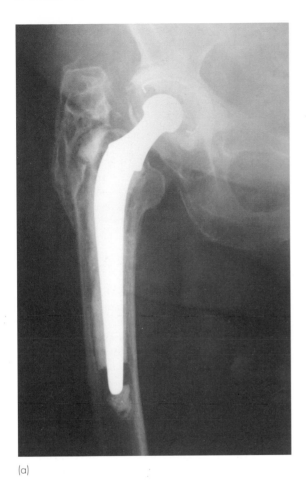

(a)

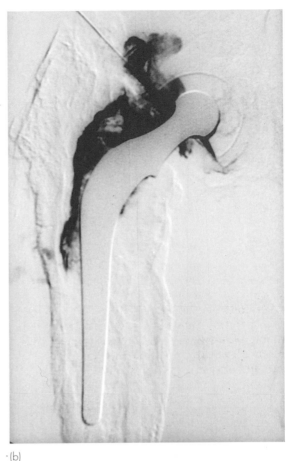

·(b)

FIG. 16.8 (a) X-ray of an infected total hip replacement, showing loosening of the prosthesis, with bone destruction (b) a subtraction arthrogram of the same hip confirming the presence of loosening with the dye tracking down the femur.

muscularly for 12 hours is satisfactory. At the time of hip revision surgery antibiotics can be incorporated in the bone cement. This provides an effective concentration for slow release around the prosthesis.

MANAGEMENT OF ESTABLISHED INFECTION AFTER TOTAL JOINT SURGERY

Once the prosthesis has become infected and chronic osteomyelitis is established, the prosthesis and its cement act as a foreign body not unlike a sequestrum (Fig. 16.8), and they should therefore be removed. This is a first stage procedure – excision arthroplasty. Antibiotic-impregnated cement beads are left in the cavity. These beads are subsequently removed at a second stage, and a new prosthesis is inserted.

INFECTION AFTER OPEN FRACTURES

Open fractures are by definition potentially contaminated with bacterial infection (see Chapter 2). There is a 'golden period' of 6 hours to perform debridement of the wound. Dead skin, fat, muscle and loose fragments of bone are excised, and the wound copiously irrigated with saline. The wound should be as clean as the surgeon's scrubbed hands. The fracture is treated by immobilization – internal or external – and the wound is left open for 48 hours. It is then inspected, and if clean, either closed by secondary suture or grafted. Osteomyelitis should then not occur (Fig. 16.9).

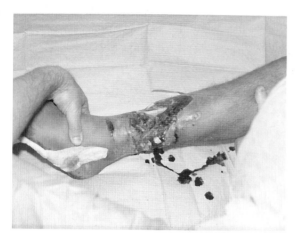

FIG. 16.9   An infected open fracture of the tibia

Summary
Bacterial infection from a variety of organisms can involve any bone or joint at any age. Early diagnosis and appropriate management with rest and antibiotics is generally rewarded with a complete cure. The price of delay and mis-management is chronic osteomyelitis, with discharging sinuses, stiff deformed joints and, in spinal tuberculosis, paraplegia. If the pathology is appreciated and if there is a high level of suspicion, chronic infection should be avoided.

EXAMPLE

Acute haematogenous osteomyelitis

Question

History   An anxious mother brought her 6-year-old son to the Accident and Emergency Department complaining that he had been fretful for 18 hours, would not eat, and refused to bear weight on the left leg.

Clinically   His skin was hot and dry. He had a tachycardia of 120/min and a pyrexia of 39.2°C. He was very difficult to examine, and was tender to palpation over all the left lower limb. The hip could be gently rotated without pain but he would not permit any attempt to flex the knee passively.

Investigations   White blood count 18 600; ESR 48 mm/h; X-ray normal. Provisional diagnosis of acute haematogenous osteomyelitis of upper tibia or lower femur.

Treatment   The left leg was supported in a plaster back-slab resting the knee. He was given intravenous flucloxicillin and fucidin.

Progress   The next morning he was sitting up in bed cheerfully eating his breakfast, with a temperature of 37.4°C. The blood culture grows *Staphylococcus aureus* sensitive to the two antibiotics. The antibiotics are continued for 6 weeks.

Answer

There should be a high level of suspicion of haematogenous osteomyelitis in the lower limb when a child presents with pyrexia of an unknown origin and a failure to bear weight.

The site of maximum tenderness is the best guide to the site of the osteomyelitis but a fretful child can be very difficult to examine.

An X-ray would be normal. Changes would not be expected for 3 weeks. A blood culture is essential to identify the organism and ensure that the bacteria are sensitive to the antibiotics.

If he had not been better within 24 hours he would have required investigation with MRI or a ^{99m}Tc biphosphonate scan to confirm the site of the lesion, and emergency surgical drainage.

17 METABOLIC BONE DISORDERS

Bone is a living structure, which is renewed every few years. The resting cells on the surface of the trabeculae are replaced by large multinucleated osteoclasts, which digest the old bone, creating a small cavity. Similarly, in cortical bone osteoclasts burrow out a tunnel. Some signal is then responsible for recruitment of osteoblasts, which begin to lay down new bone to refill the cavity. This cycle is repeated continuously. There is usually an even balance between bone resorption and bone formation.

Peak bone mass is achieved by the fourth decade of life, and then after the middle of the fifth decade, bone is lost at about 1 per cent per year. Women tend to have less bone mass than men, matching the muscle mass. Bone is lost from disuse, during a long period of recumbency, and it increases with exercise. It is also affected by the hormone status.

CALCIUM AND PHOSPHORUS METABOLISM

Calcium and phosphorus are found in two pools within the body. In one are biologically active calcium and phosphorus ions, whereas the other is a reservoir of potentially available calcium and phosphorus within the bone. The balance of bone turnover is affected by the metabolism of calcium and phosphorus, which to a large extent is controlled by the action of three hormones: parathyroid hormone, calcitonin and vitamin D.

Parathyroid hormone

Parathyroid hormone is a single-chain peptide produced by the parathyroid gland. It has three main sites of action: bone, kidney and the intestinal tract.

In the skeleton parathyroid hormone enhances the rate of bone resorption mainly by stimulating the activity of the osteoclasts and osteocytes; it also increases the production of 1,25-dihydroxycholecalciferol ($1,25(OH)2D3$) by the kidney, enhancing calcium absorption by the intestine.

Calcitonin

Calcitonin is a polypeptide hormone secreted by the parafollicular C-cells of the thyroid. It has two main actions – that on bone and on the kidney – and it also has a minor effect on the intestinal tract.

When injected it causes temporary vasodilatation of the skin and nausea from its action on the gut; it is also an analgesic.

Calcitonin acts on bone by reducing bone–blood flow. It inhibits bone resorption, reducing the circulating levels of calcium, phosphate and hydroxyproline. Osteoclast activity is inhibited and the osteocytes shrink.

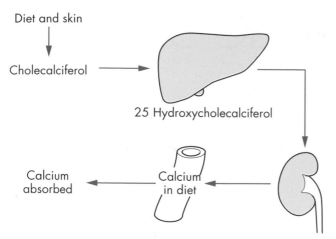

Diet and skin

Cholecalciferol

25 Hydroxycholecalciferol

Calcium absorbed

Calcium in diet

1.25 Dihydroxycholecalciferol

FIG. 17.1   The vitamin D cycle

Vitamin D (Fig. 17.1)

Vitamin D is derived from two sources: from vitamin D3 (cholecalciferol) in the skin, from which it is synthesized by ultraviolet irradiation of the precursor molecule; and from ingested food-stuffs that supply vitamin D2.

The parent vitamin D molecule is largely inactive and must be transformed by two metabolic steps before it is metabolically active. It is first converted in the liver and the gut to 25-hydroxy-cholecalciferol (25(OH)D3). Further hydroxylation takes place in the kidney to convert 25(OH)D3 to 1,25(OH)2D3, which is the active steroid hormone.

1,25-dihydroxycholecalciferol acts on the gut, bone, kidney and muscle. The active metabolite enhances intestinal absorption of calcium phosphate. The direct action of 1,25-dihydroxycholecalciferol on the skeleton is to enhance bone resorption.

The daily requirement of vitamin D is about 400 iu in children and 100 iu in adults. Oily fish contain vitamin D3. The source from sunshine is barely sufficient in the UK, thus dietary supplement is essential.

OSTEOMALACIA AND RICKETS

Osteomalacia and rickets are the result of a deficiency in vitamin D. There is a delay in mineral-

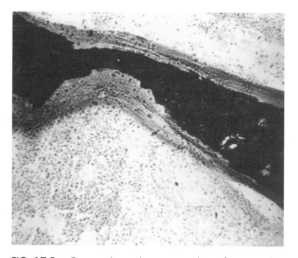

FIG. 17.2   Osteomalacia showing new bone formation that is unmineralized

ization of new bone as the organic matrix is laid. Rickets occurs in children. It affects the epiphyses, and appears clinically as abnormal skeletal growth. There is an enlargement of the membrane bones of the skull, with widening of the epiphysis and flaring of the ribs to produce the 'rickety rosary'. The long bones tend to bend under the body weight, with a bow leg deformity.

Osteomalacia occurs in adults after the epiphyses are fused. There is a deficiency of vitamin D from one of several causes. Dietary deficiency or malabsorption, absence of sunlight particularly in pigmented races living in northern climes, liver and renal disease may affect all vitamin D metabolism. Osteomalacia should therefore be considered in every osteopenic (poorly mineralized) patient, especially if there is a history of risk. Looser zones on the X-ray are almost diagnostic. These are lucent lines on the concavity of the pelvic rim, pubic rami or neck of the femur, either from vascular markings or stress fracture.

The biochemical diagnosis of rickets and osteomalacia is made from a low calcium, low phosphate and raised alkaline phosphatase measurement. In osteomalacia bone biopsy is necessary in order to establish the diagnosis (Fig. 17.2).

TREATMENT

Treatment is to replace vitamin D and ensure adequate intake of calcium.

Renal osteodystrophy

The bony lesions of renal osteodystrophy have been classified into two broad types: rickets in uraemic children and osteitis fibrosa cystica assumed to be due to secondary hyperparathyroidism.

TREATMENT

The active vitamin D metabolites can be given. Intestinal calcium absorption increases, the serum calcium levels return to normal and the elevated levels of alkaline phosphatase and parathyroid hormone are reduced.

HYPERPARATHYROIDISM

Hyperparathyroidism has been classified into primary, secondary and tertiary.

Primary hyperparathyroidism

Primary hyperparathyroidism is usually due to an adenoma of one of the parathyroid glands. Carcinoma is rare. An increase in parathyroid hormone causes a loss of calcium and phosphorus in urine. Backache and vague pains may be the only initial symptoms. Later there may be bone destruction and vertebral collapse. There is subperiosteal resorption of bone, particularly in the index and middle fingers. Later, bone cysts may form, particularly in the long bones. Spontaneous fractures may occur through these cysts and this condition is known as osteitis fibrosa cystica or von Recklinghausen's disease.

TREATMENT

Treatment consists of removal of the parathyroid lesion.

Secondary hyperparathyroidism

In patients with chronic renal disease or malabsorption, hypercalcaemia can also occur and it is then associated with hyperplasia of the parathyroid glands. Other examples of hypercalcaemia are malignant disease from bony metastases, particularly in patients with carcinoma of the breast, myelomatosis, thyrotoxicosis and vitamin D intoxication.

Tertiary hyperparathyroidism

In some forms of renal disease there may be a severe loss of calcium in the urine and the level of serum calcium is then maintained by compensatory hyperplasia of the parathyroid gland; this is secondary hyperparathyroidism. If, however, the renal failure worsens, the patient is treated by renal dialysis and a stage may be reached when eventually secondary hyperparathyroidism becomes autonomous and can persist even after renal transplantation. This is tertiary hyperparathyroidism.

OSTEOPOROSIS

Bone is osteoporotic when it is reduced in amount but normal in quality. There is a reduction in mass per volume, but this is not considered to be pathological. Rather it is physiological and the result of ageing.

After the menopause, women tend to have a brief postmenopausal dip in bone mass, and then like men, their bone continues to decrease by about

1 per cent per year. Because the peak bone mass in women is less than in men, in later life their bone strength can be seriously diminished. Should these patients fall, they are at risk of sustaining fractures of the wrist, spine and hip.

There are several risk factors for osteoporosis:

- thin individuals
- early menopause
- steroids
- anorexia nervosa
- smoking
- alcohol
- hysterectomy
- partial gastrectomy
- no children.

It can be influenced by hormonal imbalance: hyperthyroidism, hypopituitarism and hypogonadism.

Osteoporosis is a major cause of skeletal failure in the elderly, with fractures of the hip now accounting for about 10 per cent of the orthopaedic bed occupancy in the UK.

CLINICAL EXAMINATION

The osteoporotic patient has usually lost height as a result of microfractures of the thoracic spine and thoracic kyphosis. They may have had a previous wrist fracture. Conventional X-rays are insensitive for the diagnosis of osteoporosis. There is a 40 per cent loss before the X-ray films look osteopenic. Other conditions should be excluded, including myelomatosis, metastases, osteomalacia and renal osteodystrophy.

PREVENTION

Preventive strategies depend on first maintaining the bone strength, and second preventing falls. Women at risk of developing severe osteoporosis in later life can be identified at the menopause. Their bone mass is at the lower end of the spectrum of normality. Sensitive methods of measuring bone mass are dual energy X-ray absorptiometry (DEXA) of the hip or spine and broadband ultrasound attenuation (BUA) across the heel bone.

Patients at risk are then offered cyclical hormone replacement therapy to maintain bone mass. Other drugs used to maintain bone mass are calcitonin, and the biphosphonates. A healthy lifestyle is advisable, with regular exercise, adequate nutrition, and no smoking or alcohol abuse.

PAGET'S DISEASE

Sir James Paget described this condition in 1877, which he called osteitis deformans. It is thought to have a viral aetiology. The bone is disorganized, with expansion of the cortex, osteolytic areas and irregular trabecular patterns. There is an increase in bone turnover. The bone may be weakened and deformed or may fracture.

The disease is rarely found in people under the age of 40 years. It may affect any bone but it particularly involves the tibia, skull and pelvis. There may be pain with an increase in local temperature due to the high blood flow to the bone. Often, however, there is an asymptomatic enlargement of the skull with bowing of the long bones such as the radius and tibia, or kyphosis of the thoracic spine. These changes are due to the remodelling of the bone.

COMPLICATIONS

- Fractures: complete or partial or fissure fractures. Immobilization leads to hypercalciuria and occasionally to hypercalcaemia.
- Heart failure because of the increased blood flow to the bones, causing the cardiac output to be raised, leading to right-sided heart failure.
- Osteosarcoma: in this condition, which affects about 1 per cent of patients with Paget's disease, the prognosis is extremely poor and the average survival time is about 18 months.
- Deafness and blindness from auditory or optic nerve entrapment.
- Spinal stenosis may also occur, leading to cauda equina compression.

INVESTIGATIONS

Biochemical features include a raised alkaline phosphatase, raised urinary hydroxyproline and an increase in bone collagen turnover measured using calcium kinetic studies. Histological changes show increased density of bone with increased osteoblastic activity. There is also an increased number of giant multinucleated osteoclasts.

Radiologically, there is both new bone formation and increased density, and also areas of lysis. There is deformation of the bony structure. These changes produce the so-called 'cotton wool' appearance of the skull and bowing of the tibia and femur (Fig. 17.3), which can be associated with microfractures on the convex border. The patchy

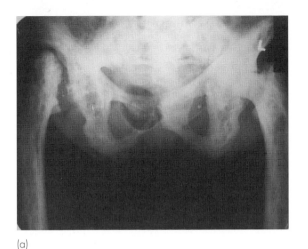

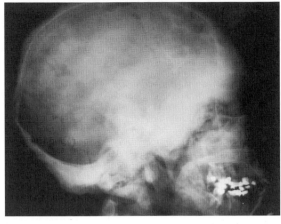

(a)   (b)

FIG. 17.3   Paget's disease: (a) of the pelvis and femora, and (b) of the skull

osteolytic lesion can be distinguished from myelomatosis because in Paget's disease, the whole bone is expanded and often deformed.

Bone scanning with radionuclides can be used to demonstrate increased activity in the bone, and this technique has been used to quantify the effects of different forms of treatment.

TREATMENT

Pain can be relieved by analgesics. Biphosphonates are given orally. The relief of bone pain is matched by a fall in alkaline phosphatase levels. It can induce osteomalacia.

Calcitonin inhibits bone resorption, thereby reducing the abnormally raised bone turnover. As a result, cellular activity becomes more orderly and healing is also seen in skeletal X-rays. Calcitonin is given subcutaneously for a period of weeks. No serious side effects have been noted.

Paget's bone is often very vascular and profuse bleeding is a major hazard. It can be reduced to some extent by a preoperative course of biphosphonates.

TREATMENT OF COMPLICATIONS

Fractures

The rate of delayed and non-union of fractures of the femur has been reported to be as high as 40 per cent, suggesting that fractures in Paget's disease do not heal at the normal rate. Internal fixation is needed for all long bone fractures that have been

displaced, but may well present considerable technical problems because of the deformity of the bone and the poor fixation that may be achieved using screws.

Osteoarthritis

The hip joint is frequently involved in Paget's disease, and osteoarthritis is a common complication. Total hip replacement may be required. The structure of the bone makes this a difficult procedure. Hemiarthroplasty is advisable in patients who have sustained a subcapital fracture of the neck of the femur or total hip replacement if the acetabulum is involved.

Spinal stenosis

Decompression of the spine may be necessary in patients who have developed a spinal stenosis from bone overgrowth in Paget's disease. Calcitonin is effective in reducing the compression on the cauda equina.

VITAMIN C DEFICIENCY (SCURVY)

A deficiency in vitamin C produces a characteristic bone lesion as a result of failure of bone formation. Cartilage proliferates and calcifies but does not form bone, and osteoclastic activity continues but bone is not replaced. Haemorrhages are common, and as the cortex thins it fractures easily.

Ascorbic acid is required for the hydroxylation of proline. Vitamin C deficiency impairs collagen formation, affecting not only bone but also the skin and the teeth. Infantile scurvy may occur in babies.

TREATMENT

Fresh fruit, which contains vitamin C, or vitamin C supplement, is given.

ECTOPIC CALCIFICATION

Ectopic calcification can be:

■ Local – associated with tuberculosis, trauma or myositis ossificans; it can also occur after total hip replacement and be particularly trouble-some. Its risk is diminished by giving perioperative NSAIDs.

■ Metastatic – due to a generalized increase in mineralization throughout the body.

■ Regional and neurological – ectopic bone will occur in the limbs below the level of a paraplegia, but not above.

Summary
Patients with poor bone mineralization should be investigated for metabolic bone disorders – hyperparathyroidism and osteomalacia – but the most common cause is age-related osteoporosis. Wrist and spinal fractures are inconvenient, but hip fracture is a serious health problem with high morbidity and mortality. Protection with hormone replacement therapy is appropriate for perimenopausal women at risk.

EXAMPLE

Osteoporosis

Question

History A 56-year-old housewife attended a fracture clinic having sustained a Colles' fracture.

Previous history She fractured the opposite wrist 3 years before. She smokes 15 cigarettes a day, and had an early menopause at 45 years of age.

Investigations Blood biochemistry was normal. DEXA scan of her hip was on the tenth percentile and ultrasound measurements on the fifteenth percentile.

Prophylactic treatment After discussing the risks and benefits she started on cyclical hormone replacement therapy (HRT).

Answer

Colles' fracture is an 'osteoporotic-related' fracture.

A previous wrist fracture, smoking and an early menopause suggest that she may be at risk of osteoporosis.

Blood investigations exclude metabolic bone disease. DEXA and ultrasound confirm that she is osteoporotic.

HRT protects from fracture of the spine and hip. It protects the cardiovascular system, but slightly increases the risk of carcinoma of the breast and uterus.

18 NEOPLASMS

New growths of the locomotor system may be conveniently subdivided into those affecting bone, and those affecting soft tissue. In each case they may be benign or malignant.

BONE NEOPLASMS

Neoplasms originating in bone may arise from osseous tissue, from cartilaginous cells associated with the epiphyses, or from the blood-forming elements contained in red bone marrow.

BENIGN BONE GROWTHS

Osteoma

Osteoma is a benign growth arising from the osseous tissue. It is comparatively uncommon and usually occurs in the membranous bones of the skull, in which it produces a smooth swelling that is dense and hard (ivory osteoma). It hardly ever causes symptoms unless it grows inwards, compressing, for example, the brain or involving the structures of the inner ear.

Osteoid osteoma (Fig. 18.1)

Osteoid osteoma is an innocent lesion that consists of a small nidus of osteoid tissue and can occur anywhere in the skeleton. In a major long bone it occurs typically in the cortex, which becomes thickened and dense, tending to obscure it in X-rays. It occurs also in cancellous bone surrounded by a ring of sclerosis. It is an uncommon tumour that usually occurs in young adults, and the main clinical feature is persistent deep boring pain, which is worse at night, and can be relieved by aspirin. There is localized tenderness. Radiologically, there is an area of sclerosis with a small rounded or oval central area of rarefaction.

Treatment consists of complete excision of the rarefied and sclerotic area.

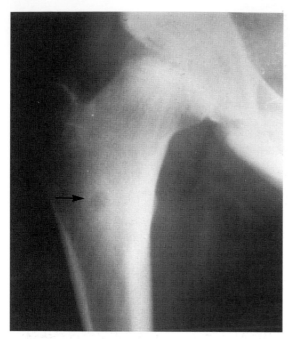

FIG. 18.1   Osteoid osteoma

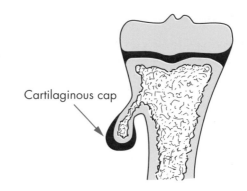

FIG. 18.2   Exostosis

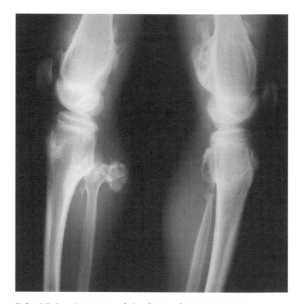

FIG. 18.3   Exostosis of the femur, fibula and tibia

Osteoblastoma

Osteoblastoma is a benign bone-forming tumour that occurs in children and young adults between the ages of 10 and 20 years. About one-third of cases affect the spine, particularly the posterior arch. Other sites include the tibia and femur and also flat bones. The lesion is larger than 1.5 cm, and consists of a sclerotic area surrounding a well defined lytic centre.

Treatment is by curettage and bone grafting.

Osteochondroma (exostosis)

Osteochondroma is a growth that arises from rests of epiphyseal cells that are left upon the bone surface, and as a result they continue to grow until the parent epiphysis fuses. With growth of the bone, the epiphyseal line moves away from the lesion, and the exostosis itself forms a pedicle that points away from the end of the bone from which it originated. If examined before bone growth has ceased, a cartilaginous cap will be found covering the surface farthest away from the pedicle (Fig. 18.2). The cartilage cap is said to ossify when the epiphyseal disc does, but the cap often persists into adult life, when it is crowned by a bursa.

Osteochondromata may be solitary or multiple (Fig. 18.3). When multiple, the condition is known as diaphysial aclasia.

COMPLICATIONS

Sometimes an exostosis is fractured; occasionally there are damaging pressure effects upon neighbouring structures such as peripheral nerves or vessels. Malignant change is rare in single exostoses but low-grade chondrosarcoma sometimes occurs in diaphysial aclasia, such that the onset of pain or enlargement of the lump after skeletal growth has ceased should be viewed with suspicion.

TREATMENT

Simple excision of the exostosis through its pedicle gives good results if the bony mass is causing symptoms or is increasing in size, but often no treatment beyond observation at intervals is necessary.

Chondroma

Chondroma is a true benign tumour composed of cartilage cells arising in a bone, although it originates from the epiphyseal cartilage. It is most common in the 'short' long bones of the hands in which it tends to occupy the medulla and is known as an enchondroma. Occasionally it occurs in flat bones, such as the ilium, from which it bulges outwards forming an ecchondroma. These tumours have a fairly even distribution and can be found in any age group.

Clinically, enchondromata in the bones of the hand often pass unnoticed unless thinning of the cortex leads to fracture. A chondroma in a major long bone may appear as a chondrosarcoma, having undergone malignant change. This should be suspected if a cartilage tumour in an adult starts to grow.

Multiple cartilaginous masses in the major long bones from failure of columns of epiphyseal cartilage to ossify is referred to under dyschondroplasia or Ollier's disease (Chapter 12). Multiple chondroma associated with angioma is Maffucci's syndrome.

TREATMENT

If an enchondroma is causing cortical erosion of a major bone, it should be curetted out and the cavity filled with cancellous bone graft. However, usually no treatment is required. Spontaneous fracture appears to stimulate new bone formation, so that often not only does union occur but also regression of the tumour follows.

OTHER GROWTHS AND CYSTS IN BONE

Simple (unicameral) bone cyst (Fig. 18.4)

Unicameral bone cyst is a condition, usually found in children between the ages of 5 and 10 years but rarely in adults, in which a central cyst forms in the substance of a bone, typically the upper metaphysis

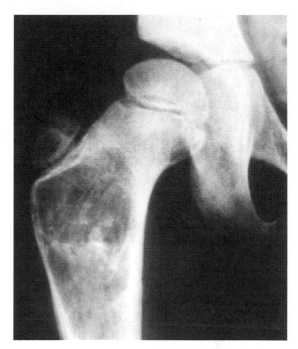

FIG. 18.4 Unicameral bone cyst

of the humerus. It is often discovered by chance, but in major long bones it may lead to a pathological fracture. It usually expands the metaphysis but, if the bone grows more quickly than the cyst enlarges, the cyst becomes separated from the epiphyseal plate by normal bone (i.e. the cyst looks as though it has moved down the shaft). The thin bony walls may have trabecular thickening, and their lining is usually very scanty and thin. The fluid contents are yellow and clear, unless sanguineous from fracture.

If the wall of the cyst fractures, the cyst may fill with bone, but this follows much less often than is generally supposed. In any event, the fracture should be allowed to heal; if thereafter the cyst persists, it may be curetted or filled with bone graft. Injection of methylprednisolone into the bone cyst has been shown to be equally effective. Although innocent, the cyst sometimes recurs, but it gradually subsides after puberty.

Aneurysmal bone cyst

Aneurysmal bone cyst occurs rather later than the simple cyst, that is, in older children and young adults. Its usual sites are the long bones and the vertebrae, especially the lamina and the spinous and transverse processes, when it may cause neurological complications. It is a cause of vertebral collapse.

Also unlike the simple cyst, it is eccentric, roughly spherical and up to about 10 cm in diameter. It destroys neighbouring tissues by compression and looks sinister in X-rays although it is in fact innocent. It has a thin bony shell. The contents of an aneurysmal bone cyst are blood with strands extending into it from a scanty lining, often containing giant cells, which may cause confusion with giant-cell tumours. Pain is slight and pressure symptoms may be the first to draw attention to it. It can usually be cured by curettage, with or without insertion of cancellous grafts, but venous-type bleeding may create difficulties unless fully anticipated. The condition is unrelated to an aneurysm, being fancifully named on a supposed resemblance to a 'blow-out'.

Non-ossifying fibroma (metaphyseal fibrous defect)

Non-ossifying fibroma is a benign fibrous tissue tumour that is found in children and young adults, being rare after the age of 30 years. It is usually seen in the femur, tibia and fibula, and may be multiple. It occurs as well defined, eccentric radiolucent lesions, often scalloped in appearance.

In young children the lesions disappear with remodelling. No treatment is required for these defects.

INTERMEDIATE GROWTHS

Giant-cell tumour of bone

Giant-cell tumour of bone is characteristically a tumour of young people, being rare under the age of 15 years, but always after skeletal maturity,

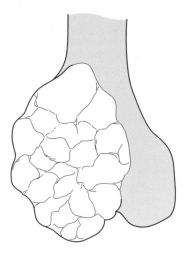

FIG. 18.5   Giant-cell tumour of the bone

affecting the ends of long bones, commonly the lower end of the femur, upper end of the tibia and often the lower end of the radius. It extends right up to the articular cartilage. Like the aneurysmal bone cyst, it is eccentric and rounded. A very thin shell, which may collapse, is filled with a maroon-coloured vascular tissue containing giant cells in a stroma of oval cells (Fig. 18.5). The X-rays often show trabeculation, but this may also be seen in simple cysts (Fig. 18.6). Pain is the chief symptom.

The condition is readily distinguished from simple cyst by the age of the patient with absent epiphyseal plate and the strictly epiphyseal situation. Distinction from aneurysmal bone cyst may depend on biopsy, and distinction from the histologically similar bone tumour of hyperparathyroidism depends upon the special characteristics of this tumour: clinical evidence of general disease,

Left   Right

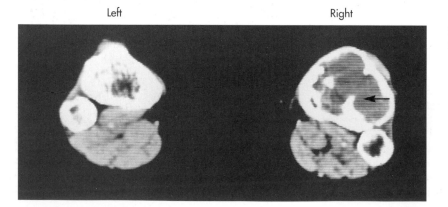

FIG. 18.6   CT of giant-cell tumour of the right tibia

often multiplicity of bone change, X-ray evidence of porosis and biochemical evidence of disturbed mineral metabolism.

Treatment is by thorough curettage and packing with bone graft. Recently preoperative arterial embolization and intraoperative bone grafting or bone cement insertion has been introduced. A recurrent growth should be excised and replaced by either massive bone grafting or major prosthetic replacement; deep X-ray therapy induces radiation sarcoma.

Unlike other lesions containing giant cells ('giant-cell variants'), which are virtually all innocent, giant-cell tumours are capricious – usually they are innocent but about 10 per cent become malignant fibrosarcomas or osteosarcomas and proceed to metastasize to the lungs.

MALIGNANT TUMOURS OF BONE

Malignant tumours of bone may be either primary, arising in the bone itself, or secondary metastatic deposits from a malignant growth elsewhere.

Primary malignant bone growths

OSTEOSARCOMA

Osteosarcoma is the most common primary malignant new growth of bone after myeloma and arises from osteoblasts. It may appear at any age, but is most frequently seen at between 10 and 20 years of age. It is extremely malignant. The tumour arises from the metaphyses of long bones and usually is found in the lower end of the femur (Fig. 18.7), the upper end of the humerus and the upper end of the tibia.

Histologically, the tumour consists of masses of poorly differentiated round or spindle cells and often with elements of connective tissue such as cartilaginous, myxomatous or fibrous tissue, interspersed with sinusoidal blood spaces. Although eventually the growth bursts through the periosteal lining and spread into the surrounding soft tissues, the epiphyseal line appears to provide a barrier to its spread within the bone.

Clinical features

The presenting symptom is pain of a constant aching nature, and this in turn may draw attention to bony swelling. Later, as the growth progresses and destruction of normal bone increases, pathological fracture may occur. Metastatic spread is by the bloodstream, and often takes place at quite an early stage. The lungs are mainly affected, but spread to other bones sometimes follows.

The prognosis is not good, although 50 per cent of patients survive 5 years with current treatment.

Investigations

Radiography

There will be signs of bony destruction within the diaphysis, with erosion of the bony cortex at first restricted to one side. Evidence that the periosteum has been raised is visible at the margins of the lesion, where new bone forms beneath it (Codman's triangle). The quantity of new bone, if any, visible in the medulla and outside the bone cortex will vary according to whether the growth is predominantly osteolytic (bone destructive) or osteoblastic (bone forming). Sometimes characteristic strands of bone radiating vertically from the cortex (sun-ray spicules) may be seen (Figs 18.8 and 18.9).

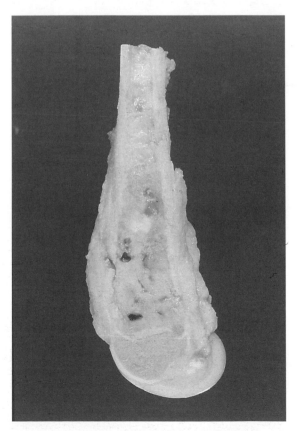

FIG. 18.7   Pathology of osteosarcoma of the femur

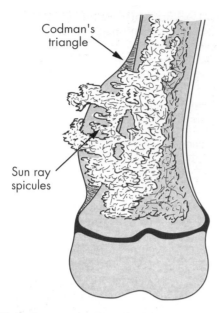

FIG. 18.8   Diagram showing osteosarcoma

X-ray of the chest and CT scanning should be undertaken at the same time, for evidence of pulmonary metastases.

Blood investigations may be required to exclude an infective lesion of bone.

An open biopsy will be needed to confirm the nature of the condition, before radical treatment is carried out.

Differential diagnosis

Infective lesions of bone may produce a clinical and radiological picture similar to that for osteosarcoma. Other bony neoplasms such as chondrosarcoma, giant-cell tumours or a carcinomatous metastatic deposit in bone from a primary growth elsewhere may require to be excluded.

Treatment

Immediately the diagnosis has been made by open biopsy, preoperative chemotherapy is commenced and is continued in high doses for 10 weeks. The agents used include high-dose methotrexate in combination with doxorubicin, cyclophosphamide

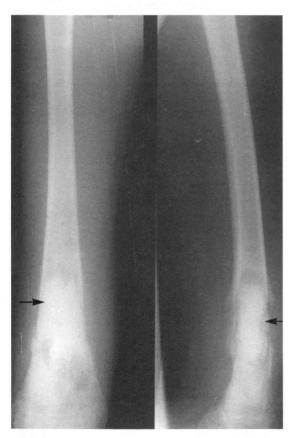

FIG. 18.9   X-ray of osteosarcoma of the femur. There is bone destruction; new bone formation and periosteal reaction with Codman's triangle

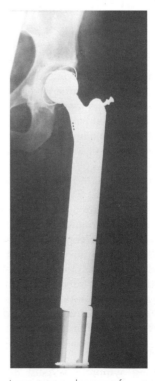

FIG. 18.10   Large joint replacement for osteosarcoma

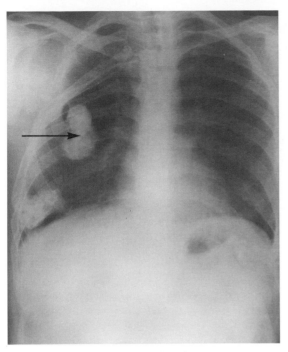

FIG. 18.11   Secondaries in the lung from osteosarcoma

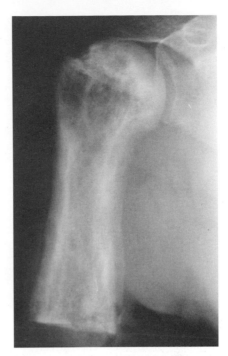

FIG. 18.12   Paget's osteosarcoma of the humerus

and cis-platinum (cisplatin). Citrovorum rescue factor (folinic acid) will also be used.

At 10 weeks the tumour is excised surgically with wide margins. If possible a custom-made prosthesis is then inserted (Fig. 18.10); alternatively, an amputation is performed.

If lung metastases develop (Fig. 18.11), they can also be treated by chemotherapy and resection of the affected lobe of the lung.

PAROSTEAL SARCOMA

A variation of osteosarcoma is a parosteal osteosarcoma. This also is found in long bones, particularly the lower femur or upper tibia. The X-ray shows the tumour to be attached to the cortex by a broad base, but there is no continuity between the medullary cavity and the tumour.

It is a less aggressive tumour than osteosarcoma and carries a much better prognosis. After resection and chemotherapy the survival rate is 80 per cent at 5 years.

PAGET'S DISEASE AND OSTEOSARCOMA

In patients with Paget's disease affecting long bones in particular, about 1 per cent develop an osteosarcoma (Fig. 18.12). It is a particularly virulent form of the disease, with most patients dying from pulmonary metastases within 18 months.

CHONDROSARCOMA

Chondrosarcoma is on the whole rather less malignant than osteosarcoma. It occurs in middle adult life and is rarely found in those under the age of 20 years. It arises from the ends of the major long bones or from flat bones such as the pelvis or scapula. Chondrosarcoma may arise in a preceding enchondroma such as in dyschondroplasia (Ollier's disease) or appear in previously normal bone. Pain or other evidence of enlargement of a cartilaginous mass in an adult should lead to a strong suspicion of malignant change.

Metastasis may be very late, and the tumour may cause swelling over the affected bone, and the latter may grow to a large size. Radiologically, the tumour is destructive and sometimes the calcification characteristic of a mass of cartilage is lost (Fig. 18.13).

Treatment

Resection of the tumour with wide margins is indicated, and if possible it should be replaced by

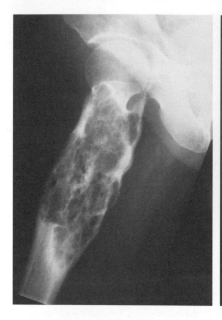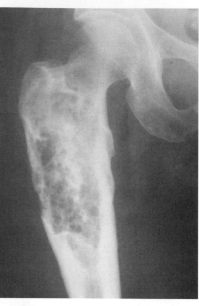

FIG. 18.13   Chondrosarcoma of the femur

a custom-made prosthesis. Alternatively, amputation of the affected limb is performed. Because of their slow growth, chondrosarcomas show a poor response to radiotherapy.

FIBROSARCOMA

Fibrosarcomas occur in adults of all ages, usually developing towards one end of the shaft of a long bone, notably the femur and tibia. Complaint is of pain, usually followed by a palpable swelling. X-ray appearances are often indefinite, and depend on destruction of trabeculae of cancellous bone or of cortex. Except that wide local resection may succeed in cases of highly differentiated tumours, the treatment is amputation; fibrosarcomas are resistant to irradiation. Most tumours show limited differentiation and have a poor prognosis.

EWING'S TUMOUR

Ewing's tumour is a highly malignant round-cell tumour presumed to be an endothelioma. It is found in children and young adults aged between 5 years and the late 20s and is first observed in a long bone or the innominate bone, but usually involves other bones early, either by metastasis or, more likely, because of its multicentric origin. It forms an endosteal destructive tumour, often with a subperiosteal reaction (Fig. 18.14). This may present an 'onion-skin' stop-and-go ossification, but this is exceptional and not peculiar to Ewing's

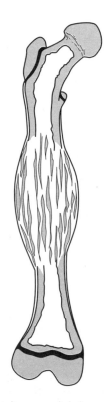

FIG. 18.14   Malignant endothelioma (Ewing's tumour)

tumour. The tumour is drawn to the attention of the patient by pain, tenderness, sometimes swelling and occasionally pathological fracture. The child may have a fever, be anaemic and have a raised white cell count and ESR, which suggest clinically an infective lesion. Diagnosis rests on a biopsy, when a distinction has to be made from other round-cell neoplasms (reticulum cell sarcoma, malignant lymphoma and metastases, including neuroblastoma) and also from osteomyelitis.

Treatment

The prognosis for Ewing's tumour has improved with the introduction of chemotherapy. The drugs used are a combination of vincristine, cyclophosphamide, actinomycin D and doxorubicin, and are administered in cycles of 10 weeks or so for up to 2 years. Radiotherapy is also used, particularly in adult patients and in children with lesions of the upper extremity. As in the lower limb, serious growth disturbances will result.

Surgery is indicated for easily resectable tumours or for those with pathological fractures. There is also a place for amputation of the lower limbs if disabling leg length discrepancy is produced by radiotherapy.

MULTIPLE MYELOMA (MYELOMATOSIS)

Multiple myeloma is a malignant neoplastic condition characterized by multiple foci of plasma cells in the red bone marrow. The outcome is uniformly fatal, although the rate of progress varies considerably and, with treatment, advancement can be delayed, sometimes for several years.

Pathologically, there are multiple foci of bone destruction, often appearing as small punched-out areas, involving chiefly ribs, sternum, vertebrae, skull and pelvis, together with the upper ends of the femora and humeri. Histologically, sheets of cells resembling rather immature plasma cells can be seen.

Clinical features

The patient is usually a middle-aged adult, and pain is the common presenting symptom. This may be a widespread ache, due to the multiple bony deposits, or of sudden onset at a single site, due to pathological fracture, particularly in the back as a result of collapse of a vertebral body. Later, bone marrow destruction leads to severe anaemia. Renal failure and paraplegia may impair the prognosis.

Investigations

Apart from the punched-out areas visible on X-rays of bone containing red bone marrow, routine urine testing usually reveals a substance that appears as a cloud when the urine is heated, but redissolves when boiling point is reached; this is due to the presence of a group of closely related proteins (Bence-Jones protein).

Blood tests will show a great increase in the ESR, a rise in gamma globulin with a myeloma band visible on electrophoresis, so an ESR of more than 100 mm/h in a patient aged over 40 years with bone pain is highly suggestive of myeloma. Sternal puncture, to obtain a specimen of red bone marrow, will reveal a great increase in plasma cells.

Treatment

Local lesions respond well to radiotherapy, which, in the case of pathological fractures of long bones, may be combined with internal fixation. General measures to prolong life consist of the use of cytotoxic drugs (e.g. cyclophosphamide or melphalan) and the administration of steroids in large doses. Anaemia may be controlled by repeated blood transfusions.

SOLITARY PLASMACYTOMA

Solitary plasmacytoma is an atypical variety of myelomatosis, in which a single tumour arises in a bone from the plasma cells in its marrow. After an interval it usually spreads, and the picture changes to typical multiple myelomatosis. Occasionally, if seen early, arrest of the disease may be achieved by an intensive local course of radiotherapy.

MALIGNANT LYMPHOMA

Malignant lymphoma is a malignant tumour of haemopoietic tissue that is found throughout all age groups except the very young. It affects any bone, but attacks the pelvis and femora more often. Its radiographic appearance is similar to that of Ewing's tumour. Many other areas of lymphoid tissue are affected but, if bone is the only site, there is a better prognosis than when this malignant condition is generalized.

Secondary (metastatic) malignant bone growths

Metastatic bony deposits arising from primary carcinomata at certain sites are common, and indeed are the major cause of malignant disease of

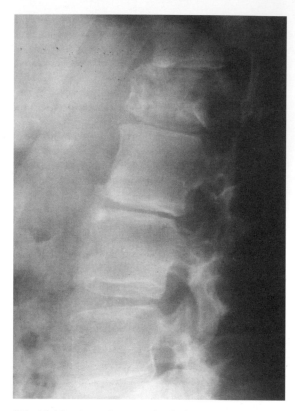

FIG. 18.15   Secondaries in the lumbar vertebrae from a patient with carcinoma of the breast

the bone, far outweighing the incidence of primary bone tumours. Usually they occur late in the disease but, occasionally, notably in carcinoma of the bronchus, a pathological fracture through a secondary deposit may be the first sign of the disease. Bony metastases are always blood-borne, and therefore occur most frequently where there is red bone marrow – in the vertebrae, pelvis and the upper ends of the femur or humerus. The common primary sites are the breast, bronchus, prostate, kidney, thyroid and gastrointestinal system.

TREATMENT

In the large majority of cases, treatment is palliative, and consists of local radiotherapy and internal fixation of pathological fractures where possible. When X-ray suggests that a fracture is imminent, prophylactic intramedullary nailing of the femur or humerus should be employed. The general spread of the disease may be slowed down by the use of cytotoxic drugs.

SOFT-TISSUE NEOPLASMS

On the whole, in the locomotor system, serious neoplastic disease is less common in soft tissues than in bone.

Fatty tissue

LIPOMA

Lipomata are common tumours occurring anywhere in the body where fatty tissue is present. Subcutaneously they form a soft, painless, lobulated nodule. Deeper, they are not so easy to recognize but their slight relative translucency in X-ray films may help. Very occasionally, there are mild pressure effects on neighbouring structures. Treatment is indicated only if symptoms warrant surgical intervention.

LIPOSARCOMA

Very rarely in liposarcomatous, malignant change occurs, in which case an indurated lump is found. Diagnosis depends upon biopsy results, and very wide excision is indicated.

Musculotendinous tissue

True tumours of muscles and tendons are rare. Very occasionally, a malignant new growth of striated muscle – *rhabdomyosarcoma* – occurs. It is highly malignant and metastasizes rapidly.

Synovial tissue

New growths arising from synovial tissue may affect either joints or tendon sheaths.

VILLONODULAR SYNOVITIS (BENIGN GIANT-CELL SYNOVIOMA)

Benign giant-cell synovioma are benign, arising from the synovial tissue of joints or tendon sheaths, usually in the hand and especially the flexor sheaths of the fingers. They cause local lobulated swellings that are often confused with ganglion.

Treatment consists of complete excision. Occasionally, they may recur.

SYNOVIAL SARCOMA (MALIGNANT SYNOVIOMA)

Synovial sarcoma is a highly malignant growth arising from synovium, usually of a major joint such as the knee; it produces a firm fleshy mass that spreads widely in the surrounding soft tissues, but rarely invades the bone. It is composed of ill developed fusiform cells, among which are spaces suggesting attempts to form synovial cavities.

Clinically, an indurated swelling at or near a joint is the main feature. Movements are often largely unaffected. Pulmonary metastases occur early, and the prognosis is poor. X-rays in some cases show calcification within the tumour.

Treatment

Where possible, amputation offers the best hope of a cure; if, however, this is difficult, wide excision coupled with large doses of radiotherapy may be indicated, although the tumour is commonly radio-resistant.

Nervous tissue

NEURILEMMOMA (SCHWANNOMA)

Neurilemmoma is the most common of all peripheral nerve tumours, which can be removed without loss of function of the nerve in which it originated. It is an encapsulated slow-growing tumour that arises from the neural sheath, consisting mainly of Schwann cells. The treatment is enucleation after a wide incision.

NEUROFIBROMA

Neurofibroma is a tumour arising from the fibrous tissue lining of the peripheral nerve. It forms a firm swelling, but usually the conduction of the nerve from which it arises is not affected unless it is situated in an area in which space is restricted. They need not be removed, as they are benign.

NEUROFIBROMATOSIS (VON RECKLINGHAUSEN'S DISEASE)

Neurofibromatosis is not to be confused with von Recklinghausen's disease affecting bone, which is associated with parathyroid hypertrophy (Chapter 17).

This is a condition in which there are multiple neurofibromata, with patches of skin pigmentation (café-au-lait patches). It is hereditary, and the skin pigmentation is often first seen in early childhood. It is associated with severe kyphoscoliosis (Chapter 12) and is a rare cause of club feet. A neurofibroma can exert pressure on the spinal cord or cauda equina, in which case it may result in cord or nerve root irritation. About 5 per cent of neurofibromata undergo malignant change.

Treatment

Only excision of the individual neurofibromata that are causing symptoms should be undertaken. No treatment for the overlying general disease is possible.

Blood vessels (haemangioma)

Haemangioma are probably not true tumours but a local congenital anomaly of small blood vessels, which fail to become fully differentiated. There are two types, depending upon the size of the blood spaces:

- capillary haemangioma, in which there is a mass of fine vessels, which if near the skin, causes a red blotchy area;
- cavernous haemangioma, in which large blood cavities are present, causing a swelling. In these case, firm pressure over the mass causes it to disappear and it then fills up again when the pressure is released.

Because diffuse haemangiomas cause an increase in local blood flow, if they are situated in a growing limb, epiphyseal overgrowth may occur.

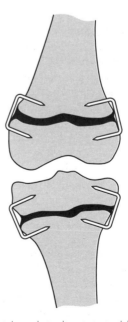

FIG. 18.16   Epiphyseal stapling to retard bone growth

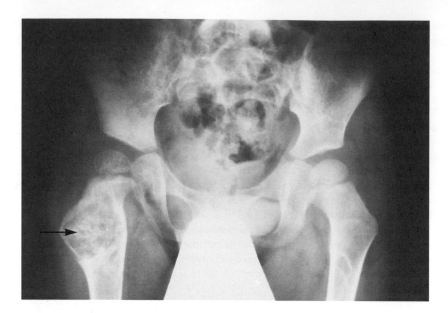

FIG. 18.17 Fibrous dysplasia of the femur

TREATMENT

Treatment may be difficult. Capillary haemangiomata on the skin surface may require excision for cosmetic reasons. Cavernous haemangiomata may sometimes also be excised, but this can be difficult; alternatively, embolization may arrest their progress.

Overgrowth in a limb may sometimes require epiphyseal arrest by stapling (Fig. 18.16).

Idiopathic inflammatory histiocytosis

EOSINOPHILIC GRANULOMA

Eosinophilic granuloma is a local condition, found in children between the ages of 5 and 10 years, in which a granulomatous deposit is present in bone, filled with eosinophils. Occasionally, several deposits are present. Affected bones are usually the skull, vertebrae, ribs, pelvis, femora or humeri. Attention is often drawn to the condition by the occurrence of a pathological fracture. Treatment is often unnecessary, but chemotherapy may hasten resolution. Sometimes in a young child, gross collapse of a vertebral body gives symptoms very like those of spinal tuberculosis.

LETTERER–SIWE DISEASE

Letterer–Siwe disease has its onset mainly in infants and in children below the age of 2 years. It is characterized by the wide dispersion of histiocytes throughout the body, particularly in the spleen, lymph nodes, bone marrow and liver. The skeletal lesions may be clinically silent or the effect of the destructive lesions in the bone may be apparent, particularly in the skull.

In most cases of Letterer–Siwe disease the condition runs a fulminating course, the affected child usually dying within a month or two of the diagnosis.

HAND–SCHÜLLER–CHRISTIAN DISEASE

As with Letterer–Siwe, Hand–Schüller–Christian disease affects the whole body, but in an older age group, mainly 5–10 year olds. The skull is chiefly involved and the patient may have diabetes insipidus, exophthalmos and calvarial deposits.

The generally advocated treatment for the bone lesions of this disease is radiotherapy.

FIBROUS DYSPLASIA (Fig. 18.17)

Fibrous dysplasia is a congenital disorder of unknown aetiology. It may be polyostotic or monostotic. There is a proliferation of osteoclasts, with bone destruction and replacement by fibrous tissue. There is no biochemical change apart from a raised alkaline phosphatase level. The monostotic form is more common, affecting the femur, ribs, tibia and facial bones. Albright's syndrome is fibrous dysplasia with pigmented skin lesions and precocious puberty or other endocrine changes as a result of the involvement of the pituitary fossa.

Biopsy of the lesion is followed by treatment comprising packing the defect with bone graft.

MALIGNANT FIBROUS HISTIOCYTOMA

Malignant fibrous histiocytoma is a rare malignant condition of uncertain origin that is found throughout adult life. It usually occurs in the long bones, and on X-ray shows evidence of bone destruction; the histological features are variable, and may be difficult to distinguish from fibrosarcoma. The outlook is variable.

MOLECULAR BIOLOGY AND BONE TUMOURS

Recent advances in molecular biology are beginning to provide useful information on bone tumour predisposition, diagnosis and behaviour.

Tumour predisposition

Approximately 10% of childhood osteosarcoma and soft tissue sarcoma is due to an autosomal dominant inherited cancer predisposition. The two most common familial malignant traits responsible are hereditary retinoblastoma (in which osteosarcoma is the most common malignancy after retiniblastoma) and Li-Fraumeni cancer family syndrome (in which bony and soft-tissue sarcoma cluster together with leukaemia, breast cancer, brain and adrenocortical malignancies). Germ-line defects in the Rb gene (in familial retinoblastoma) and p53 gene (in Li-Fraumeni syndrome) can be found in 50% of individuals exhibiting the familial trait. At this stage the challenge is to determine whether our acquired knowledge of increased cancer risk can lead to earlier detection and treatment of malignancy.

Tumour diagnosis

Since the biological behaviour of bone tumours varies greatly from one type to another, optimal treatment relies upon accurate histological diagnosis. This is not always straightforward. Advances in cytogenetics provide additional data which may assist in tumour classification. Characteristic chromosome translocations, for example, occur in Ewing's sarcoma, malignant Schwannoma synovial sarcoma and extraskeletal myxoid chondrosarcoma, some of which appear to be highly specific.

Tumour behaviour

Proven features of prognostic significance include tumour grade, size and local or distant metastases. Modern molecular and immunological techniques have allowed the identification of oncogenes, tumour suppressor genes, host and tumour proteins which are also of prognostic significance. Current debate centres on whether some of these factors are of independent significance, with clinical application affecting management decisions.

EXAMPLE

Malignant growths

A 14-year-old girl presents with a swelling near to her left knee. She noticed the swelling a few weeks previously and it had recently started to become painful.

Questions
- What is the likely diagnosis?
- What is the treatment?

Answers
- Clinical examination reveals a tender swelling over the lower end of the femur on the inner side. There is only a small effusion (collection of fluid) in the knee joint.
- The differential diagnosis in this age group is osteosarcoma, osteomyelitis, a fracture, osteochondroma or a bone cyst.
- X-rays reveal a florid lesion arising from the left femur with Codman's triangle visible.
- The diagnosis is now most certainly osteosarcoma.
- The patient is referred to a bone tumour centre for open biopsy, staging of the tumour, chemotherapy, resection of the lesion and, if possible, a large joint replacement.
- The outcome is currently about 50 per cent 5-year survival.

19 NEUROMUSCULAR DISORDERS

Neurological conditions requiring orthopaedic assistance are those primarily affecting the locomotor system. In the majority, permanent changes have already occurred and the main problems are preservation of function and the correction of deformities. The spinal cord extends from the atlas to the upper border of the second lumbar vertebra. Thirty-one pairs of spinal nerves spring from the spinal cord at intervals along its length, each nerve having an anterior and a posterior root. The anterior horn cells lie within the anterior grey columns. Paralysis is of two types – spastic, involving the upper motor neurons, in which the causative lesion is in the central nervous system, either the brain or the spinal cord, or flaccid, involving the lower motor neurons, in which the lesion is in the peripheral nerves, the nerve roots, or the anterior horn cells in which the peripheral motor nerves have their origin.

UPPER MOTOR NEURONE DISORDERS

Spastic paralysis

Spastic paralysis may occur in four ways:

■ Paraplegia – in which, as a result of some lesion in the spinal cord, both lower limbs are affected, the extent of involvement depending upon the level.

■ Quadriplegia – in which all four limbs are involved, as a result of a lesion either high in the cervical part of the cord or at the base of the brain (also called 'tetraplegia').

■ Hemiplegia – in which two limbs on one side are affected. This is usually due to some condition in the cerebral cortex, which may also cause facial weakness on the opposite side.

■ Monoplegia – in which a single limb is involved. This also is usually due to a lesion in the brain itself, but can result from a condition affecting only half the spinal cord, though this is uncommon.

If the lesion affects the spinal cord, there will be sensory and motor loss, whereas in brain lesions, as the sensory and motor areas are unrelated, there is motor paralysis alone.

In spastic paralysis, all muscle groups in the involved area are in a state of spasm, with the result that deformities are liable to occur because, in opposing muscle groups, one side is more powerful. Thus, in the foot, the calf muscles are stronger than the anterior tibial muscles, so an equinus deformity occurs. In the knee, the hamstrings have a greater mechanical advantage over the quadriceps, with the result that flexion deformities are common. In the hip, the adductors and flexors also have a greater than normal advantage over the abductors and extensors. Similarly, in the wrist and hand, flexion deformities occur, the forearm becomes pronated, the elbow loses full extension and the shoulder is held adducted.

Cerebral palsy

Cerebral palsy is the motor manifestation of unchanging brain damage sustained in infancy or childhood. The damage may be due to some maternal upset, or as a result of a prolonged and difficult labour, in which cerebral anoxia is a feature. Postnatally, severe jaundice is a frequent cause, and in later childhood cerebral palsy may follow encephalitis or meningitis.

The clinical picture depends upon the site and extent of cerebral damage. Cerebral palsy may be:

- Spastic, which may occur as hemiplegia, double hemiplegia (i.e. a tetraplegia or quadriplegia), monoplegia or diplegia (which is a paraplegia of cerebral origin).
- ataxic
- dyskinetic
- mixed.

The incidence of spastic hemiplegia appears to be reducing whereas ataxic and dyskinetic, though less common, are remaining about the same in number. Patients with ataxic, dyskinetic and the mixed cerebral palsy are more the province of the paediatric neurologist and will not be considered further.

Some degree of mental handicap may be present in children with spastic cerebral palsy, but is not usually anything like as severe as in the dyskinetic or ataxic child. However, other associated motor problems may be apparent in the spastic, such as a speech defect.

CLINICAL FEATURES

Attempts at sitting, standing and walking will be delayed, and at the time when a normal baby would be taking these steps, uncoordination of movement, with rigidity in the affected limbs, becomes obvious. In the hemiplegic patient, the limbs on the affected side assume a characteristic appearance. In the arm, the elbow is flexed and the wrist is flexed and pronated. In the leg, the foot is in rigid equinus, with the knee flexed, and the hip both flexed and

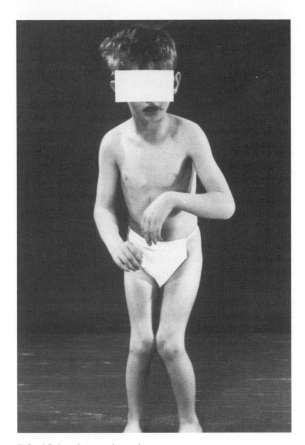

FIG. 19.1   Spastic hemiplegia

adducted. When both legs are involved, walking may be almost impossible because hip adductor spasm causes the legs to cross each other ('scissors gait') (Fig. 19.1).

In the athetoid patient, constant involuntary movements affecting the face and all four limbs increase when any purposeful action is undertaken, such that in severe cases the patient is almost unable to do anything for themselves.

TREATMENT

As the brain damage is irreversible, a cure is impossible and treatment needs to be directed towards assisting the patient to overcome their disabilities by re-education and training. In the severely affected spastic child of fairly normal intelligence, specialized schools for the physically handicapped obtain excellent results. In these schools speech, hearing defects and education can all be catered for, making the child's management a team event.

Orthopaedic treatment is concerned with individual lesions, and it is important to keep in mind that the basic defect is in the brain and that over enthusiastic correction of individual deformities may upset the overall pattern and thereby impair, rather than improve, function.

CONSERVATIVE TREATMENT

Conservative treatment is undertaken in schools for physically handicapped children, in which realistic goals are set for improvement in each child's mobility and activities of daily living. Physiotherapy by passive mobilization is performed to minimize the degree of deformity, which is due to a combination of reduction in the elasticity of the muscle combined with differential rates of growth of the bones and muscle. Orthoses and serial plaster casts are used to overcome the degree of spasticity. Clearly, though, these orthoses or serial casts should not be applied with such force as to cause pain or pressure sores.

SURGICAL MANAGEMENT

Orthopaedic surgery has an important role in the management of cerebral palsy. The prime purpose is to correct fixed deformity. Therefore surgery is directed mainly towards the spastic hemiplegic patient. The principle is to improve function of the limb. This is mainly achieved by tendon release, particularly in the upper limb, in the patient with 'thumb in palm' or lower limb tight tendoachilles.

In an equinovarus deformity of the lower limb, subtalar fusion can be used to stabilize the joint and control the varus deformity.

In the hip, open release of the adductor muscles, combined if need be by division of the obturator nerve, is sometimes of value in releasing adductor spasm, and flexion deformity of the hip can be improved by psoas release. Subluxation of the hip joint can occur if the child is walking with aids. If unaided, an internal rotation gait will result. If the child does not walk at all, an acquired dislocation of the hip will result. Prevention is the best form of treatment, passive stretching being the most important. If subluxation has occurred, muscle release will be of benefit, often combined with a femoral osteotomy. In true dislocation, extensive muscle release; neurectomy; combined with femoral and pelvic osteotomy should be considered, and the decision to undertake such major surgery must depend on the overall condition of the child.

In the knee there may be hamstring spasticity or contracture and knee-joint flexion, which may be related secondarily to a passive stretching. Serial plasters should overcome these contractures but, if they are fixed, the hamstrings may be released.

Cerebrovascular accident

The most common cause of an upper motor neuron lesion in the adult is a cerebrovascular accident, the incidence being 2 per 1000 of the population. Although the principles of treatment are the same as for spastic hemiplegia in a child, frequently there are associated diseases and the patient's age must also be considered. Nevertheless, progressive deformity will ensue unless it is specifically prevented. Flexion and adduction deformities occur in the hip and may even lead to dislocation of the hip joint.

Intense physiotherapy, including passive stretching, early mobilization and appropriate orthoses are the mainstay of treatment of the effects of the hemiplegia.

Surgical treatment is applied far less frequently than in the child with cerebral palsy because there are real risks of further cerebral infarcts if an operation is performed under general anaesthesia. However, surgery can help and the principles are the same. Overactive muscles are weakened either by tendon lengthening or by denervation, and in selected patients weak muscles can be enhanced by tendon transfer.

MIXED UPPER AND LOWER MOTOR NEURONE DISORDERS

Spina bifida

Originally, in early fetal life, neurological tissue appears as a flat plaque, which later becomes infolded to form a tube; the vertebral column develops in a similar manner.

Arrest of this process can occur at this stage. In many normal individuals, radiological examination of the lumbosacral region reveals failure of fusion of the laminae in the fifth lumbar of first sacral vertebra. This is known as spina bifida occulta. Occasionally, when it is a little more marked, a bony defect may be palpable clinically, and a minor tuft of hair may be present at that site. In such individuals there may be tethering of the sacral nerve roots to the defect, leading to pes cavus and clawed toes as growth proceeds.

If the bony defect is more extensive, the contents of the spinal canal are exposed on the surface. This may take two forms. In one, a meningeal sac may be present, the nerve roots lying within it, but the cord is not involved. This is known as a meningocele, and is a failure of the vertebrae to fuse. In the second form, if the cord is involved and remains in the primitive state as an open plaque on the back, it is known as a myelocele. In this case, cerebrospinal fluid leaks on to the surface. Commonly, there is an associated hydrocephalus due to obstruction to the outflow of cerebrospinal fluid from the fourth ventricle by a tongue of cerebellum protruding into the foramen magnum. This is known as the Arnold–Chiari malformation.

The incidence of children born with spina bifida is on the decrease at least in part because of early intrauterine detection of this disease by the presence of alpha-fetoproteins and the use of ultrasound. The cause of spina bifida is partly genetic and partly environmental.

MANAGEMENT

Once the newborn infant has been diagnosed as having open spina bifida, they should be referred to a regional centre where, after evaluation, the defect is closed by the neurosurgeon within the first 24 hours. The procedure involves excision of the sac and closure of the skin. If the child then develops hydrocephalus, a ventriculoperitoneal shunt is inserted to allow drainage of the cerebrospinal fluid into the peritoneum. At this stage the child is seen by the orthopaedic surgeon for an assessment of their lower limb abnormalities.

When nerve tissue is involved, functional impairment will result. This varies in severity up to complete flaccid paraplegia with sensory loss and urinary and faecal incontinence.

As a result of muscle imbalance, various lower limb deformities commonly occur. When the upper lumbar roots alone survive, unopposed action of the iliopsoas muscle causes the hips to dislocate. If the lower lumbar roots remain intact in the hip, flexion contractures follow, in association with paralytic dislocation; in the knee the unopposed quadriceps causes hyperextension; and in the foot ankle dorsiflexors lead to a calcaneovarus deformity. Also, because of sensory loss, trophic ulceration and fractures often complicate the picture.

TREATMENT

Spina bifida occulta requires no specific treatment.

Lower limb deformities and paralysis are controlled by suitable apparatus, assisted in certain cases by surgery. Paralytic dislocation of the hip may be controlled by the application of a splint at birth, such as a Pavlik harness, which is left in place for 12 months. At this stage adductor and psoas release may be undertaken to obtain a functional but dysplastic result. In some patients an innominate osteotomy may be undertaken. Other procedures include lengthening the flexor tendons of the knee and a supracondylar osteotomy. In the foot, soft-tissue release, calcaneal osteotomy and elongation of the tendo Achillis are occasionally performed.

SPINAL DEFORMITY

One-half of the total number of myelomeningocele patients will develop a spinal deformity, which may be a long thoracolumbar scoliosis possibly combined with a severe angular kyphosis. Bracing is required early, and definitive spinal surgery is undertaken between the ages of 10 and 12 years. The surgery, which is extensive and specialist in nature, involves a two-stage anterior and posterior spinal fusion with instrumentation.

ORTHOTICS

Children with lesions at the level of T12 or L1 will not have any hip control and will require knee–ankle–foot orthosis with a pelvic band in order to remain upright. Lesions below this level will need knee–ankle–foot orthosis, and indeed ankle–foot orthosis will be necessary for lesions down to S1.

Associated with the orthopaedic problems there may be the following problems.

- Genitourinary, due to lack of urethral sphincter control. A catheter or urinary device will be needed, perhaps with a sphincterectomy for active control.
- Bowels: training of the bowels is often adequate.

LOWER MOTOR NEURONE DISORDERS

Anterior poliomyelitis

Anterior poliomyelitis is a viral infection of the anterior horn cells. Since the advent of active immunization, it has become rare in most western countries, but it is still a cause of permanent motor paralysis in developing countries, and epidemic outbreaks may occur. These epidemics are rather more common in late summer or autumn than in winter months.

The virus enters through the alimentary tract and spreads via the bloodstream to the anterior horn cells in the central nervous system. Initially there is a round-cell infiltration of the affected areas, with local oedema, thereby impairing the function of the anterior horn cells. Later this may resolve, with recovery of function, or the anterior horn cells may be destroyed, leading to permanent paralysis.

In certain cases, the central nervous system is unaffected, the patient having merely a 'summer cold'. During the stage of active infection, the virus is excreted in the faeces, so the non-paralytic case is liable to be a carrier of the disease.

As the old name 'infantile paralysis' implies, the age of onset if often early childhood, though in recent years it has become more common in later childhood and early adult life.

CLINICAL FEATURES

The course of the disease may be subdivided into three phases:

■ The stage of activity, corresponding to when the virus is producing active infective changes.
■ The stage of recovery, when the anterior horn cells affected by the virus, but which survived its attack, resume function.
■ The stage of residual paralysis, which is permanent, and is linked with the number of anterior horn cells that have been destroyed by the disease.

INVESTIGATIONS

During the stage of activity, lumbar puncture will reveal an increased cell content in the cerebrospinal fluid.

The extent of initial paralysis, and its subsequent progress should be assessed regularly by a muscle chart, using the Medical Research Council grading. The power in each muscle is tested, and placed in one of six categories.

0 = No contraction whatever.
1 = Flicker of contracture insufficient to produce any movement.
2 = Active movement possible, if the effects of gravity are eliminated.
3 = Active movement possible against gravity.
4 = Active movement weaker than normal, though possible against resistance.
5 = Normal muscle power.

COMPLICATIONS

Apart from chest problems occurring when there is respiratory paralysis, three main complications are found in poliomyelitis.

■ Vascular: widespread muscle paralysis leads to vascular stagnation, which causes coldness, cyanosis and chilblains, and may be troublesome.
■ Shortening of the limb: because of the diminished blood flow in the affected limbs, epiphyseal growth is liable to be retarded in young children.
■ Deformity: when there is partial paralysis, normal muscle balance about a joint is upset and the less affected muscles will tend to pull the part out of alignment. At first this can be passively overcome, but eventually fibrosis follows, and a fixed deformity occurs.

TREATMENT

In the acute stage with muscle pain, rest is necessary in normal postures and heat is useful in relieving pain. As soon as pain has settled, the joints are put regularly through their full normal range of movement and graduated muscle re-education may begin. In the intervals between treatment the limbs should be held in physiological position because deformities readily occur.

The treatment of the established paralysis may be conservative or operative.

Conservative

Conservative treatment entails using external appliances to replace the paralysed muscle and to correct any deformity (Fig. 19.12).

Operative

Surgical measures may be directed towards muscles and tendons or bones and joints. Operations upon muscles may take the form of a tendon transfer, in which the tendinous insertion of a functioning muscle, which may therefore be causing a deformity, is transferred and made to act in the direction of its paralysed opponent. When there is a fixed deformity, the muscle attachments may be divided so that the deformity can be overcome. This is most

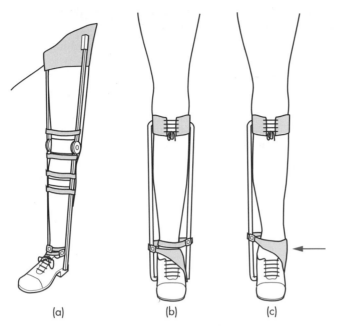

FIG. 19.2 (a) Full-length caliper with knee lock: a knee–ankle–foot orthosis; (b) double below-knee iron; (c) outside iron and inside 'T-strap' to control valgus deformity of ankle: an ankle–foot orthosis

(a) (b) (c)

frequently employed to correct flexion contractures of the hip and knee.

In the upper limb, tendon transfer is useful at several sites. Thus a paralysed biceps muscle may be replaced by detaching the origin of part of pectoralis major from the chest wall and reinserting it into the upper arm. Wrist and finger extensors may be replaced by attaching the tendon of flexor carpi ulnaris into the extensor digitorum and pollicis longus tendons. Opposition of the thumb may be restored by transferring the flexor digitorum sublimis of the ring finger realigned through a pulley to the head of the first metacarpal.

In the lower limb, hip abduction and extension may be improved by transfer of the iliopsoas tendon into the greater trochanter of the femur. Quadriceps power may be improved if the biceps femoris or semitendinosus tendons are reinserted into the patella. Eversion or inversion deformities at the ankle may be corrected by transferring either a peroneal tendon to the inner side or tibialis anterior or posterior to the outer side of the tarsus, respectively. Claw toes may be corrected by transferring the long flexor tendons to the extensor expansion on the dorsum, and a dropped first metatarsal by moving the extensor hallucis tendon to the metatarsal neck. However, it must be stressed that the effect of tendon transfer must be considered carefully before the operation. It is easy

to remove a deforming force and transfer it, only to produce the reverse deformity. The aim is to balance the muscle action.

Operations upon bones and joints usually take the form of arthrodesis, in which, by stiffening one flail or deformed joint, the remaining muscle power may be employed to utilize some other part of the limb. Thus, in the upper limb, fusion of a flail shoulder enables the scapulothoracic group of muscles to move the arm as a whole. In the hand, fusion of the first metacarpal to the second in a position of opposition, employing a bone graft to bridge the gap, is useful where sublimis tendon transfer is not possible. In the lower limb, arthrodesis of the hip and knee should be approached with caution as it may merely add to the strains imposed upon weakened muscles elsewhere or porotic bones liable to fracture. Arthrodesis of a paralysed ankle in slight equinus may be very useful if there is widespread muscle weakness in the leg, because when weight is put upon the limb, the knee is locked in an extended position provided the centre of gravity can be brought in front of the hip. Instability of the foot may be corrected by triple arthrodesis of the tarsus (Chapter 12). If there is weakness of dorsiflexion causing a drop-foot deformity, this may be corrected at the same time by cutting a wedge from the lower surface of the talus, having its base anteriorly so that, when the foot is horizontal, the ankle articular surface is in a plantar-flexed position. Sometimes arthrodesis of both the ankle and subtalar joints (pantalar arthrodesis) may be useful in providing stability when the foot is completely flail. Claw toes may be corrected by interphalangeal arthrodesis instead of the flexor to extensor tendon transfer already described. Arthrodesis of joints should not be employed until growth is reaching maturity, or growth may be interfered with, especially in the long bones, by premature fusion of epiphyses.

TREATMENT OF COMPLICATIONS

Apart from deformities resulting from muscle imbalance, the management of which has already been discussed, the two main complications occurring in poliomyelitis are those due to vascular

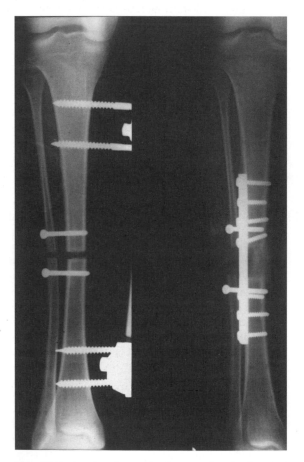

FIG. 19.3   Leg lengthening by bone graft with plate and screws

stagnation, which affect mainly the lower limbs, and shortening due to impaired epiphyseal growth when the disease occurs in young children.

If chilblains and other effects of vascular stagnation in the legs are troublesome, occasionally lumbar sympathectomy is carried out. Also, in the lower limbs, discrepancy in length may, in selected cases, be corrected by arresting epiphyseal growth on the normal side by placing metal staples across the epiphyseal cartilages of the lower femur and upper tibia (see Fig. 18.16) or by the process of leg lengthening, using a leg lengthening device, in which the femur or tibia is divided and then lengthened gradually (Fig. 19.3).

Spinal muscular atrophy

Spinal muscular atrophy is a group of disorders in which there is degeneration of the anterior horn cells and also of the motor nuclei of the cranial nerves. It is inherited as an autosomal recessive with an incidence of 1 per 10 000 live births. There are three main clinical groups.

■ Severe (Werdnig–Hoffman's disease), in which there is weakness of all muscles with a typical development of a frog-leg posture, head lag, virtual absence of arm movements and weakness of respiratory muscles. There may be bulbar paralysis making feeding and breathing difficult, and the child frequently dies from pneumonia.
■ Intermediate: in this group the onset is usually in the first year of life, and most of these children can lift their heads, hands and legs, and can stand for brief periods of time. This disease may remain static after a period of progressive weakness. The children have bulbar paralysis, and facial or respiratory muscle weakness, although they may show fasciculations and wasting of the tongue. As they get older, skeletal deformities become more apparent, particularly scoliosis, which is a neuropathic scoliosis and affects the whole spine. These children spend a great deal of time in a wheelchair and contractures can develop in the upper and lower limbs.
■ Mild: this is Kugelberg–Welander disease and is the mildest form of spinal muscular atrophy. It is detected in children between the ages of 5 and 15 years. The child presents with difficulty in walking and climbing; proximal muscle groups are most frequently affected, more so than the distal groups. The progress of this disease is slow and the children continue to walk up to

the age of 30 years. Later there is weakness of the shoulders and arms, and, eventually, they are confined to a wheelchair.

INVESTIGATIONS

Electromyography shows characteristic fibrillation at rest and a decreased interference pattern.

Muscle biopsy shows characteristic atrophy of muscle fibre types.

MANAGEMENT

Children with the intermediate type of spinal muscular atrophy usually benefit initially from spinal bracing and later from spinal fusion with instrumentation in order to correct and control the curve.

Peroneal muscular atrophy (Charcot–Marie–Tooth disease)

Charcot–Marie–Tooth disease is a form of hypertrophic neuropathy in which there is motor and sensory impairment, and it is inherited as an autosomal dominant. The child usually presents in the first decade of life with abnormalities of gait and pes cavus. The gait is clumsy and the child frequently trips because of the associated foot drop that occurs from the peroneal muscular weakness. The peroneal muscles are affected early, as are the intrinsic muscles of the foot, to produce the cavovarus deformity.

MANAGEMENT

The cavovarus deformity may be corrected by soft-tissue release, tendon transfer or a wedge resection and arthrodesis. Clawing of the toes can be corrected by tendon transfer.

MUSCULAR DYSTROPHIES

Duchenne muscular dystrophy

Duchenne muscular dystrophy is a progressive disorder of childhood and is inherited as a sex-linked autosomal recessive (i.e. it is passed on to boys from unaffected mothers). Between 2 and 3

per 10 000 newborn males suffer from Duchenne muscular dystrophy. A child with this dystrophy usually goes through the normal childhood milestones. However, when he starts to stand and tries to walk the muscle weakness becomes apparent and he frequently falls and has a waddling gait. There may be pseudohypertrophy of the muscles, particularly of the calf. As the child gets older he acquires a broad-based stance with hyperlordosis of the lumbar spine and frequently develops contractures of the calf muscles and flexion of the hip. The muscle weakness and developing contractures soon make walking impossible and the child may then be confined to a wheelchair for the rest of his life. The child with Duchenne muscular dystrophy dies in his late teens from cardiac and respiratory complications.

INVESTIGATIONS

The muscle enzyme creatinine phosphokinase is always high in Duchenne muscular dystrophy.

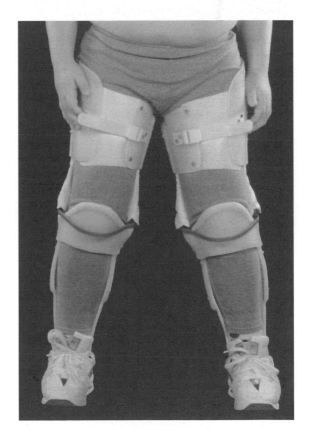

FIG. 19.4 Knee–ankle–foot orthosis for patient with Duchenne muscular dystrophy

Muscle biopsy is an essential investigation and shows the changes characteristic of Duchenne muscular dystrophy, in that there is increased fibrosis and central nuclei are present within the muscle fibres.

MANAGEMENT

As Duchenne muscular dystrophy is incurable, the management is aimed at improving the quality of the child's life. Contractures may be corrected by surgical release, and mobilization is encouraged by the use of lightweight knee–ankle–foot orthoses to enable the child to stand (Fig. 19.4). Eventually, even after a period of assisted mobilization, the boy with Duchenne muscular dystrophy will spend the remainder of his life in a wheelchair.

Facioscapulohumeral muscular dystrophy

Fascioscapulohumeral muscular dystrophy is inherited as an autosomal dominant and it occurs in between 3 and 10 patients per 1 000 000 of the population. Usually the patient presents between the second and third decade with weakness of the facial and scapular muscles. This results in the patient being unable to close their eyes completely, to whistle or to drink through a straw, and also causes winging of the scapula.

INVESTIGATIONS

Electromyography reveals the characteristic myopathic or denervation patterns of this disorder.

MANAGEMENT

The winging of the scapulae can be controlled by operation, but this is often not necessary as the patients manage reasonably well without any surgical interference.

BRACHIAL PLEXUS INJURIES

Birth injuries

Birth injuries to the brachial plexus occur in infants as a result of difficult delivery. They are due to

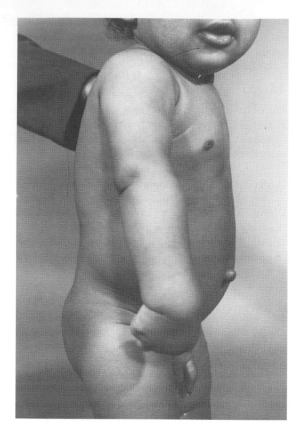

FIG. 19.5   Erb's palsy

tractional forces applied to the baby's head when it is laterally flexed to one side with the shoulder on the opposite side pulled downwards. They are slightly more common in a breach presentation than in a normal delivery.

UPPER ARM TYPE (ERB'S PALSY) (Fig. 19.15)

Erb's palsy is the most common form of birth injury. It affects the upper trunk of the plexus composed of the fifth and sixth cervical nerve roots. It causes the shoulder to be adducted and the arm internally rotated, the elbow extended and the wrist pronated and flexed. It is usually fairly obvious as soon as the baby is born.

LOWER ARM TYPE (KLUMPKE'S SYNDROME)

Klumpke's syndrome is a less common type of birth injury and is due to an adduction strain pulling the lower trunk of plexus composed of the eighth cervical and first thoracic nerve roots. It causes a claw-hand deformity due to paralysis of the intrinsic muscles. The sympathetic trunk is also often affected, causing narrowing of the pupil and recession of the eyeball on the affected side (Horner's syndrome). This type is less likely to be noticed at birth and may only be observed when the baby fails to grasp objects in the normal manner.

MANAGEMENT

Some spontaneous recovery usually occurs.

TREATMENT

Treatment consists of daily passive movements; splints are rarely used. Reconstructive surgery may be performed using tendon transfer, particularly the triceps to biceps and the wrist flexors to extensors, which may, in later life, be combined with arthrodesis to improve function. Early nerve repair is also practised in certain centres.

Closed injuries to the brachial plexus in adults

Injuries to the brachial plexus occur particularly in young men after motor cycle accidents. Invariably they are traction injuries and are the result of the head being forced laterally at the moment of impact. These lesions are frequently associated with other injuries such as fractures or injuries to the head, chest or abdomen. With a few patients there is complete avulsion of the brachial plexus. In complete lesions of the brachial plexus certain factors such as pain, presence of Horner's syndrome or evidence of cervical meningoceles on myelography indicate a poor prognosis for recovery.

CLINICAL PRESENTATION

Frequently a brachial plexus lesion is not obvious immediately after the accident, as there may be many other injuries that the patient has sustained. There may be considerable variations and, although the patient may present with a flail limb from a complete brachial plexus lesion, recovery to some degree may still occur.

INVESTIGATIONS

Histamine test

Histamine is injected into the skin and the development of a wheal and flare indicates an intact spinal arc. Hence, a positive axon reflex is diagnostic of a preganglionic lesion, and a postganglionic lesion is one with an interrupted reflex.

Myelography or MRI

This may reveal a meningocele, a herniation from the dura of the spinal cord. The presence of meningocele indicates a poor prognosis, as the roots have been pulled out of the cord to produce this effect. MRI provides more information than a myelogram on the state of the cord.

TREATMENT

The treatment of a complete brachial plexus injury was historically to arthrodese the shoulder, amputate the arm and fit a prosthesis.

With improved microsurgical techniques it is now possible, in specialist centres, to re-anastomose the individual lesions of the brachial plexus, and the results are encouraging. However, lesions of the brachial plexus are disastrous for the young men concerned and every available method should be employed to ensure that individuals return to a useful existence in the community, so that they can earn a living and maintain their independence.

EXAMPLE

Brachial plexus injuries

An 18-year-old man is involved in a road traffic accident, sustaining a brachial plexus lesion to his right (dominant) arm.

He has no other injury.

Questions
- How do you assess the severity of the lesion?
- What is the prognosis?

Answers
- Careful examination of the flail limb is important, including if possible motor and sensory assessment, along with MRC muscle grading.
- If the lesion is complete, it suggests all the nerves of the brachial plexus are involved, that is, from C5 to T1.
- MRI is the most useful investigation, demonstrating the state of the nerves and the spinal cord.
- Electromyography (EMG) and nerve conduction studies (NCV) along with the histamine test later on, are also useful studies combined with X-rays of the affected area, to demonstrate a fracture.
- Current treatment is to refer the patient to a specialized centre, in which nerve repair and grafting is undertaken.
- The prognosis obviously depends on the success of the surgery that may have been performed.
- However, if unsuccessful these injuries have a poor prognosis, because of severe pain and loss of the use of the dominant arm in a young man at the beginning of his career.

AMPUTATIONS

Broadly, amputation is indicated if the presence of the limb is a menace to life or if replacement by a substitute offers the best prospect of functional (and sometimes cosmetic) improvement. In the lower limb in which stability and the transmission of relatively simple movement are the chief requirements, replacement by a prosthesis can be very effective. But in the upper limb, the complicated functions of the hand and, above all, tactile sensation make effective prosthetic replacement more difficult.

Except in an emergency, at least one other consultant should be asked to see the patient before an amputation, the full implications of which should be explained to the patient. The help and advice of a limb-fitting surgeon before the operation and after it can be extremely helpful. Earliest possible activity, especially with a temporary prosthesis, is very important, especially in elderly patients, but immediate postoperative fitting of a prosthesis has largely lost its attractions and the provision of the prosthetic device is usually delayed for about 10 days. Most of the patients have peripheral vascular disease, with such serious complications as involvement of the opposite limb, coronary or cerebrovascular disease and their complications, and a short expectation of life. Their social care is consequently very important.

INDICATIONS

Trauma

Part of the limb may be so obviously damaged that its survival is impossible, in which case immediate amputation cannot be avoided. Alternatively, after attempting to save the limb, it may become clear that the damaged part cannot be made use of and the patient will be better off with an artificial limb.

Vascular insufficiency

If there is severe peripheral vascular disease with gangrene, amputation at a site above the level where reasonable circulation is still present may be necessary to save life, to relieve pain and to enable the patient to lead a more normal life with an artificial limb.

Malignant new growths

Amputation for many primary neoplastic conditions may be the only hope of saving the patient's life.

Other indications

If a patient has a useless limb as a result of either gross congenital deformities or muscle paralysis, occasionally an amputation at a carefully planned site may enable the patient to be supplied with an artificial limb that is more use to them than their own limb.

OPERATIVE TECHNIQUE

A clear distinction must be made between, on the one hand, amputations in cases of infection or contamination as in road accidents or in military or civil strife (provisional amputation) and, on the other hand, 'clean' amputations (definitive amputation).

Provisional amputation

Provisional amputation demands the greatest reasonable preservation of all visible and uncontaminated tissue without immediate closure of the wound. In order to prevent retraction, it is permissible to hold the tissues over a gauze pack with a few lax sutures, but otherwise skin traction is necessary. Some days later, the pack is removed and the wound closed by delayed primary suture. 'Guillotine' amputation in its literal sense is seldom necessary or justifiable. Later, after further assessment and when the area is surgically clean, a definitive amputation may or may not be indicated.

Definitive amputation

In the absence of sepsis or potential sepsis, the chief consideration with definitive amputation is the provision of the best possible function, with or without a prosthesis, consistent with adequate removal of pathological tissue. Certain sites of election in such circumstances have been deter-

mined from experience. With major amputation in the lower limbs, end-bearing is a great advantage and can be achieved if the amputation is below the knee joint, through the tibia. Above the knee region, most weight has to be transferred through the ischial tuberosity and the disability is much greater. In planning skin flaps, these should mainly be chosen so that they will carry the best circulation. They should be full thickness skin, subcutaneous tissue, deep fascia and muscle. Divided fascia and muscle are sutured over the cut end of the bone to prevent retraction. A tourniquet is used if possible except in cases of peripheral vascular disease.

Great care must be taken in the ligation of important divided vessels and with haemostasis in general. Care is taken that cut ends of nerves are so placed that the tender terminal amputation neuromata are well removed from sites of pressure and friction. Suction drainage is usual.

COMPLICATIONS

The operation of major amputation is liable to the complications of any surgical operation – shock, haemorrhage, sepsis – and special attention should be paid to the danger of carrying out an emergency amputation before shock has been properly treated. After amputation, sensory phenomena are often referred to the absent member, or part of it, and is often displaced – the phantom limb. Sometimes these sensations are painful, and occasionally very painful. The pain may be resistant to treatment, but improvement has been obtained from a large variety of procedures, including percussion, neurectomy and transcutaneous electrical stimulation. Use of a prosthesis helps rather than hinders.

Stripping of periosteum at the end of the stump can lead to a terminal ring sequestrum if sepsis is present.

LOWER LIMB AMPUTATIONS

Hindquarter amputation

Hindquarter amputation is a most drastic operation in which not only is the whole lower limb removed but, in addition, the ilium (or most of it), ischium and pubis on the affected side. It is carried out only in the treatment of primary malignant disease involving the upper femur or pelvic bones. The fitting of an artificial limb is difficult because the only bony points upon which weight can be taken are the stump of the pubic symphysis anteriorly and the ala of the sacrum on the affected side posteriorly.

Disarticulation of the hip

In disarticulation of the hip, the lower limb is removed through the hip joint. It also leaves considerable disability because the prosthetic limb must incorporate an artificial hip and knee. Weight is transmitted to the artificial limb through the pelvis, the patient in effect sitting on the socket of the limb on the affected side.

Above-knee amputation

Above-knee amputation is the most common major amputation. At this level, the aim is to provide a conical stump, having good muscle power, which can be inserted into the socket of the artificial limb, thereby providing power to move the limb, although weight is borne at the top, through the ischial tuberosity. Because little or no weight is taken directly on the end of the stump, equal skin flaps are cut, leaving a terminal scar. If possible, the femur should be divided between 26 and 30 cm from the top of the greater trochanter.

Below-knee amputation

In below-knee amputation, the length of the stump is governed by the prosthesis. If the stump is too short, it may be liable to slip out of the socket when the knee is actively flexed. If it is too long, because the tibia is subcutaneous, an adherent, painful scar may remain. The ideal length is 14 cm from the knee joint, though somewhat shorter stumps may be effective if this length is impossible to obtain. In order to obtain a conical stump, the fibula should be divided about 2.5 cm higher than the tibia and the tibia bevelled in front. In cases of vascular insufficiency a long posterior full-thickness flap gives the best vascularity, and its use has diminished the need for through-knee and above-knee amputations. The prosthesis, supported by a suprapatellar strap, takes weight from the tibial condyles, patella and the patellar ligament, the so-called patellar tendon-bearing prosthesis.

Syme's amputation

Syme's amputation is of the foot and ankle joint, through the broad lower end of the tibia and fibula, which is covered by a heel flap comprising the tough soft tissue from behind and below the calcaneum, giving a bulbous stump that is end-bearing with or without a prosthesis. In the operation the flaps are cut, the ankle disarticulated, the calcaneum carefully dissected from the heel flap without impairing its circulation, and then the thickest part of the lower end of the tibia and fibula is sawn through. Great care is necessary in siting and fixing the heel pad squarely on the end of the stump.

Tarsal amputations

If the forefoot has been severely crushed, a useful stump may be obtained by amputation through the base of the metatarsals or at the metatarsotarsal junction (Lisfranc's amputation). A large plantar skin flap is used, so that the suture line is not in a weight-bearing area. A suitable sponge-rubber inset, can be fitted into an ordinary lace-up shoe.

Midtarsal disarticulation has been virtually abandoned.

For severe toe deformities, disarticulation of all toes may be sometimes employed to assist the fitting of acceptable shoes.

UPPER LIMB AMPUTATIONS

Forequarter amputation

Forequarter amputation is a very radical procedure in which the whole upper limb is removed, including the clavicle and scapula. It is employed only in the treatment of malignant disease. The fitting of a prosthesis after operation, even for cosmetic appearances alone, is almost impossible. A pad can replace the scapula, so that clothing remains in place.

Disarticulation through the shoulder

As with forequarter amputation, disarticulation through the shoulder is usually reserved for the treatment of malignant disease. If possible the humeral head is retained *in situ*, and amputation performed at the level of the surgical neck, to give a rounded contour upon which to suspend the prosthesis. In the case of primary malignant disease of the humerus itself, however, this may not be possible, as it is desirable to remove the whole bone.

Above-elbow amputation

In above-elbow amputation, a stump of 20 cm from the acromion is preserved if possible in order to fit a prosthesis. This amputation may be undertaken in patients with complete lesions of the brachial plexus.

Below-elbow amputation

Amputation through the elbow has no place, as it is essential for the prosthesis to be able to bend at elbow level. In below-elbow amputation, the stump must be long enough to move the artificial hand.

Occasionally, after traumatic bilateral amputation of the upper limbs, the Krugenberg procedure can be performed. In this the radius and ulna are separated, leaving a 'V' with which the patient may be trained to grasp objects; it has the additional advantage that tactile sensation is preserved.

Amputations through the hand

Because the preservation of tactile sensibility is most important, amputations through the hand should be as conservative as possible, preserving any portion of a digit that can be salvaged. This applies particularly to the thumb, and for this reason no standard procedure is described.

Amputations of digits

Amputations of stiff, painful fingers may be carried out at any level. But in the case of the middle, ring and little fingers, if the whole digit must be sacrificed, removal of the metacarpal bone as well, thus obviating a gap, improves both the cosmetic and the functional results.

In the case of the thumb, any portion should be preserved. If the whole thumb must be removed, it may be possible by dividing the second metacarpal near its base, deepening the cleft between it and the third metacarpal and then rotating it through 90° to replace the lost part. This is known as pollicization of the index finger.

PROSTHETICS AND ORTHOTICS

Prosthetics

UPPER LIMB

Indications for upper limb prosthetics are now generally due to congenital abnormalities and as a result of trauma. Obviously it will occasionally be necessary to acquire an upper limb prosthesis after tumour surgery.

The type of prosthesis available are body-powered (Fig. 20.1), externally powered (Fig. 20.2) and cosmetic. In the hand various forms of prosthesis have been developed to provide a functional cosmetic hand.

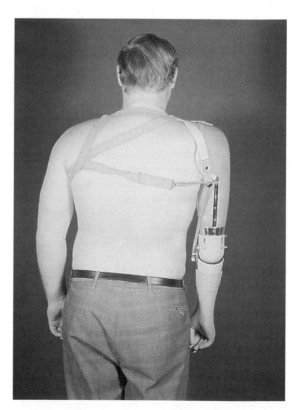

FIG. 20.1 Body-powered upper limb prosthesis

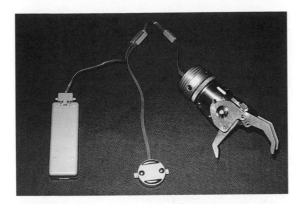

FIG. 20.2 Externally powered upper limb prostheses

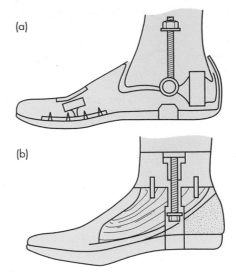

FIG. 20.4 The prosthetic foot. (a) Conventional ankle foot assembly; (b) the SACH (solid ankle cushion heel) foot

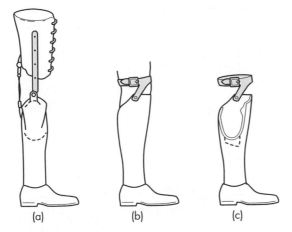

FIG. 20.3 Prostheses for below-knee amputees: (a) conventional; (b) patellar tendon-bearing prosthesis (PTB); (c) section through PTB prosthesis to show socket

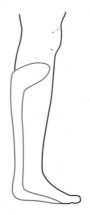

FIG. 20.5 Polypropylene drop-foot splint

LOWER LIMB

In the lower limb, however, prostheses are in greater demand, especially after vascular disease and trauma.

A below-knee amputation can be fitted with a prosthesis, which can be patellar bearing (Fig. 20.3).

For the foot a solid ankle, cushion heel is a simple modular device that is stiff and has a solid rubber foot allowing for some spring in motion (Fig. 20.4).

Orthotics

The aim of an orthotic appliance is to

■ control movement;
■ resist deformity;
■ correct the deformity if possible;
■ redistribute forces;
■ provide weight relief;
■ assist in movement.

There are several types available, usually made of light-weight material including a drop-foot splint for the lower limb (Fig. 20.5); a four poster collar for the cervical spine (Fig. 20.6) and a halo body device (Fig. 20.7), especially useful after an injury to the neck; and some form of temporary lumbosacral support for the lumbar spine. Other braces available for the lumbar spine include the Jewett and Taylor braces (Fig. 20.8).

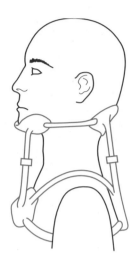

(a)

FIG. 20.6   (a) Diagram of four poster collar; (b) patient wearing a four poster collar for a cervical spine injury

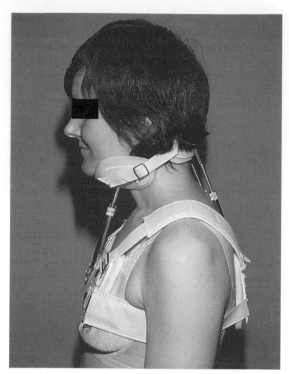

(b)

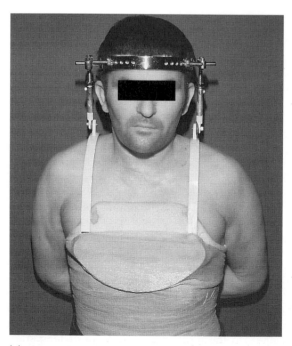

(a)

FIG. 20.7   A halo-body device for a cervical fracture

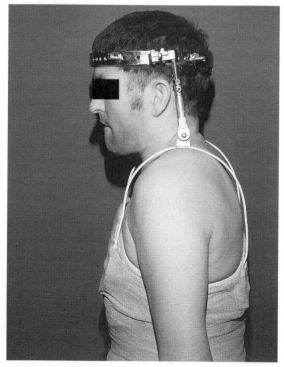

(b)

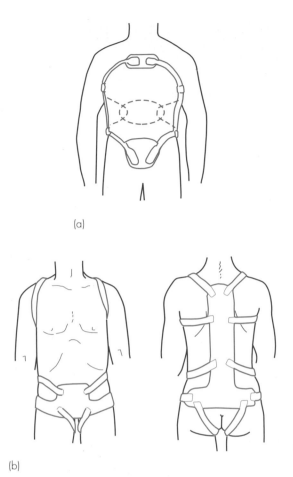

(a)

(b)

FIG. 20.8 (a) Taylor brace; (b) Jewett anterior hyperextension brace

Summary

Amputations
Amputations are performed for trauma; vascular impairment for bone tumours, and occasionally for gross congenital deformities.

The most common type of lower limb amputation is an above knee, usually for impairment of the circulation.

Digits of the hand may require amputation, especially if the finger is painful or stiff.

Prostheses
Upper limb prostheses are now becoming increasingly sophisticated and include external power sources.

In the lower limb the conventional below knee prosthesis is usually patellar-bearing and the foot piece is the solid ankle cushion heal (SACH).

Orthosis
In the neck a four posterior collar is required for a stable cervical spine fracture, whilst in the lumbar spine a three point brace is appropriate for a similar type of fracture.

Orthosis can also be supplied for the upper arm, forearm, hand, hip and foot.

EXAMPLE

Questions
A 46-year-old postman is admitted with an open comminuted fracture of the middle third of the tibia. There is a large contused and contaminated wound. The foot is cold and pulseless.

■ What is your management plan?
■ If it is decided to amputate, how is this done?
■ What sort of a prosthesis will be provided?

Answers
■ Resuscitate him and seek a second opinion about wisdom of attempting to save the leg, re-establishing the blood supply, or amputating the leg.
■ In view of the gross contamination perform a provisional amputation, excising all the dead tissue and preserving long skin flaps. Hold the tissues over a loose pack of gauze. Inspect at 48 hours and perform a definitive amputation at the optimal site (14 cm from the knee joint), when the sepsis has been eradicated.
■ A patellar tendon-bearing prosthesis is ideal, taking weight on the tibial condyles, patella and patellar tendon, and not on the stump itself.

INDEX